WOMEN'S SEXUAL DEVELOPMENT

Explorations of *Inner Space*

The female child under all but extreme urban conditions is disposed to observe evidence in older girls and women and in female animals of the fact that an inner-bodily space—with productive as well as dangerous potentials—does exist.

The influence of women will not be fully actualized until it reflects without apology the facts of the "inner space" and the potentialities and needs of the feminine psyche.

—E. H. Erikson, 1968
Identity, Youth and Crisis

WOMEN IN CONTEXT: Development and Stresses

THE WOMAN PATIENT —MEDICAL AND PSYCHOLOGICAL INTERFACES
Volume 1: Sexual and Reproductive Aspects of Women's Health Care
Edited by Malkah T. Notman and Carol C. Nadelson

BECOMING FEMALE: PERSPECTIVES ON DEVELOPMENT
Edited by Claire B. Kopp

WOMEN'S SEXUAL DEVELOPMENT: EXPLORATIONS OF INNER SPACE
Edited by Martha Kirkpatrick

WOMEN'S SEXUAL DEVELOPMENT

Explorations of *Inner Space*

EDITED BY
Martha Kirkpatrick, M.D.

PLENUM PRESS • NEW YORK AND LONDON

Library of Congress Cataloging in Publication Data

Main entry under title:

Women's sexual development.

(Women in context)
    Includes index.
    1. Women—United States—Sexual behavior—Addresses, essays, lectures. 2. Feminin-
ity (Psychology)—Addresses, essays, lectures. 3. Women—Psychology—Addresses, essays, lectures. I. Kirkpatrick, Martha. II. Series.
HQ29.W674   155.3′33   80-15486
ISBN 0-306-40375-7

© 1980 Plenum Press, New York
A Division of Plenum Publishing Corporation
227 West 17th Street, New York, N.Y. 10011

Printed in the United States of America

Contributors

Paul L. Adams, M.D. • Professor and Vice-Chairperson, Department of Psychiatry and Behavioral Sciences, University of Louisville and Louisville Veterans Administration Medical Center, Louisville, Kentucky

Christine Adams-Tucker, M.D. • Fellow in Child Psychiatry, Department of Psychiatry and Behavioral Sciences, University of Louisville, Louisville, Kentucky

Mildred Ash, M.D. • Psychiatrist and Psychoanalyst in Private Practice, Palo Alto, California

Cori Baill, B.S., R.N. • Phipps Psychiatric Clinic, The Johns Hopkins Hospital, Baltimore, Maryland

Elizabeth K. Canfield • Health and Family Planning Counselor, University of Southern California, Los Angeles, California

Virginia Lawson Clower, M.D. • Training and Supervisory Analyst, Adult and Child Psychoanalyst, New Orleans Psychoanalytic Society and Institute, New Orleans, Louisiana

Carol Downer • Director, Feminist Women's Health Center, Los Angeles, California; Chair, Federation of Feminist Women's Health Centers

Laura Edwards, B.A. • Editorial Assistant to Dr. Lawrence

Rudolph Ekstein, M.D. • Clinical Professor of Medical Psychology, University of California Medical School, Los Angeles, California; and Training and Supervisory Analyst, Los Angeles Psychoanalytic Institute and Southern California Psychoanalytic Institute, Los Angeles, California

v

Susanna Isaacs Elmhurst, M.D., F.R.C.P. • Associate Clinical Professor of Child Psychiatry, University of Southern California Medical School, Los Angeles, California; Training Analyst, Institute of Psychoanalysis, London, England

Eleanor Galenson, M.D. • Clinical Professor of Psychiatry, Mount Sinai School of Medicine, New York, New York; Member, New York Psychoanalytic Society and Institute

Sharon Ordman Geltner, Ed.D. • Social Studies Teacher, Los Angeles Unified School District, California

Joshua Golden, M.D. • Director, Sexual Dysfunction Clinic, Department of Psychiatry, University of California, Los Angeles, California

Allen Lawrence, M.D. • Director, Caring Parenthood Center, and Center for Caring Medicine, Los Angeles, California; and Private Practice, Obstetrics/Gynecology, West Los Angeles, California

Myrna I. Lewis, A.C.S.W. • Psychotherapist in Private Practice, Washington, D.C.

John Money, Ph.D. • Professor of Medical Psychology and Behavioral Sciences and Associate Professor of Pediatrics, The Johns Hopkins University and Hospital, Baltimore, Maryland

Priscilla Oaks, Ph.D. • Associate Professor of American Literature, Department of English, California State University, Fullerton, California

Barbara Ponse, Ph.D. • Psychotherapist in Private Practice, Los Angeles, California

B. F. Riess, Ph.D. • Adjunct Professor of Clinical Psychology, New School for Social Research, New York, New York

Margo Rila, D.A. • Faculty, The Institute for Advanced Study of Human Sexuality, San Francisco, California

Herman Roiphe, M.D. • Associate Clinical Professor of Psychiatry, Mount Sinai School of Medicine, New York, New York; Member, New York Psychoanalytic Society and Institute

Elizabeth J. Roberts, M.A. • President, Population Education, Inc.; and Executive Director, Project on Human Sexual Development, Cambridge, Massachusetts

Lynne Rubin, M.N., Ph.D. • Obstetrics and Gynecologic Nurse Practitioner in Private Practice, Los Angeles, California

Judith Steinhart, D.A. • Clinical Assistant Professor, Department of Health Sciences, State University of New York, Stony Brook, New York; and Department of Health Sciences, Brooklyn College, City University of New York, Brooklyn, New York

Robert J. Stoller, M.D. • Professor of Psychiatry, University of California School of Medicine, Los Angeles, California

Preface

This is not a textbook nor an encyclopedia; rather, it is a collection of papers representing a variety of points of view on contemporary issues, controversies, and questions about female sexual development. The editor has a point of view, not a point of view as to which of the various authors' positions presented in this book is correct, or even the most useful, but a point of view about the format of such a book; namely, that the definitive answers, and the experts who will provide them, are not yet identified. Therefore, many voices should be heard from different areas of expertise, training, experience, and background. Inevitably there are contradictions and disagreements. There should be. Several authors who were asked to provide short discussions for papers found themselves unable to answer in less than an additional paper. The editor welcomed this response. This is an area full of ancient myths, new discoveries, and alternate perspectives. It is hoped that the book reflects these ambiguities and controversies and that it will stimulate as many questions as it provides answers.

You will find represented in this volume, and its forthcoming companion volume on women's sexual experience, authors not generally found together between the covers. When useful and where possible, a discussion or an addendum to a paper has been included by an author who approaches the subject from a different base of information or experience. Some names are familiar to those acquainted with the literature, while others are not. The list of contributors includes a brief description of the background of each author.

You will find represented social workers, psychiatrists, psychoanalysts, sociologists, psychologists, nurses, educators, feminist activists, male, female, and old and young and in between.

Female sexuality has been a subject of worship and wonder, inspiring endless fascination and debate among men—not mankind, but men. Woman's psyche was studied first by gynecologists, since her mysterious power lay in the activities of her uterus; her mind was a flimsy sidecar. Psychiatrists often seemed to agree. While women have, for the most part, reflected the definitions and descriptions men gave them, they have had a secret knowledge not available to science. This knowledge about womankind is handed down in the women's subculture when female bonds are strong and are supported by the rituals of society. The breakup of the extended family and the idealization of the isolated nuclear family; increased mobility geographically, culturally, and socially; the loss of ritual and community; and the power of the media which have portrayed women as only rivalrous with other women for "the man"—all have fragmented women's cultural bonds. The women's movement has produced an euphoric reunion, a healing network of concern and respect among women. From this position of strengthened identity, women have begun to write about themselves, this time not in secret, as in the tradition of women's diaries, nor only for each other, as in the 19th-century tradition of love letters, but in scientific, literary, and news publications for all to see!

This book reflects some of these new points of view and some opposing ones as well. The guiding principle of the editor is the belief that uncertainty and a questioning approach are necessary characteristics of intellectual integrity and are to be cultivated and sponsored as the only protection against cultism and bigotry. New thoughts and attitudes are fertilized, developed, and given life by the coming together of opposites, or at least differences, in a productive, sometimes loving, mental intercourse. In that sense, I hope you will find this to be a "very sexy" book.

Many have participated in this love-in, especially Dr. Karen Blanchard, Dr. Patricia Parsons, Dr. Anne Seiden, and Ms. Carole Morgan, who helped develop the concept, read papers, and supported my flagging efforts; Ms. Molly Lewin, who gave freely of her expert editorial advice and wisdom; and Ms. Elayne Mitchell for support and help far beyond the call of administrative and secretarial duties.

MARTHA KIRKPATRICK

Los Angeles, California

Contents

Chapter 1

"Roll, Jenny Jenkins, Roll"

*Little Girls and Maidens in American Folksongs—
An Analysis of Sexual Attitudes*

Priscilla Oaks

Introduction

The sexual patterns of woman's life from birth to early maturity are
not only illustrated in folksongs but influenced by them as reflectors of
cultural attitudes and norms. Handed down from generation to generation and traditionally anonymous, folksongs are conservative and
perpetuate by both inclusion and omission what a society holds valid
and proper.

This essay focuses on the folksongs that inform the young years of
a woman's life, from the time of her birth through her puberty. What
do the songs say about growing up female in America? The childhood
songs to be discussed here are culturally derivative and conservative.
Late puberty, the period of courtship and womanhood, is the time
when women begin to sing out with their own voices, reflecting not
only the roles prescribed for them by American society, but the melo-
dies and words created from their own vital female experiences. Then
mothers sing to their daughters with bitter wisdom and friend sings to
friend about the private truths learned and handed on among women
for themselves.

But first, what is a folksong? It is impossible to be incorrect about
this as there are as many definitions of the word as there are experts in
the field. One folklorist insists that the "folk" must be illiterate; another imposes the criterion of age on a song; a third gives emphasis to
anonymity.

PRISCILLA OAKS, Ph.D. • Associate Professor of American Literature, Department of
English, California State University, Fullerton, California. Copyright 1979.

1

For this essay, two flexible and interrelated definitions will suffice. Burl Ives (1953) wrote: "Folk music becomes a part of the *people,* the *folk,* who molded it and made it their own by imposing their individual and collective mark upon it. This is the essence . . . *a people using music as their own personal expression."* Jan Brunvand (1978) stated: *"Folksongs* consist of words and music that circulate orally in traditional variants among members of a particular group" (p. 152). A folksong does not have to be hoary with age, either. Lomax and Lomax (1941) believe that a folksong can be contemporary and of immediate significance. Nor, in the opinion of others, does it have to be anonymous.

In preparing this crosscultural study, it has been necessary to make several broad assumptions in order to proceed in a very neglected area with few bibliographic aids.

First, we assume that folksongs are artistic endeavors and that, as such, they may be looked at as artifacts reflecting cultural attitudes.

Second, we assume that a nonethnocentric or multiple viewpoint is necessary if one is to appreciate and understand folksongs from a woman-oriented or feminist point of view. As each culture develops its own cohesive value system and sets up its own "norms," it is easy to adopt a unilateral or ethnocentric viewpoint toward others,[1] which is a main reason that studies of womansong or focus on women in folklore are so neglected in male-dominated American society.

Third, we assume that women have a separate and viable subculture where they live with other women when they are not interacting with the patriarchal American main culture.

The folksongs produced in this woman's culture reflect its values and "norms" and must be interpreted from that perspective.

The songs used in this essay are still sung today and were culled from the most popular anthologies of American folksong as well as from inclusive scholarly collections. Like many other products of women's achievement, the songs barely cast a shadow in the volumes in which they repose. They will not be found in the standard table of contents under such categories as "Work Songs" or "Heroes," or historical catchalls, such as "Developing America," although women worked, sang songs while they did, and were and are heroic and pioneering in spirit.

Indeed, the first group of songs to be discussed, lullabies, are

---

[1] Ethnocentrism is "an attitude or outlook in which values derived from one's own cultural background are applied to other cultural contexts where different values are operative" (Levine, 1972, p. 1). An ethnocentrist tends to regard other cultures as "incorrect, inferior or immoral" and to look at his or her own group with "pride and approval" and at other group value systems with "contempt and hatred" (Levine, 1972, p. 1).

work songs, as any mother with a fretful baby knows. As sung by women, they reflect a variety of attitudes and are variable in tone. Those sung by a slave woman with a white nursling are very different from both those of a Native American mother, and the tunes of a young farm girl at a dance who must watch all the babies in the sleeping room.

The next group, nursery rhymes, are less variable and more socially stringent and instructive. As tunes and words that one remembers all one's life, they are important determinants to the little girl of what her adult attitude toward herself should be.

When she finally enters school, circle games and play songs allow for some originality and are variable, but they still reflect a conservative and traditional orientation. Programming toward a passive sexual role and marriage as the ultimate goal in a woman's life starts at a very early age, as is evident in both these sets of songs.

With puberty come kissing games, courtship songs, and a growing sense of identity with a sexual self (not discussed in this chapter). This developing sexuality in the girl causes anxiety. And it is here also that folksongs show the beginnings of rebellion against cultural norms. Support for these attitudes can be found in songs sung by mothers giving advice to their daughters. Female bonding also begins to show the growing girl that she has a feminine subculture to rely upon for support.

Besides this attitudinal shift, two major themes or topics appear in the song lyrics, manifesting themselves as metaphors: women as food and women as nature, more specifically domesticated into women as gardens. Both of these themes have different emphases in the various sets of songs, but they are so manifest that they ought to be studied further in a crosscultural and interdisciplinary context.

INFANCY

"Probably the first music heard by any little boy or girl is a crooning lullaby song sung by a mother, a grandmother, or a big sister" (Hofmann, 1952). The word itself is heavy with *l* sounds and *Lully-lu* is often used in lullabies, "which are incantations to persuade children to sleep and also little proofs of joy in them" (Drinker, 1948, p. 27).

Whether the songs are "little proofs of joy" or not, they are universal. Sometimes they even contain the mother's recollections of her childbirth experience:

Peace, my child, be still and sleep, my love, my tiny one
Pain I learned from you, learned such pain as only God and I can ever
 know, and she who stayed beside me and saw you born.
Peace, my child, and cease to weep. Peace, my child, be still.

(Drinker, 1948, p. 46)

Perhaps the first "lullaby" an infant hears, besides the mother's heartbeat *in utero,* are the sounds a woman makes while giving birth, if she has not been too drugged to respond.

How this sound affects the neonate can only be theorized about, but certainly cultural attitudes toward birth influence the mother and her mothering, as do attitudes toward singing. Sophie Drinker (1948) described with many illustrations the power singing has to ease childbirth in her book *Music and Women*: "Among the Fans of Africa, the business is so important that a special enchantress hides in the bushes near the place of confinement and chants and chants an elaborate melody for hours. Even the pregnant woman sings" (pp. 22–23).

Many times the birth singing is wordless, a sighing, wailing sound that imitates as sympathetic magic the laboring woman's cries of pain: "The mother's sound may be re-enforced by the beating of drums, timed to strengthen the rhythmical contractions of birth" (Drinker, 1948).

Control by women over their own giving of birth has become increasingly popular in this country and with that control, contemporary American birth songs:

> O my woman's work is just begun,
> breathe nice and slow.
> staring moon-eyed at the wall, until the tightness goes.
> Well I know I'll love that little babe no matter when she come,
> hope it's sooner and not later—O yes hurry little one.
> (Cheney, 1976, pp. 130–132)

Like birth singing, lullabies are also work songs. The baby must be kept quiet while the Native American mother does her other chores:

> No-ni-hi-e, no-ni-hi-e, Go to sleep, my child,
> Go to sleep, my babe, Go to sleep, my child,
> While your mother works. (Hofmann, 1952)

Sometimes the woman is a southern mammy tending a white baby:

> Hush, li'l baby, don' say a word,
> Mamma's gonna buy you a mockingbird.
> If that mockin' bird don' sing,
> Mamma's gonna buy you a diamond ring. (Lomax, 1941, p. 95)

Often the mother is tired and dreams of extra helping hands:

> Duérmase mi niño, duérmase mi sol,
> duérmase, pedazo de mi corazón.
>
> María lavaba, San José tendía,
> eran los pañales que el niño tenía.

(Go to sleep my baby, go to sleep my sunshine,
go to sleep, little piece of my heart.

The Virgin Mary is washing, Saint Joseph was hanging out to dry; these
were the diapers that the baby had.) (Paredes, 1976, p. 120)

Not every baby is so loved. Misery at home, a drunkard husband
and poverty, too much work—all these can make mothers resent their
children. "Rockabye Baby on the Tree Top," the most familiar of all
Anglo-American lullabies has a frightening ending: "When the bough
breaks the cradle will fall/ And down will come cradle, baby, and all"
(Opie and Opie, 1951, p. 61).

This Creole mother living in the bayous of Louisiana wants a bit
of freedom and she fantasizes it:

Fais, dodo, mon fils, Crabe dans calalou;
Fais dodo, mon fils, Crabe dans calalou.

Papa, li couri la rivière, Manan, li couri pêcher crabe.
(Go to sleep, my son, Crabs are in the pot;
Got to sleep my son, Crabs are in the pot.
Paw, he's gone to the riverside, Maw, she's gone off
a-catching crab.) (Lomax, 1941, p. 97)

Perhaps, as in this next example, the mother has taken her freedom and gone off to dance at the church social, leaving a daughter or a
sitter with her baby. Or she may be the one taking care of all the
babies at a quilting bee:

What'll I do with this baby-o? (Repeat 3 ×)
If he won't go to sleepy-o?
Wrap him up in a tablecloth (Repeat 3 ×)
Throw him up in the fodder-loft.

Dance him north, dance him south,
Pour a little moonshine in his mouth.
Everytime the baby cries
Stick my finger in the baby's eye!
That's what I'll do with the baby-o. (Cheney, 1956, p. 128)

Certainly many of these lullabies are unsentimental and reflect a
variety of moods that, from a woman's point of view, are realistic. The
infant may not understand the words, but he or she will feel the emotion, the female emotion, for lullabies are singularly womansongs.
This last one is handed down from mother to daughter:

Sway away away to sleep
Little daughter, go to sleep
Oh, sway away, away, away,
Away, away,
Swinging away, oh,
Little daughter, go to sleep. (Bierhorst, 1974, p. 17)

Tender, rhythmic, and repetitious, the baby in her tree cradle probably went promptly to sleep at the sounds.

THE LITTLE GIRL

Children hear songs and stories long before they can read and
write and are exposed through them to the sexual roles and personalities favored by their culture. In societies with a continuous oral tradition, most of the songs children learn are communal adult songs sung
at festivals and rituals that are not necessarily created especially for
them. Children take part in these rites and customs as they grow
older.

The Anglo-American child who learns to read and write at about
the age of six is also subject to her oral traditions before that time. As
a toddler, she already knows by heart many nursery rhymes and
counting or clapping games. Here, in these verses, she learns the
traditional and conservative attitudes of her culture about women. She
absorbs them as her mother and sisters absorbed them, without thinking about their relevance and values and what they will mean in determining her future life. Thus, in urban and rural white America, a little
girl learns that it is proper to be good, clean, and passive; to stay at
home in her rightful role as a woman; to occupy herself with household tasks; and above all, to avoid the dangerous outside world.

The little girl learns, also, certain relevant connections between
women and food. Women are associated with food in nursery rhymes
in many ways. Food itself means life and safety. Eating gives comfort
and pleasure. Food is always important to a little child and is a topic
easily understood; the relationships between women and food can,
therefore, be taught early as a basic series of lessons in sexual conformity. An examination of *Mother Goose*, that venerable set of nursery
rhymes brought to the United States from England, bears out the connection between the two and demonstrates that it is a matter of life
and death.[2] Food is presented as a symbol of reward or punishment in
this collection of truly anonymous folksongs. Be good and you will be
given nourishment. Act bad, and, if you are a female, you will be
eaten by a male.

But first of all, implicit in the Mother Goose rhymes related to
food is the concept that it is the man who "brings home the bacon":

[2] There are many other collections of Mother Goose songs, each of which offers a slightly
different version of the same verse in the true folk tradition. A scattering of sociological
and psychological analyses has been made of these nursery rhymes; a larger number of
political analyses have been made in attempts to show that Mother Goose rhymes contain code words for political people and acts.

> The king was in the counting house,
> Counting out his money,
> The queen was in the kitchen,
> Eating bread and honey. (Benet, 1943, p. 7)

Husband and wife are here shown in their most elite social roles. The power and the control belong to the king. It is "his" money. Indeed, he has so much of it that it is in a separate house or bank. But the role of the queen is no different from that of a peasant woman. She is in the kitchen (some versions say "parlor"), consuming the most basic of foods. Later, she might bake some tarts. Perhaps she baked the pie of 24 blackbirds mentioned in the song in which the maid has her nose pecked off while she is hanging out the wash. Since scrubbing clothes clean is another approved activity for women, one wonders what the maid did to be so assaulted by the blackbirds.

Other songs show that without a man, a woman is starving and fuddled. Old women—probably widows, are forced to live in shoes or keep for protection dogs that they can't feed—:

> There was an old woman
> Who lived in a shoe;
> She had so many children
> She didn't know what to do. (Benet, 1943, p. 42)

The queen is safe as long as she pleases the king. She is as much his possession as is his money. Here is a less regal Mother Goose excerpt that says the same thing, adding the offer of a bribe. Curly Locks may be put on a status pedestal, in this case, a cushion, if she consents:

> Curly Locks! Curly Locks! Wilt thou be mine?
> Thou shalt not wash dishes nor yet feed the swine,
> But sit on a cushion and sew a fine seam,
> And feed upon strawberries, sugar, and cream. (Benet, 1943, p. 18)

Ironically, Curly Locks may not have to feed garbage to the pigs or clean up after dinner, but the reward offered for her acquiescence to passivity, for becoming a little poodle-headed pet, is certainly a temptation to gluttony.

And, of course, here is the most famous munching "sitter":

> Little Miss Muffet
> Sat on a tuffet,
> Eating her curds and whey. (Benet, 1943, p. 39)

Miss Muffet, however, is not perched on a cushion but on a tuft of grass in the dangerous freedom of out-of-doors:

> Then came a great spider,
> And sat down beside her,
> And frightened Miss Muffet away. (Benet, 1943, p. 39)

Compare this ending to a similar eating jingle, but one that involves a boy, not a girl:

> Little Jack Horner
> Sat in a corner
> Eating a Christmas pie.
> He put in his thumb
> And pulled out a plum
> And said: "What a good boy am I!" (Benet, 1943, p. 55)

Jack Horner enjoys his holiday treat and feels, moreover, that he deserves it. His is not a role of passive anxiety, but one of action and self-confidence. After he pokes around messily with his fingers for the plum, since a boy does not have to keep as clean as a girl, he ends his song in happy self-praise at his success.

Miss Muffet has no such ability to control her environment. It does not occur to her to lift her little foot and squash the bug. Instead, she probably runs back into the house and may not even finish her snack, which is certainly no Christmas pie, but plain food, not much fancier than cottage cheese. This is reminiscent of an ancient Chinese folksong from the *Shih Ching*, which clearly spells out the roles set for the two sexes:

> Boys shall have beds, hold sceptres for toys,
> creep on red leather,
> bellow when they would cry
> in embroidered coats. . . .
>
> Small girls shall sleep on floor and play with tiles,
> wear simple clothes and do no act amiss,
> cook, brew and seemly speak,
> conducing to the family's quietness. (Birch, 1965, p. 15)

Little girls are scheduled for the Spartan life, dedicated to serving the family, not to acting out their personal needs. Nor are they to covet delicacies such as plums or oranges:

> Dingity, diddley, my mammy's maid,
> Stole oranges, I'm afraid;
> Some in her pocket, some in her sleeve,
> She stole oranges, I do believe. (Benet, 1943, p. 29)

Other songs about eating show an even more dangerous aspect, that of cannibalism. This threat is everywhere, whether you are small and unimportant, as little girls may feel, or compensating by trying to be sweet. Take these two separate songs:

> There was an old woman called Nothing-at-all,
> Who rejoiced in a dwelling exceedingly small;
> A man stretched his mouth to its outmost extent,
> And down at one gulp house and old woman went. (Benet, 1943, p. 76)

> What are little girls made of, made of?
> What are little girls made of?
> Sugar and spice, and all that's nice;
> And that's what little girls are made of, made of. (Benet, 1943, p. 16)

If you are composed of the same ingredients that go into a dessert, there's no relief from the threat of being eaten, even in heaven, where Saint Peter stands at his gate "waiting for a buttered cake" (Benet, 1943, p. 30). Possibly these songs acquaint a girl with the concept of generous motherhood so, that in the future, she can sit Baby Diddit "on her lap and give him some pap" (Benet, 1943, p. 64). Give all, including your anonymous self, to the devouring masculine world of Baby Diddit, whose symbolic name sums up his accomplishment-oriented lifestyle.

In contrast, little boys are tough and inedible, an unappetizing menu composed of "frogs and snails and puppy dogs' tails" (Benet, 1943, p. 16). Nor do they have to be neat and tidy, another condition set on little girls as shown by another two rhymes, the first of which cautions against commerce:

> See, saw, Margery Daw,
> Sold her bed and lay upon straw,
> Was not she a dirty slut,
> To sell her bed and lie in dirt? (Benet, 1943, p. 18)

> Little Polly Flinders,
> Sat among the cinders,
>   Warming her pretty little toes!
> Her mother came and caught her,
> and whipped her little daughter
>   For spoiling her nice new clothes. (Benet, 1943, p. 18)

Punishment is swift in social censure and whippings. The rewards for good and controlled passive behavior direct the small girl toward her future role of becoming a sex object and vying for masculine approval:

> Charley loves good cakes and ale,
> Charley loves good candy,
> Charley loves to kiss the girls
> When they are clean and handy. (Benet, 1943, p. 18)

This behavior leads to marriage, although the danger of cannibalism does not stop with possession:

> Peter, Peter, pumpkin-eater,
> Had a wife and couldn't keep her;

> He put her in a pumpkin shell,
> And there he kept her very well. (Benet, 1943, p. 58)

If Peter happens to be myopic some night at dinnertime, this runaway and imprisoned wife is in deep trouble.

Little girls, therefore, learn from their nursery rhymes to be clean and sit still. They are to stay indoors, away from the dangers of large spiders; put the kettle on, like Polly; and take it off again, like Sukey. They can stay by the fire and spin, but never like Cross-Patch should they draw the latch. They must always be open and available, "clean and handy" for glamorous, outgoing males to kiss and later marry:

> Bobby Shafto's gone to sea,
> Silver buckles at his knee,
> Will he return and marry me?
> Bonny Bobby Shafto! (Opie and Opie, 1951, p. 90)

The question is rhetorical, if wistful. Yes, Bobby Shafto (note his phallic name) will marry this female who knows her place. She is not a wild one like Peter's wife. Yet!

The necessity for such tight control over female destiny is proper. Little girls must learn at a young age that females are inadequate and never do anything right. At least, not in *Mother Goose*. Little Betty Blue loses her shoe and Little Bo Beep loses her sheep, then can't figure out how to find them. The Queen of Hearts has her tarts stolen, a situation full of seductive significance because they have been stolen by the Knave of Hearts and obviously belong to the King. Old Mother Hubbard is unable to feed her dog and the Old Woman Who Lived in a Shoe is equally unresourceful. Like the Queen of Hearts, she has been too permissive sexually, which, in her case, resulted in so many children "she didn't know what to do." The punishment for misplaced passion in *Mother Goose* is starvation and harassment.

It is not surprising that these poorly functioning females become frustrated, bad-natured, and antisocial. Cross-Patch draws her latch and Jumping Joan stays alone and does not seek out others when nobody's with her.

Some of the women, particularly the older ones, become vicious to those in their care. The old libertine in the shoe with her passel of brats is so unable to maintain peace and quiet that she:

> Gave them some broth
> Without any bread,
> Then whipped them all soundly
> And sent them to bed. (Benet, 1943, p. 42)

A thin diet and a depriving one.

Similarly, another old woman, a spinner by occupation, took her calf and threw it over the wall. Her strength is used destructively. A nice man lends his pony, Dapple-Gray, to a lady who whipped and slashed him and "rode him through the mire" (Benet, 1943, p. 39). And who knows whether or not the cow with the crumpled horn received that crimp from the maiden all forlorn after her fight with Mary, Mary, quite contrary?

Little boys and men in nursery rhymes don't have these emotional problems. They are creative and active. Little Boy Blue, who loses his sheep like Bo Beep when he falls asleep, gets them back by blowing his horn. Jack, besides gobbling pie and leading Jill up a hill, builds a house and jumps over a candlestick. Johnny rides to Banbury Cross and is a drummer. Daddy goes a-hunting. Doctor Foster goes to Gloucester. The crooked man is able to walk a crooked mile. And even that village idiot, Simple Simon, manages to get to the fair alone. One old man survives decently in the wilderness and another goes about in the misty moisty weather, protected by his leather clothes. Whereas the women are limited to mother and queen and lowly maid roles, the men, besides having musical hobbies, are shown in a large number of professions: farmer, blacksmith, lawyer, doctor, barber, fisherman, miller, lord mayor, and, of course, king.

The men, not subject to the same frustrations, also have good temperaments and are sociable. The miller is jolly, King Arthur is a goodly king, and the best ruler of all, Old King Cole, that "merry old soul," (Benet, 1943, p. 46) likes to give parties.

The sociosexual role of females in nursery songs is summed up succinctly in the familiar counting rhyme with which so many children learn their numbers:

> Thirteen, fourteen,
> Maids a-courting;
> Fifteen, sixteen,
> Maids in the kitchen;
> Seventeen, eighteen,
> Maids in waiting;
> Nineteen, twenty,
> My plate's empty.
>   (Opie and Opie, 1951, p. 333)

GIRLHOOD

When the toddler develops into a schoolchild, a period of separation between the sexes takes place. American girls and boys go their individual ways in their play and singing games until early puberty or prepuberty, when they come back together again for kissing games. Boys are especially adamant about excluding girls:

> Pinch, punch, join in the ring,
> Pinch, punch, no girls in. (Opie and Opie, 1969, p. 17)

Like the nursery rhymes, and just as ancient in origin, girls' play and game songs are narrow in scope, preoccupied with domestic activities and courtship. In nursery school and the early grades, girls like to act out service songs such as "This Is the Way We Wash Our Clothes," "Dame, Get Up and Bake Your Pies," and "Don't You Hear My Needle Sing, Zing!" which tells about stitching for brother and knitting for daddy. (Landeck and Crook, 1969, pp. 36–37).

In preparation for being attractive to boys, many of the girls' songs show a preoccupation with appearance and dress:

> Mary wore her red dress, red dress, red dress,
> Mary wore her red (or blue or green) dress
> All day long. (Landeck and Crook, 1969, p. 15)

In succeeding verses, Mary wears her red hat, shoes, and gloves and ends up baking a red cake, about which the folklorists who collected the verses, appended a commentary: "If the baby don' go to sleep by now, you can jes' keep on an' on th'ough all de ingreemunts o' de cake." (Landeck and Crook, 1969, p. 15). Although this song is now used as an acting-out game for school, it originally helped little black southern girls with their baby-sitting, necessary while their mothers worked. In the last verse, Mary turns into a red bird. How many of these little girls must have wished they could fly away!

In the middle school grades, circle games become popular with both sexes, many of them derivatives of ancient songs still circulating in Europe. As a result, the same patriarchal value system of the nursery rhymes appears, and women are shown as sexual objects dependent on men. The girls' songs are preoccupied with courtship and weddings, but there is clear anxiety in some of them:

> Here I bake, here I brew
> Here I make my wedding cake,
> Here I mean to break through. (Players link hands)
> Open wide the garden gate,
> The garden gate, the garden gate;
> Open wide the garden gate,
> And let me through. (Opie and Opie, 1969, p. 238)

This song is ambiguous because it contains two contrary actions within it. In the center of the ring, the girl does her cooking and brewing. Then she tries to escape, suddenly seeing the circle as a garden, a potent sex symbol of the pubescent female. Marriage, of course, implies sexual intercourse. Can this song act out the fears of a prepubescent girl about her adult life to come?[3]

---

[3] Young American girls do not have such deep fears about their futures as Mexican girls, and readers interested in prepubescent sexual anxieties that are actively expressed

A second circle song directs a girl to dry her tears and resolve her anxiety and depression by learning the arts of adult sexual seduction:

> Little Sally Walker, sitting in a saucer, (sometimes Sally Waters)
> Rise, Sally, rise,
> Wipe your weeping eyes.
> Put your hands on your hips,
> Let your back-bone slip,
> Shake it to the east,
> Shake it to the west,
> Shake it to the one you love best,
> Mama say so, papa say so,
> That's the way to shake it if you want a beau. (McIntosh, 1974, p. 86)

Nothing could be more explicit than this pelvic rotation exercise.

Jump-rope games are similarly preoccupied with the opposite sex and courting:

> Mother, may I go out?
> All the boys are waiting,
> Just to take me out.
> Some will give me candy,
> Some will give me kisses,
> Behind the garden gate. (Note the garden again.)
> I don't want any candy,
> I don't want any cake.
> But I want (boy's name) to kiss me
> Behind the garden gate. (Opie and Opie, 1969, p. 101)

And here is another with a pun on pies:

> Strawberry shortcake, gooseberry pie,
> Tell the initials of your honeypie. (Opie and Opie, 1969, p. 110)
> (Say A, B, C, etc.)

Another one, also preoccupied with thoughts of eating, shows a girl passively accepting payment for sexual favors, training for adult women's work to come:

> Johnny gave me apples,
> Johnny gave me pears,
> Johnny gave me fifteen cents
> And kissed me on the stairs. (Botkin, 1944, p. 792)

---

should read Inez Cardozo-Freeman's article, "Games Mexican Girls Play," in Claire R. Farrer (Ed.), *Women and Folklore*, Austin: University of Texas Press, 1975, pp. 12–24. (Previously published in the *Journal of American Folklore*, 1975, *88*:347 (January–March): "Everything that keeps a woman suppressed is bound up in values that are determined by men," Ms. Cardozo-Freeman wrote (p. 15). But some of the games girls play "give expression to the feelings of hostility, fear, and frustration that the Mexican woman endures in her culture" (p. 15). Some of the games act out rape, betrayal, abandonment, and death, and they predict, as Ms. Cardozo-Freeman concluded, "a very dreary adulthood indeed" (p. 22).

Other jump-rope songs, sometimes used also for ball bouncing and leg-over games, show more assertive images in fantasizing adult dating behavior, which includes drinking coffee, tea, and wine. Some sound self-confident enough to be satiric or downright sassy. But it is the boys who still initiate sexual actions, such as being "stuck on" a girl or giving her "kisses":

> I love coffee,
> I love tea;
> How many boys
> Are stuck on me?
> (Count until there is a miss.) (Botkin, 1944, p. 792)

> Cinderella dressed in yellow
> Went uptown (or downtown) to meet her fellow.
> How many kisses did he give her?
> (Count until there is a miss.) (Botkin, 1944, p. 791)

> Mary's mad,
> And I am glad,
> And I know what will please her:
> A bottle of wine
> To make her shine,
> And a sweet little boy to squeeze her. (Botkin, 1944, p. 791)

Again, the boy is the actor. An insulting, satiric version of this song shows recognition of miscegenation taboos:

> Mary's mad,
> And I am glad,
> And I know how to please her:
> A bottle of ink
> To make her stink
> And a little nigger to squeeze her. (Botkin, 1944, p. 799)

Another set of songs goes beyond kissing and squeezing to rehearse the sequences of adult sexual activity in terms of external facts:

> First comes love,
> Then comes marriage;
> Then comes Edith
> With a baby carriage. (Botkin, 1944, p. 800)

Another goes into fuller details, while yet another expresses the old adage of sexual payment: "How many diamonds will he buy (count) . . . ?" (Opie and Opie, 1969, p. 109).

Not all the songs are so carefree. As in the first circle game, the next reflect anxiety about the future. The singer seems to shrug off adult courtship problems, which include the threat of widowhood. But the conditional *should*, used, according to linguists, by women and other subservient people more frequently than dominant ones, contradicts the stance:

> I should worry, I should care,
> I should marry a millionaire;
> He should die, I should cry,
> I should marry another guy. (Botkin, 1944, p. 797)

The next recognizes adult sexual competition between women, which isolates them from one another. Again the stance is tough, and note the garden metaphor again, but the ending is cruel and weak. The girl rejects responsibility toward her friend and blames the male:

> If you don't like my apples,
> Then don't shake my tree;
> I'm not after your boyfriend,
> He's after me. (Botkin, 1944, p. 799)

These prepuberty songs rehearse the patterns that girls ought to follow in courtship and marriage when they become older. The boys will offer candy and diamonds and other material goods, and the girls must learn to compete with each other and to bargain in socially proper ways. Therefore they must appear romantic and receptive rather than shrewd and assertive about selling themselves on the marriage market.

There is anxiety in the prepubescent girl and fear as shown by some of these songs, but there is still acceptance of the cultural values concerning women as sexual objects, and these feelings are not, therefore, worked out.

Only one group of sexually oriented play songs of middle-school children show the young girl free to express anxieties and resentments; those are the songs dealing with her mother. Many versions exist of the next song about a new sibling who gets neatly wrapped up and done away with symbolically as a load of excrement. Sending the "fudge" out "the back door" with her singing voice must give the young girl a lot of pleasure as she bounces her ball and sings:

> Fudge, fudge, tell the judge,
> Mama has a newborn baby.
> Wrap it up in tissue paper,
> Send it down the elevator.
> First floor, second floor . . . eight floor,
> And out the back door.
> (Opie and Opie, 1969, p. 110. See also Botkin, 1944, pp. 794, 801)

As direct interest in the opposite sex starts, both older girls and boys participate together in kissing games with dialogues about love and marriage. According to folklorists, kissing games have increased in popularity over the past 50 years. The following games are played in a circle group, where often a handkerchief or a piece of paper is dropped behind a favored person by "It," causing him or her to be chased and kissed:

> A tisket, a tasket,
> A red and yellow basket,
> I sent a letter to my love
> And on the way I dropped it. (Opie and Opie, 1969, p. 200)

A more complicated kissing game involves a girl's choosing a partner, who is then captured with her by the group. They sing to the boy:

> Then hug 'er and kiss 'er sweet,
> My honey, my love, my heart's above—
> Then hug 'er nice, and kiss 'er twice,
> Below Galilee. (Botkin, 1944, p. 811)

A number of play songs go through the motions of selecting a husband or a wife. "I Am a Rich Widow" recalls ancient marriage games of selection and involves a mother trying to marry off her daughter:

> I am a rich widow, I live all alone,
> I have but one daughter, and she is my own.
> Daughter, oh, daughter, go choose a man,
> Choose you a good one, or else choose none. (Linscott, 1962, p. 20)

At the opposite end of the range of women's possible marital roles is a similar circle game, "Here Stands an Old Maid Forsaken," which also advertises financial comfort in exchange for a husband:

> Here stands an old maid forsaken
> She's of contented mind;
> She's lost her own true lover,
> And wants another as kind;
> She wants another as kind, sir.
> I'll have you all to know,
> She's very well provided for,
> With forty-five strings to her bow.
> With forty-five strings to her bow! (Linscott, 1962, p. 16)

This Diana needs no Cupid with such a well strung "bow" and "contented mind."

"Paper of Pins" and "Lazy Mary" are two circle dialogue games in which a catalog of presents is reeled off—in the first by a boy and in the second by a mother—until the girl or Mary accepts the offer. In "Paper of Pins," the girl refuses pins (jewelry), a red dress with gold embroidery, and variously, silk gloves, shoes, horses (especially in the Southwest), or the boy's hand and heart. Only when the key to the boy's chest of gold is offered does she accept. The boy then turns her down with great disapproval:

> Oh, ho, ho, ho, now isn't that funny,
> You don't want me, but you want my money,

> And you'll not marry, marry, marry,
> And you'll not marry me.

The directions for this song involve pantomime:

> As the boy offers the key to his money, the girl listens adoringly. But the
> boy's expression slowly changes to scorn, while she advances with out-
> stretched arms, which he refuses. . . . . As he continues, the girl hides her
> face with her hands and turns away crying. (McIntosh, 1974, pp. 88–89)

When heart and hand go with a financial offer, that is the cue for the
acceptance of a contract.

In "Lazy Mary," the daughter will not get up, and the mother
bribes her all day with various foods until she offers her "a nice young
man," which produces the desired results. (Linscott, 1962, p. 33) A
shift is noticeable here. Sex has become more interesting than eating!

Other circle games such as "On the Green Carpet," and "Poor
Mary Sits A-Weeping" deal similarly with the importance of a
woman's having a sweetheart, the assumption always being that marriage is the suitable role for a woman and that she is brokenhearted
without a man.

The last courting song, "Jenny Jenkins," is interesting because it
uses color symbolism: red stands for sin, blue, for faithfulness, and
white for purity. Again, it is a dialogue song between a boy and a girl
in which "by asking the girl what dress she intends to wear, the
young man hopes to learn something of her attitude toward him."

> Will you wear red,
> Oh my dear, oh my dear,
> Will you wear red,
> Jenny Jenkins?
>
> No, I won't wear red,
> It's a color I dread,
> I'll buy me a fol-de-rol-de, til-de-tol-de,
> Seek a double us-a-caus-a,
> Roll, Jenny Jenkins, roll. (Scott, 1967, pp. 48–49)

Playing with him, Jenny Jenkins goes off into nonsense syllables as
she tells him that she won't wear green, "it's a shame to be seen," nor
white, "cause the color's too bright," nor blue, "cause the color's too
true." Finally she leaves him in complete doubt by concluding coyly,
as if she understood none of the symbolism involved: "Now what do
you care, so I don't go bare?" (Scott, 1967, pp. 48–49). And this jaunty,
teasing song demonstrates, any young girl singing it is now ready for
the most important game of her life, the drama of courtship.

REFERENCES

Benet, W. R. *Mother Goose, A comprehensive collection of the rhymes.* New York: Heritage Press, 1943.

Bierhorst, J. *Songs of the chippewa.* New York: Farrar, Straus & Giroux, 1974.

Birch, C. (Ed.). *Anthology of Chinese literature: From early times to the fourteenth century.* New York: Grove Press, 1965.

Botkin, B. A. (Ed.). *A treasury of American folklore.* New York: Crown Publishers, 1944.

Brunvand, J. H. *The study of American folklore: An introduction* (2nd ed.). New York: W. W. Norton, 1978.

Caraway, G., and Caraway, C. (Eds.). *Freedom is a constant struggle: Songs of the freedom movement.* New York: Oak Publications, 1968.

Cheney, J., Deihl, M., and Silverstein, D. (Eds.). *All our lives: A women's songbook.* Baltimore: Diana Press, 1976.

Drinker, S. *Music and women.* New York: Coward-McCann, 1948.

Hofmann, C. (Ed.). *War whoops and medicine songs.* Boston: Boston Music Company, 1952.

Ives, B. *The Burl Ives songbook.* New York: Ballantine, 1953.

Landeck, B., and Crook, E. *Wake up and sing: Folk songs from America's grass roots. . . .* New York: William Morrow and Company, 1969.

Levine, R. A., and Campbell, D. T. *Ethnocentrism: Theories of conflict, ethnic attitudes and group behavior.* New York: John Wiley & Sons, 1972.

Linscott, E. H. (Ed.). *Folk songs of old New England.* Hamden, Connecticut: Archon Books, 1962.

Lomax, A., and Lomax, J. A. *Our singing country.* New York: McMillan, 1941.

McIntosh, D. S. *Folk songs and singing games in the Ozarks.* Carbondale: Southern Illinois University Press, 1974.

Opie, I., and Opie, P. *Oxford dictionary of nursery rhymes.* Oxford, England: Clarendon Press, 1951.

Opie, I., and Opie, P. *Children's games in street and playground.* Oxford, England: Clarendon Press, 1969.

Paredes, A. *A Texas-Mexican cancionero: Folksongs of the lower border.* Urbana: University of Illinois Press, 1976.

Reynolds, M. *The Malvina Reynolds songbook.* Berkeley, Calif.: Schroder Music Company, 1974.

Scott, J. A. *The ballad of America: The history of the United States in song and story.* New York: Grosset & Dunlap, 1967.

Chapter 2

The History of Female Sexuality in the United States

Myrna I. Lewis

The course of sexuality for the American female has gone through re-markable changes, from the variety of sexual customs found in early colonial days to the repressions of the 19th century and the liberaliza-tion of attitudes and behavior in the 20th century. Some of what has happened has been done to women—through cultural training, medi-cal influences (e.g., 19th-century physicians' attributing a number of female medical problems to sexual "excess"), and the impact of male expectation and interpretation of female sexuality. But at least a share of female sexual behavior has been determined by females themselves, acting in what they felt were their best interests considering the choices available at the time. This is especially clear in the 19th cen-tury, as we shall see.

Colonial Women

When females began arriving as colonists in North America, as many as 1 million American Indian females were already here. The sexual customs of Indian women varied tremendously, but in general, unmarried girls had considerable sexual freedom, while married women were expected to remain faithful to their husbands. As Indian women were joined by European colonial women, both bond servants and free, and by African women brought as slaves, North America represented a mixture of sexual customs for women that was fascinat-ing in its diversity. But European cultural values were soon imposed

Myrna I. Lewis, A.C.S.W. • Psychotherapist in Private Practice, Washington, D.C.
This chapter is condensed from the author's forthcoming book *Women in American Soci-ety: A Summing Up,* to be published by C. V. Mosby and Company, St. Louis, Missouri.

legally and socially wherever possible, with these values, in turn, dominated by the New England Puritans in the northern colonies. Gradually an "American" point of view toward female sexuality evolved.

THE NEW ENGLAND COLONIES. Marital sex for the Puritan Calvinists was a necessary evil, tolerated in order to conceive children and avoid nonmarital sexual temptations. Early marriage for girls, at age 17 or 18 was common, providing a practical method of limiting fornication and illegitimate pregnancies. Like any other human pleasure that the Puritans allowed themselves, sex within marriage was to be conducted with restraint, and care was taken that it did not interfere with religious duties. One minister warned, ". . . sometimes a man hath a good affection to Religion, but the love of his wife carried him away. . . . This is an inordinate love" (Cotton, 1658).

Puritan clergymen fought a desperate fight against "inordinate" sexuality, presenting women as dangerous embodiments of Eve, the temptress. Frequently these warnings took on hysterical tones, as in the exhortations of Cotton Mather's father to colonists to avoid the perils of "gynecandrical" dancing (unmarried men and women dancing together): "This we affirm to be utterly unlawful, and . . . it cannot be tolerated in such a place as New England without great Sin" (Mather, 1684). Any sexual practices between unmarried persons were strictly forbidden. In seeming contradiction, until we remember that marital sex was taken for granted, a man could be stripped of church membership because he "denied Conjugal fellowship unto his wife," refusing sex for two years (Records, Boston, n.d.). A woman could also obtain annulment or, more rarely, divorce if her husband was impotent or withheld sex from her.

Many Puritans were unable to meet their own exacting sexual standards. Premarital sex, adultery, illegitimacy, rape, and, to a lesser extent, homosexuality were widespread, and only prostitution, identified with the later gradual change from a rural to an urban culture, was absent from the roster of common illegal sexual practices. The Puritans were one of the few cultural groups that expected equal sexual abstinence outside of marriage for both men and women. Women generally received the more severe punishments for disobeying. In a few communities, like early Plymouth, female adulterers were sentenced to wear the scarlet letter *A* on their dresses for the rest of their lives; more often they were severely whipped, fined, or imprisoned. Males, on the other hand, were more likely to be fined or sentenced to standing locked in the pillory. If a child was conceived and the father could be identified, he was required to support it.

THE MIDDLE COLONIES. A much more relaxed sexual standard prevailed in the middle colonies, particularly New York and Pennsylvania, where premarital sex was an accepted social custom among groups like the Pennsylvania Dutch. The only sexual practice outside of marriage that consistently received severe punishment was miscegenation. "Bundling," the practice of young unmarried men and women lying in bed together partially or fully clothed while they conversed, was a popular custom in a number of colonies. Bundling occurred primarily between courting couples in homes where firewood and candlelight were scarce, but rural colonists with a scarcity of extra beds offered similar hospitality to traveling strangers. Lively debates arose as to whether bundling encouraged sexual contact and illegitimate pregnancies, and though it undoubtedly did, the practice continued in the middle colonies and in some rural New England communities until about 1800.

THE SOUTHERN COLONIES. Sexuality for women in the southern colonies was influenced by slavery and the fact that the less sexually strict (at least toward males) Anglican Church of England rather than Puritanism was the dominant religious influence. A sexual double standard existed between white men and women, with many men openly keeping black and white slave and servant women as mistresses. Adultery for males was socially acceptable in even the most fashionable circles. In contrast, white upper-class women were expected to be "pure" and faithful to their husbands, as slave and servant women provided convenient sexual services for the white men who controlled them. The ostensible reason for the double standard was to avoid "confusion of progeny" for purposes of inheritance. But more clearly, neither slave and servant woman nor their upper-class mistresses had the legal protection or the social sanctions to object to the situation effectively.

"MRS. GRUNDY." A new force arose toward the end of the 18th century with the expansion of the middle class and an accompanying concern with propriety, conformity, and social acceptability. This force was symbolized as "Mrs. Grundy," the nosy neighbor, that is, an increasing worry about what "others" would think and how they would judge one's behavior, especially one's sexual behavior. "Respectability" began to vie with and even replace religion as the central ruling factor in people's lives. The sexuality of women, already dangerous in theological terms, began to be unacceptable socially even in marriage. The new ideal was the sexless, ethereal female who was dismayed and shocked by the baseness and animality of physical sex.

THE 19TH CENTURY

The first public discussion of female sexuality began in the United States in about 1830, when books on "sexual physiology" and "sexual hygiene" began to appear. Written largely for a middle-class audience by white middle-class Protestant clergymen and physicians, many of these books presented the 19th-century American female as "congenitally incapable of experiencing complete sexual satisfaction and peculiarly liable to sexual anesthesia" (Ellis, 1903). A statement by Dr. William Acton, one of the most widely quoted sex experts of his time in England and America, is typical:

> As a general rule, a modest woman seldom desires any sexual gratification for herself. She submits to her husband, but only to please him; and, but for the desire of maternity, would far rather be relieved from his attention. (Acton, 1865)

This point of view appears so repeatedly that one is forced to take a serious look at what happened to make women acquire the reputation for such extreme passivity and sexlessness.

INFLUENCES ON FEMALE SEXUALITY. One factor was a change in the social attitudes toward women. By the middle of the 18th century, female labor was no longer so desperately required in a variety of occupations as it had been earlier, and the mark of a successful family became the housebound wife, removed from the world of industry, commerce, and trade. Acting within their newfound leisure, American women began to imitate what they surmised to be the behavior of polite society in Europe. Relations between men and women in the growing middle class became stiffly formal and proper as the two sexes backed themselves into rigidly separated roles. Peculiar signs of affectation appeared in the language to signal a "refined" approach to physical functions: *legs* became *limbs, breasts* were called *bosoms, pregnant* became *enceinte, masturbation* was the solitary vice, and so forth (Rugoff, 1971). Increasing prosperity in the nation brought a preoccupation with fashion, manners, and "taste," as the female descendants of rough adventurers, colonists, pioneers, and settlers began to enjoy some of the luxuries of "gentlewomen" and "ladies of culture." A lack of interest in sex was an important feature in the repertoire of the newly delicate American female.

Another element in sexual restraint was the fact that although American women had been producing children at an astonishing rate during the colonial era, a movement was afoot that began giving them ideas about controlling the number and timing of their pregnancies. Thomas Malthus and his followers had raised the specter of the world population's outstripping its own food supply, inspiring the beginning of the modern birth-control movement. The dangers of overpopulation in America's wide-open space were hardly an impressive argument for American women, but the concept of limiting and spacing births must have had enormous appeal to them from a purely personal standpoint. In the 19th century, as in all of previous history, childbirth was a perilous, often life-threatening occasion, and the large colonial families of as many as 15 or 20 children sapped the energy when they did not extinguish the life of the mother. A well known 19th-century female writer observed:

> Mothers . . . bear children with such rapidity that a second babe comes out before the first is out of arms; . . . if there is any hope for America, . . . a woman must be recognized as holding her motherhood entirely in her own hands, to accept or reject as she thinks best. (Duffey, 1876)

But how were women to begin limiting pregnancy? Malthus himself advised sexual restraint and late marriage as the only ethical ways to control births. A few other methods were available but largely unsatisfactory. Coitus interruptus, or withdrawal of the penis from the vagina prior to ejaculation, was condemned by most medical advisers, interestingly enough, as dangerous to women's health and temperament. The "rhythm method" was totally unreliable, since 19th-century experts could not agree on the average time of ovulation—most thought it occurred at menstruation. Abstinence, therefore, was the only sure method of birth control, and much of the popular sexual-advice literature urged couples to practice periods of restraint ranging from having intercourse once a month to once a year. For those who could not manage this, another curious choice was available: "karezza," or intercourse without male orgasm (Stockham, 1896). Karezza was promoted as a technique with several advantages: men could demonstrate sexual love to their wives, practice birth control, and benefit spiritually and physically from the conservation of their sperm. The 19th-century interest in "spermatic economy" was an old idea dating back to as early as the 5th century B.C. and a treatise theorizing that even a small discharge of semen could weaken a man (Hippocrates, 1952). Karezza naturally appealed to women, since they could have prolonged intercourse without pregnancy (although some pregnancies occurred from sperm in the preejaculatory lubrication), but for obvious reasons, it never became popular with men.

A further interesting influence on female sexuality was the belief that simultaneous orgasm on the part of both partners increased the possibility of conception (Napheys, 1869). It follows that some women must have held back orgasm as a birth control technique. How widespread this theory was is unclear, but judging from the number of eminent physicians in the latter part of the century who took considerable pains to refute it, it must have been fairly well accepted.

Venereal diseases also had a profound effect on the behavior of women. Syphilis and gonorrhea were rampant in the latter half of the 19th century, with estimates that as many as 30% of men and women eventually contracted a venereal infection. Many men had affairs during marriage in addition to the high proportion who had sexual experiences before marriage. Since these experiences were often with prostitutes who were already infected, the dread "social diseases" were spread from husbands to wives and passed on to their children. Silver nitrate to prevent blindness in babies born to mothers with gonorrhea was not available until 1884. Progress of any kind in the treatment of syphilis had been stymied for 300 years until the discovery of Salvarsan in 1904. Sulfa drugs were introduced in 1936. But the risk and fear of venereal disease continued in the United States until after 1945, when the introduction of penicillin was accompanied by a greater public willingness to acknowledge and control the diseases.

Other physical ailments and diseases took a toll on women. Nonvenereal infections of the vagina with a discharge known as "the whites" were common and difficult to treat. Many women and girls had "the whites" chronically, or at least periodically, and it was believed that this condition, as well as urinary tract infection, was related to or aggravated by sexual contact. Tuberculosis, a disease epidemic in the United States from the mid-19th century on, was assumed to be connected with "sexual excess" as one of its causes. Women particularly were warned of this possibility since the death rate for young females was often twice that of males (Ehrenreich and English, 1973). Numbers of other physical conditions as well were blamed on "sexual excess," as the fledgling medical profession struggled to explain and cure the diseases of women.

The "Self-Abuse" Phobia. Probably the greatest impediment of all to healthy sexual expression in females was the 19th-century horror of masturbation (also called *self-abuse, self-pollution,* or the *solitary vice*). The idea that masturbation could cause disease was a rather new one, traceable to an anonymous 18th-century pamphlet called "Onania: or, The Heinous Sin of Self-Pollution, and All Its Frightful Consequences in Both Sexes Considered, Etc." (1737). Before the 18th century, masturbation in females seems to have been ignored, in contrast with the long history of negative attitudes toward male masturbation. This was true primarily because the "loss of seed" in males was the focus of concern. However, the author of "Onania" and subsequent writers introduced the notion that masturbation had other dire effects, for example, placing a drain on the nervous energy of the body, damaging the mind, and upsetting the body's balance through orgasm. Concerned parents began guarding their daughters as closely as their sons. An unfortunate semantic confusion between masturbation and venereal disease, which had already begun in the 16th century, added to the growing fears.

Writers of advice books began elaborating on the ills of masturbation, eventually depicting it as even more dangerous for females than for males. Hysteria, incurable jaundice, stomach cramps, prolapse and ulceration of the womb, and clitoral rashes were some of the female consequences. In addition, tuberculosis, chlorosis (chronic anemia due to menstruation), dyspepsia, spinal disease, headache, epilepsy and other "fits," impaired eyesight, heart palpitations, diabetes, incontinence of urine, vaginal infections, inflammation of urinary organs, and even death were all at one time or another blamed on masturbation. In 1845, young ladies were warned of "lunatic" asylums where

> alcohol is considered prime minister in working insanity and masturbation second in rank, but the temperance revolution is about to dispose the premier and then masturbation will be "by merit raised to that bad eminence." (Gregory, 1845/1974)

Young girls were subject to an immense number of restrictions (evidently often ignored) to help them avoid masturbatory temptations. Reading novels, listening to "passionate" or "voluptuous" music, wearing heavy hair pieces and wigs, and lacing oneself too tightly into a girdle were all suspected as inducements of the feared practice. Even the French bidet and the treadle sewing machine were possible culprits in seducing females into "venereal excitement." A well-received book among the medical profession in 1908 advises guarding young girls against remaining in bed unless asleep and warns that they should not sleep on their backs nor stay in the bathroom any longer than is absolutely necessary. Spicy food, alcohol, coffee, tea, cocoa, and horseback or bicycle riding were to be avoided, "nor should [girls] be given opportunity for daydreaming" (Talmey, 1904/1908). In spite of all of these precautions, a physician observed with alarm: "Women do practice the vice with a frequency which is almost incredible" (Robinson, 1938).

Scoldings and physical restraint were the most common preventive techniques, but both English and the American physicians not infrequently took other approaches with those females declared incorrigible. A surgical procedure known as clitoridectomy (removal of the clitoris) and the cauterization (burning or blistering) of the spine, thighs, or genitals were two accepted procedures. The clitoridectomy was introduced in England in 1858 by Isaac Baker Brown, a respected London surgeon who later became president of the Medical Society of London (Brown, 1866). Although he was eventually expelled from the

English Obstetrical Society for his work and condemned by a majority of American doctors, clitoridectomy and cauterization continued to be used on thousands of females in America for many years (Dawson, 1912). Even baby girls were considered dangerous to themselves: in 1905 a toddler of two and a half year had her clitoris removed (Sachs, 1895), and a major pediatric textbook mentions such practices as late as 1936 (Holt, 1897/1936).

In light of later findings that self-exploration and masturbation in early childhood are important in enabling females to learn to respond easily and pleasurably to sexual stimulation, the massive repression of masturbation in the 19th century explains a good part of whatever sexual difficulties the Victorian female had. Meanwhile, the aftereffects of this repression still remain today.

THE OTHER VICTORIANS. It is important to point out that American women were apparently not an easy lot to repress. The New England Puritan sexual ethic was confronted by a female population that was geographically strung out along the entire eastern coastline and represented a rambunctious and headstrong collection of personalities. The sheer variety of cultures from which women came and the need for their active participation in settling the New World made their control difficult. In the latter part of the 18th century and early 19th century, when it looked as though large numbers of women were finally settling into more traditional female roles, the birth control movement, the women's suffrage campaign, the Free Love Movement, and finally the need for female labor in factories began to counterbalance the influence of John Calvin, the Mathers, and "Mrs. Grundy."

Evidence of interest in sex from women themselves has to be gathered from between the lines of what they wrote, for women expressed themselves in the formal terminology of the times. But it is not difficult to believe, for example, that Abigail Adams was alluding to her sexual as well as her affectionate feelings toward her husband when she wrote to him: "I dare not express to you at three hundred miles' distance, how ardently I long for your return. . . . The idea plays about my heart, unnerves my hand whilst I write" (Donovan, 1966). The tremendous 19th-century female interest in romantic novels undoubtedly had a sexual basis in addition to a romantic, sentimental motivation. In describing these novels, Duffey (1876) remarked, "The ideas are presented in a voluptuous guise, purposely shaped to inflame the blood and make sin attractive and excusable."

An impressive assortment of medical literature from the 19th century speaks more directly of a strong sex drive in women as well as a healthy capacity for orgasm (Degler, 1974). For example, one physician wrote of treatments for "female impotence" with the assumption that this was an aberration that need not be tolerated. *The Physical Life of Women*, one of the leading guides for women, divides female sexuality into three categories:

1. The smallest group: those who have no sexual feelings.
2. A larger group: those who have "strong passion."
3. The vast majority of women: those "in whom the sexual appetite is as moderate as all other appetites" (Napheys, 1869).

Necessary Conditions. In view of the numerous forces mentioned earlier that clearly operated against female sexuality, what were the conditions that made the enjoyment of sexuality possible for at least some 19th-century women? A mutually monogamous relationship with a man probably helped, since the woman was thereby protected from venereal disease. Fortuitous escape from oppressive surveillance of her early physical self-explorations was probably another factor, as well as lack of access to or a simple ignoring of the sexual advice manuals of the day. Good health or a minimum of contact with physicians who advocated female sexual restraint for a whole variety of physical ailments was no doubt beneficial. And finally, some method of controlling pregnancies was surely important. Although few of the available birth control methods even at the end of the century were foolproof, women were obviously making some progress in limiting pregnancies, since birthrates were falling. A few of the advice manuals began to reflect the greater possibilities for female sexual enjoyment, for example, ". . . it is her duty to her husband, her children and herself, to heartily enjoy with her husband sexual intercourse and to keep herself in such condition that she may enjoy it" (Hanchett, 1887).

THE 20TH CENTURY

EARLY 20TH-CENTURY THEORISTS ON FEMALE SEXUALITY. The study of human sexuality began flourishing around 1890 as part of the general interest in the biological and medical sciences. The first major changes in public thinking about female sexuality came from the efforts of two European men, Havelock Ellis and Sigmund Freud. Ellis, an English psychologist and author who later became a physician, laid the groundwork for a good deal of 20th-century thought about sex in his major life work, *Studies in the Psychology of Sex,* published in seven volumes between 1897 and 1928. He introduced the general public to the revolutionary idea that women were as interested in sex as men and even had, in his opinion, a more complex and all-inclusive sexuality. Female arousal involved a much greater proportion of the body, including the clitoris (which Ellis saw as the central organ of female sexuality), the breast, the vagina, and the uterus, while male arousal focused primarily on the penis. In fact, Ellis postulated that women might be *more* psychologically interested in sex than men because of their greater physiological response and, in a phrase that produced mixed reviews from the early feminist movement in England, said, "In a certain sense their brains are in their wombs" (1903). Willing to challenge most stereotypes, Ellis nevertheless clung firmly to the Victorian belief that women were by nature passive, requiring men to take the initiative.

Sigmund Freud, the Austrian physician who founded psychoanalysis, shares with Ellis the distinction of refuting the widespread 19th-century belief that women were uninterested in sex. But Freud was far less accepting of female sexuality as healthy and natural: he found pathology lurking in every developmental phase from babyhood on. Believing with Ellis that psychologically healthy adult females are innately passive, Freud saw the sexuality of small girls as essentially masculine—that is, assertive and unintimidated—until they realize at about the age of four that they are lacking a penis. From this moment on, they are filled with "penis envy" (1925) and spend a good part of the remainder of childhood trying to adjust to the feeling of loss. Their sexuality must undergo a drastic metamorphosis. Libidinal (sexual) feelings formerly directed toward their mothers (who have no penises and are therefore declared inferior) are turned toward their fathers through the mechanism that Freud called the "female Oedipal complex" (or the "Electra complex"). The little girl fantasizes that her father will impregnate her and give her a baby to compensate for the penis she believes she has lost. When she slowly realizes this is not going to happen, she represses her sexual impulses in disappointment. Her sexuality remains largely dormant until she is ready for marriage and has found a suitable partner toward whom she feels appropriately affectionate and sexual; she is then presumably introduced, as it were, to her own sexual feelings through the act of sexual intercourse.

Freud elaborated on a particular element in this drama that has had profound effects on several generations of attitudes toward female sexuality. He felt that the female child's clitoral masturbation was a masculine activity (he equated the clitoris with an undeveloped penis), which the child must give up in order to accept her "femaleness." This renunciation takes place at age four or five, with sexual feelings returning at a much later time mysteriously ensconced in the vagina. Those not able to produce orgasms vaginally (the physiology of which Freud was never able to explain) were termed "frigid"—obstinate resisters of their fate as women—and Freud set the stage for the "vaginal" orgasm as the only sound form of female sexual expression.

Several women psychoanalysts (Karen Horney, Melanie Klein, Josine Müller) and a few men like Ernest Jones argued that Freud's views were marred by male bias and overvaluation of the penis. Horney (1926), in particular, objected: "I do not see why . . . it should not be conceded that the clitoris legitimately belongs to and forms an integral part of the female genital apparatus." But most well-known women analysts of the era—Marie Bonaparte, Ruth Mack Brunswick, Jeanne Lampl-deGroot, Helene Deutsch, Therese Benedek, and others—generally accepted and elaborated on Freud's theories. Interestingly, Freud himself reserved final judgment. In one of his last statements on the subject ("The sexual frigidity of women . . . is a phenomenon that is still insufficiently understood"), he speculated that there might be constitutional or anatomical as well as psychogenic factors (1933). Nonetheless, his theories became hardened into orthodoxy by his followers, and even today numbers of psychoanalysts, psychiatrists, and other therapists base their work with females on Freud's clitoral–vaginal transfer theory. As in Freud's time, much of the "frigidity" they seek to correct with these methods remains stubbornly unresponsive to treatment.

Sex Advice Manuals Between 1900 and 1950. The impact of the increasing interest in and the changing attitudes toward female sexuality is reflected in sexual advice manuals written for the general public. Pleasure, rather than simply procreation, began to be advocated as a goal for women in the early part of the century, only, of course, within the context of marriage. Female sexual desire, while steadily gaining acceptance, was qualified in two ways: first, it was quiescent and depended on the husband to activate it; second, it was more "spiritual" and "pure" than that found in males (Gordon, 1971). Consequently, the double standard could still be comfortably supported, since women were seen as more monogamous by their very nature.

In a tradition begun by Ellis, husbands were put to the task of learning to arouse and please their wives. The most outstanding exponent of this school was Theodoor van de Velde in his book *Ideal Marriage* (1930), one of the most popular marriage manuals of all time. The prize was the highly desirable "simultaneous orgasm," with both husband and wife reaching sexual climax at precisely the same moment. This aim put great pressure on couples to "succeed" and added a new burden for women, who had to combine this directive with the already demanding task of producing the often elusive "vaginal orgasm."

One of the most unusual advice manuals written during the

period was that of an English gynecologist, Dr. Helena Wright, in the 1930s. Wright not only gave step-by-step instructions for women on how to have orgasms through intercourse but also taught them how to masturbate, something unheard of in most professional circles.

THE FIRST FEMALE SEX SURVEYS. At the same time that psychoanalysis was emerging as a new way of looking at women, another technique came into use: the personal interview. The first known sex survey appeared far before all the others and was conducted by a female physician from 1890 to 1920. Clelia Mosher of Stanford University collected information on a small number of women born before the Civil War or shortly thereafter, and her work, which has never been published in its entirety, is the first glimpse we have of actual women talking directly about their sexual feelings and responses (Degler, 1974). Many were surprisingly frank in their enjoyment of sexuality, even though most held the typically 19th-century view that sex was primarily for reproductive purposes.

Some 30 to 40 years later, large-scale interview surveys appeared, including Katherine B. Davis's *Factors in the Sex Life of Twenty-Two Hundred Women* (1929), Robert Dickinson and Lura Beam's *A Thousand Marriages: A Medical Study of Sex Adjustment* (1931), and *Psychological Factors in Marital Happiness* (1938), by Lewis M. Terman *et al.* None was revolutionary, but all added to the growing fund of knowledge about women.

THE KINSEY REPORT ON WOMEN (1953). A breakthrough in the understanding of female sexuality occurred with the work of Alfred Kinsey and his associates at Indiana University, where some 6000 white female volunteers were interviewed about their sexual activities. Kinsey found that many sexual activities such as premarital intercourse, masturbation, and homosexuality were much more common than previously thought and that younger generations of women were more sexually active than their mothers and grandmothers had been. One of his most publicized findings—that women reached their peak of sexual functioning around age 30, while males peaked at age 16 and 17—was assumed to be a true physiological difference between the sexes. However, later evidence strongly suggests that this difference was merely a measurement of the cultural repression of sexuality in adolescent and young adult women.

One of Kinsey's most important contributions was his explanation of the findings that women, although they could masturbate to orgasm as quickly as men, failed at a much greater rate to reach orgasm through intercourse alone. Kinsey felt that the reason was simply that the clitoris was not sufficiently stimulated. In opposition to Freud, Kinsey believed that the clitoris was the primary response site for females and that female sexuality was physiologically similar to male sexuality in arousal and orgasm.

The next step was to test this theory under controlled laboratory conditions. A number of investigators, including Dickinson, van de Velde, and Kinsey, had already made direct clinical observations of female sexual response, but it remained for Masters and Johnson to conduct major experiments.

MASTERS AND JOHNSON'S STUDY OF FEMALE SEXUAL PHYSIOLOGY. The work of William Masters and Virginia Johnson in St. Louis, Missouri, in the late 1950s and the early 1960s led to a much greater clarification of a number of questions about female sexual physiology. Their laboratory observations and photographs of the physiological reactions of women and men during a variety of sexual activities, including intercourse, resulted in the publication of two books, *Human Sexual Response* (1966) and *Human Sexual Inadequacy* (1970), with the latter including a study of the psychological factors interfering with sexual response.

Masters and Johnson found the human sexual response cycle to be similar for both sexes, with vaginal lubrication in the female seen as the "neurophysiological parallel" to erection in the male as a major signal of sexual arousal. Like Kinsey, they concluded that clitoral stimulation was central to female response and demonstrated that all female orgasms, whether achieved by masturbation or intercourse, are physiologically similar. The clitoris, even during intercourse, is stimulated, since its hood is moved back and forth by the thrusting penis and the muscles in the vaginal area. Unlike other investigators, Masters and Johnson were impressed by the female capacity for a number of orgasms in quick succession (multiple orgasms) in contrast to the capacity of the male, who is limited by the need for a recovery (refractory) period after each orgasm. Although at times criticized as having a feminist or a "clitoral bias," Masters and Johnson's important work established a new way of looking at females as sexual beings in and of themselves, as fully equal partners with men rather than as mere reactors to male initiative.

NEW DISCOVERIES IN BIOLOGY. One of the most fascinating discoveries in the field of female sexuality has been in the area of biology. Psychiatrist Mary Jane Sherfey (1966) has attempted to realign current psychiatric views of women with new work in biology, particularly the modern inductor theory of primary sexual differentiation. The inductor theory, derived from endocrinology research in the 1950s, holds that male mammals, including man, develop from the female embryo and not, as had long been believed by scientists and lay persons alike, the other way around. During the first five or six weeks the human embryo is neither undifferentiated nor is it bisexual, as was thought in Freud's time; rather, it is anatomically female. Genetic sex, although established at birth, does not affect the embryo until the fifth or sixth week, when the fetal androgens begin to differentiate the males. If the fetal sex gonads were removed before the fifth week, *all* fetuses would develop as females; genetic males would be lacking only ovaries. Sherfey was quick to point out that this does not mean the female is superior; the phenomenon represents an adaptation that probably served to ensure species survival. Nonetheless, it provides a biological basis for refuting the still stubbornly held notion that females are somehow "lesser males." As Sherfey succinctly put it, ". . . modern embryology calls for an Adam-out-of-Eve myth!"

A SURPRISING SEXUAL TRADITIONALIST. In 1952, a year before the publication of Kinsey's book on female sexuality, Frenchwoman Simone de Beauvoir published *The Second Sex,* a book that provided much of the early inspiration for the new wave of American feminism appearing in the last 20 years. But de Beauvoir's attitudes toward sexuality in females were heavily influenced by traditional Freudian concepts of female passivity and the inferiority of the female genitals. She believed that the clitoris "perpetuat[ed] juvenile independence" (that is, independence from the need for a male in order to have sexual pleasure) and mourned the fact that "there is no organ that permits the virgin to satisfy her active eroticism [she has no penis]; and she has no actual experience with the one that dooms her to passivity [the vagina]." Even more interestingly, de Beauvoir questioned whether the adult woman really has true orgasms; she says, ". . . it is uncertain whether vaginal feelings ever rise to a definite orgasm . . . [the woman] may never find full deliverance." Her point of view demonstrates the continuing power of Freudian arguments through the middle of the 20th century, buttressed by societal pressures on women to remain sexually passive.

PSYCHOANALYTIC RETHINKING. The 1950s and 1960s saw some beginning restructuring of the "vaginal orgasm" theory by the psychoanalytic community. In 1960, a psychoanalytic panel on the issue of female "frigidity" was held for the first time, chaired by Helene Deutsch. She and fellow analyst Therese Benedek expressed their shock at the high incidence of "frigidity" in women and the fact that psychoanalytic and other psychotherapeutic techniques had proved so ineffective in treating it. Both questioned whether the vaginal orgasm could any longer be held out as the indicator of psychosexual maturity. Their attempts to redefine healthy sexuality for women were inconclusive, but they did represent a growing concern among some psychotherapists about the validity of old assumptions about females.

Recent Studies. In an analysis of scientific and theoretical literature, Fisher (1972) concluded that ". . . there seems to be a good reason for questioning practically every accepted idea about femininity," but in his own five-year study of 300 young middle-class wives, he resurrected the old idea of female dependence, of the need for a warm but firm father setting the stage for the daughter's later relationship with a trustworthy male who will make her feel secure enough to have orgasms. Singer (1973) brought things full circle by questioning the theory that there is only one kind of female orgasm physiologically. He postulated vulval, uterine, and "blended" orgasms.

The *Redbook* survey (1974) of 100,000 young middle-class women reported in some detail that most married middle-American women were enjoying sex more than ever. The optimism of this study contrasts with *The Hite Report* (1976), in which the American male was seen as still generally ignorant of or uninterested in what results in a successful sexual relationship with a woman. The overall tenor of all the studies, however, is that females are becoming more sexually active and more responsive than previously. Terman (1938) and Kinsey found a pattern of increasing premarital sex since the turn of the century, accelerating during World War I. A slowdown then occurred until the 1950s, after which it is generally accepted that premarital sex for girls began to increase again.

Sex Manuals from 1950 through the 1970s. In the manuals from 1950 to 1970, women are still depicted as more emotional and passive than males but having somewhat greater initiative than earlier (Gordon and Shankweiler, 1971). A growing acceptance of nonmarital sex for women and what has been called "gourmet sex," techniques for livening up sex, became apparent. Following Wright's earlier example, manuals appeared that taught women to masturbate as well as to use vibrators and to explore oral and anal sex. The "cult of the mutual orgasm" disappeared, and advocacy of successive orgasm (first one partner and then another) took its place. Sexuality for women past the age of 60 gained a greater acceptance (Butler and Lewis, 1976), as did bisexuality and lesbianism. The most obvious omission from most sex manuals was the female capacity for multiple orgasms, something that the authors apparently had not yet been able to assimilate into mutual heterosexual behavior in a manner that was not threatening to males.

Some Problems for Women. Conflicts in the 1960s and 1970s over the right to legal abortions, concern about the possibility that birth control pills and vasectomies lead to greater risk of heart attacks in both sexes, and the appearance of new strains of venereal diseases, especially herpes progenitalis, that were resistant to treatment have acted as counterforces to the general loosening up of sexual behavior for females. Religious constraints continue to affect female sexuality, with the Catholic Church maintaining its positions against masturbation and premarital sex and other major church bodies following a less condemnatory, but still traditional point of view toward sexual practices other than marital intercourse.

New sexual freedoms brought other difficulties. Many females became uncertain about their right to refuse sexual contact, especially during dating. In contrast to the women of the 19th century, many worry about what they are *not* doing sexually rather than about restraining their sexual activities. A pressure to produce orgasms exists, with some females admitting to "faking" climaxes to please or impress their partners. Many are still concerned about whether they are having the "right" kind of orgasms, especially if they require clitoral stimulation. Many men are confused or threatened by the new sexual assertiveness in women and are uncertain about how to react to the now well-documented female capacity for multiple orgasms. In summary, sexual relations between men and women are changing swiftly, with consequent emotional turmoil for both.

The Current State of Knowledge

Nearly all of the research to date on the sexuality of women has been conducted on white middle-class and upper-middle-class females. While these limits may not seriously interfere with understanding the physiology of sex, they are obviously a critical drawback to clarifying the psychology of sex as it varies from one cultural group to another.

Significant longitudinal studies of female sexuality—or for that matter, female physical health in general—following the same females from birth through old age, have not been done. As an example, females were just added in 1978 to the Baltimore longitudinal study of the National Institute on Aging, which has been studying men for 20 years. Thus, we have little idea of what happens to the individual female over the course of her life.

Physiology. The old debates about female "frigidity" or an overall lack of sexual response are about over, since it is now generally accepted that most females can learn to experience orgasms through masturbation. The issue now centers on the fact that a substantial proportion of heterosexual females, perhaps over half or more, do not regularly have orgasms through intercourse alone. Does this finding indicate that intercourse is not the optimal method of stimulation for females? Or does it mean that, as a result of cultural conditioning, females have collectively repressed or "forgotten" how to use intercourse for their own pleasure? "Militant clitorists," including many Lesbian women, have declared the penis superfluous to female enjoyment. Other female writers and researchers (Sherfey, 1973; Seaman, 1972; Hite, 1976) have documented the importance of the masturbatory experience for women while recognizing the important role that sexual intercourse plays. They share a general agreement that (1) intercourse alone does not provide many women with enough physical stimulation to reach climax; (2) intercourse is highly valued by many women as an emotional and physical experience; and (3) whether combined with clitoral stimulation or not, an orgasm during intercourse feels distinctly different from an orgasm without intercourse, in spite of the fact that all orgasms are now believed to follow similar physiological patterns.

Sherfey pointed out that the "cryptic" (hidden) female clitoral anatomy that underlies the clitoris itself has been ignored by comparative anatomists, biologists, physiologists, and physicians, and she concluded that the reason is the still widely held beliefs that the clitoris is a rudimentary organ that can be discounted. As she pointed out, an understanding of the clitoris and its entire underlying system of veins, supporting muscles, and tissue is necessary before the female orgasm can be scientifically delineated once and for all.

Many other aspects of women's sexual physiology are still barely understood, for example, the exact nature of premenstrual tension, the physiological versus the psychological components of the menopause and its sexual aftermath, the safety of prescribed hormones during and after menopause, the factors affecting female ovulation, the effects of pregnancy hormones on the capacity for orgasm, the role of the cervix and the uterus in sexual response, and the variable use that women make of pelvic muscles to build up tension toward orgasm.

PSYCHOLOGY. The psychology of female sexuality is nearly as poorly formulated now as it was in Freud's time. Throughout most of the 20th century, the belief persisted that females were more passive by nature than males. Sex was "done to" them, and they had to learn to "give in." Consequent indoctrination in passivity, along with the inhibition and punishment of masturbation in small girls and the restrictions on premarital intercourse as part of the double standard so masked the natural development of female sexuality that it is still difficult to see what is truly female and what is cultural conditioning. Young girls continue to be subjected to tremendous pressures to inhibit their assertiveness in many areas of functioning, even though new freedoms, including sexual freedoms, have opened up for them. A loving family environment in childhood, long touted as the key to healthy female sexual responses, has proved to be an important but insufficient condition for females to develop into fully sexual adults. An equally critical condition appears to be a family or cultural setting in which the inborn female capacity for assertiveness and activity is prized and supported rather than thwarted and repressed. In such an environment, the sexuality of females more easily develops its own natural course along with full growth of the personality.

There is much in female sexuality that is truly unique, especially physiologically, but inhibitions, stereotypes, and false premises must be disposed of before this uniqueness can be fully discerned.

REFERENCES

Acton, W. *Functions and disorders of the reproductive organs.* London: J. and A. Churchill, 1865.

Barbach, L. G. *For yourself: The fulfillment of female sexuality.* Garden City, N.Y.: Doubleday, 1975.

Barber-Benfield, G. J. *The horrors of the half-known life: Male attitudes toward women and sexuality in nineteenth-century America.* New York: Harper & Row, 1976.

Brown, I. B. *On the curability of certain forms of insanity, epilepsy, catalepsy and hysteria in females.* London: Hardwiche, 1866.

Butler, R. N., and Lewis, M. I. *Sex after sixty: A guide for men and women for their later years.* New York: Harper & Row, 1976. (Paperback title: *Love and sex after sixty,* Perennial, 1977.)

Cotton, J. *A practical commentary . . . upon the first Epistle Generall of John.* London: Printed for Thomas Parkhurst, 1658.

Davis, K. B. *Factors in the sex life of twenty-two hundred women.* New York: Harper & Bros., 1929.

Dawson, B. E. (Ed.). *Orificial surgery, its philosophy, application and technique.* Newark, N. J.: Physicians Drug News Co., 1912.

DeBeauvoir, S. *The second sex.* New York: Alfred A. Knopf, 1952. (Paperback: Bantam, 1961.)

Degler, C. What ought to be and what was: Women's sexuality in the nineteenth century. *The American Historical Review,* 1974, *79,* 1467–1491.

Dickinson, R. L., and Beam, L. *A thousand marriages: A medical study of sex adjustment.* Baltimore: Williams & Wilkins, 1931.

Donovan, F. *The women in their lives.* New York: Dodd, Mead, 1966.

Duffey, E. B. *The relation of the sexes.* New York: Wood and Holbrook, 1876.

Ehrenreich, B., and English, D. *Complaints and disorders: The sexual politics of sickness.* Old Westbury, N.Y.: The Feminist Press, 1973.

Ellis, A. Is the vaginal orgasm a myth? (1953). In Manfred De Martino (Ed.), *Sexual behavior and personality characteristics.* New York: Grove Press, 1966.

Ellis, H. The sexual impulse in women. In H. Ellis (Ed.), *Studies in the psychology of sex,* Vol. 3. Philadelphia: F. A. Davis, 1903.

Ellis, H. *Man and woman: A study of secondary and tertiary sexual characters.* New York: Houghton-Mifflin, 1929. (Originally appeared as an introduction for *Studies in the psychology of sex,* 1894.)

Fisher, S. *The female orgasm.* New York: Basic Books, 1973.

Freud, S. Some psychical consequences of the anatomical distinction between the sexes (1925). In J. Strachey (Ed.), *The standard edition of the complete psychological works of Sigmund Freud,* Vol. 19. London: Hogarth Press, 1961.

Freud, S. Three essays on the theory of sexuality (1905), Vol. 7, pp. 125–243. Female sexuality (1931), Vol. 21, pp. 223–243. Femininity (1933), Vol. 22, pp. 112–135. In J. Strachey (Ed.), *The standard edition of the complete psychological works of Sigmund Freud.* London: Hogarth Press, 1964.

Gordon, M. From an unfortunate necessity to a cult of mutual orgasm: Sex in American marital education 1830–1940. In J. A. Henalin (Ed.), *Studies in the sociology of sex.* New York: Appleton-Century-Crofts, Educational Division, Meredith Corporation, 1971.

Gordon, M. and Shankweiler, P. Different equals less: Female sexuality in recent marriage manuals. *Journal of Marriage and the Family,* 1971, *33,* 459–466.

Gregory, S. *Facts and important information for young women on the subject of masturbation: With its causes, prevention and cure.* Published by George Gregory, 1845. (Reprinted in *The secret vice exposed: Some arguments against masturbation.* New York: Arno Press, 1974.)

Hanchett, H. G. *Sexual health.* New York: Charles Hulburt, 1887.

Hippocrates, *On intercourse and pregnancy* (Spurious and Doubtful Works). New York: Henry Schuman, 1952.

Hite, S. *The Hite report: A nationwide study of female sexuality.* New York: Macmillan, 1976.

Holt, L. E. *Diseases of infancy and childhood.* New York: D. Appleton Century, 1936. (Originally published in 1897.)

Horney, K. The flight from womanhood: The masculinity complex in women, as viewed by men and by women. *International Journal of Psychoanalysis,* 1926, *7.*

Kinsey, A. *Sexual behavior in the human female.* Philadelphia: W. B. Saunders, 1953. (Pocketbook edition, 1955.)

Koedt, A. The myth of the vaginal orgasm. In A. Koedt, E. Levine, and A. Rapone (Eds.), *Radical feminism,* New York: Quadrangle/New York Times Book Company, 1973.

Levin, R. J. The Redbook report on premarital and extramarital sex. *Redbook Magazine,* October 1975, p. 38.

Levin, R. J., and Levin, A. Sexual pleasure: The surprising preferences of 100,000 women. *Redbook Magazine,* September 1975, pp. 51–58.

Lewinsohn, R. *A history of sexual customs.* New York: Harper and Brothers (English translation), 1958. (Original edition in German, 1956.)

Masters, W., and Johnson, V. *Human sexual response.* Boston: Little, Brown, 1966.

Masters, W. and Johnson, V. *Human sexual inadequacy.* Boston: Little, Brown, 1970.

Mather, I. *An arrow against profane and promiscuous dancing drawn out of the quiver of the scriptures.* Boston: Printed by Samuel Green, 1684.

Millet, K. *Sexual politics.* Garden City, N.Y.: Doubleday, 1970.

Moore, B. E. Panel report: Frigidity in women. *Journal of the American Psychoanalytic Association,* 1961, *9,* 571–581.

Napheys, G. H. *The physical life of women: Advice to the maiden, wife and mother.* Philadelphia: G. Maclean, 1869.

Onania: or, The heinous sin of self pollution, and all its frightful consequences in both sexes considered, 1737 (pamphlet).

Records of the First Church in Boston. (Manuscript copy in the Library of the Massachusetts Historical Society), n.d.

Robinson, W. *Woman: Her sex and love life.* New York: Eugenics Publishing Company, 1938.

Rugoff, M. A. *Prudery and passion.* New York: G. P. Putnam's Sons, 1971.

Ruitenbeck, Hendrik M. *Psychoanalysis and female sexuality.* New Haven, Conn.: College and University Press, 1966.

Sachs, B. *Treatise on nervous disorders of children.* New York: William Wood, 1905. (Originally published in 1895.)

Seaman, B. *Free and female: The sex life of the contemporary woman.* New York: Coward, McCann and Geoghegan, 1972. (Paperback: Fawcett Crest, 1972.)

Sherfey, M. J. *The nature and evolution of female sexuality.* New York: Random House, 1966. (Paperback: Vintage, 1973).

Singer, I. *The goals of human sexuality.* New York: W. W. Norton, 1973.

Stiles, H. R. *Bundling: Its origin, progress and decline in America.* New York: AMS Press, 1974. (Originally published in 1871.)

Stockham, A. B. *Karezza: Ethics of marriage.* Chicago: Stockham Publishing Co., 1896. (Reprinted in *Sex indulgence and denial, variations on continence.* New York: Arno Press, 1974.)

Talmey, B. S. *Woman: A treatise on the normal and pathological emotions of feminine love.* New York: Practitioners Publishing Company, 1908. (Originally published in 1904.)

Terman, L. M., assisted by P. Buttenwieser, L. W. Ferguson, W. B. Johnson, and D. P. Wilson. *Psychological factors in marital happiness.* New York: McGraw-Hill, 1938.

van de Velde, T. H. *Ideal marriage: Its physiology and technique.* New York: Random House, 1930.

Wright, H. *The sex factor in marriage.* London: Williams and Norgate, 1959. (Originally published in 1947.)

A Historian's Approach

SHARON ORDMAN GELTNER

After reading Myrna Lewis's "The History of Female Sexuality in the United States," I asked myself how a historian would have researched, evaluated, organized, and written this material.

Uncovering the history of female sexuality can be compared with the uncovering of the female body: both lie hidden beneath outmoded outer garments and inner garments, and between many layers of misconception, prudery, and generalized material. Recent changes in dress and the writing of history have been influenced by the feminist movement of the 1960s. To this critical interpretation of marriage, the family, and traditional child-rearing methods can be added the Marxian interpretations of the economic exploitation of women, rigid class stratification, and complex categories of role and status; the "great lady" approach, which idolizes the women who achieved the same status as men and wielded great power; and the sociological, anthropological, or psychological approach, which attempts to explain woman's sexual history in terms of roles, socialization, or a myriad of other theories.

Added to the problem of interpretation and polemics is the problem of finding appropriate sources from which to write the history. Popular images left behind in literature, drama, or social history do not necessarily reflect the actual life experiences of women as recorded in diaries or in statistical and demographic records such as fertility rates, the sexual composition of the labor force, illegitimate births, divorces, probate, and numerous other records. Finally historical events do not necessarily fall into categories by time or place.

A careful and extensive examination of sermons, church records, diaries, trials, and laws will show that the Puritans enjoyed sexual in-

SHARON ORDMAN GELTNER, Ed.D. • Social Studies Teacher, Los Angeles Unified School District, California.

tercourse and believed that it was to be enjoyed as long as it was within marriage and did not interfer with religion. Ms. Lewis examines the result—namely, children—and views the colonial woman as womb and nursery as an example of division of labor by sex. The historian needs to examine personal relationships and consider the colonial woman in more specific detail. She had an average of eight children; was married in her early to mid-20s; engaged in fornication, adultery, or other sexual offenses inside and outside of marriage; was responsible for the care and socialization of an extended family of indentured servants or apprentices; provided welfare services for the town; and assumed all of the legal, social, and moral responsibilities of the family on the death of her husband. The colonial family was a unit of production, not consumption. Marriages were considered in terms of dowry, availability of land, and the ability of the man and woman to perform domestic skills. Love was not a primary factor but would blossom after marriage and sex. Colonial town records show an abundance of "early births," children born less than nine months after the marriage. As many as one-third of the children were conceived before the wedding, but after the engagement. Seemingly an indication of promiscuity, these early births may also be interpreted as an example of great restraint, since these first pregnancies appeared long after puberty. While the colonies generally had equal fines and lashings for men and women who indulged in fornication, women generally were more frequently listed as being punished. It is hard to say whether the reason was a policy of treating women more harshly than men, as Ms. Lewis suggests, or the fact that women showed the result of intercourse in pregnancy and childbirth or that women were unwilling to name their partners.

Whether lover or wife at the time of conception, all colonial women faced the danger of a pregnancy that in at least 30% resulted in death to the child or the mother. While the high birthrate and large families support the contention of a lack of birth control, closer examination shows that prominent ministers were preaching against abortion and extolling the joys of motherhood.

Marriage, motherhood, submission, femininity, asexuality, chastity, and mindlessness were the qualities most frequently idealized in Victorian novels, etiquette books, and advice manuals for women. Here again, the careful historian needs to consider these popular stereotypical images as contrasted with hard data. Changes in production and commerce gave more alternatives to the 19th-century woman. She might be the Victorian doll depicted above, or an entrepreneur, a worker in a sweatshop, or a western pioneer, or she could be in an almshouse or a prison. The instabilities of war, the industrial system, disease, and urbanization increased the potential for unemployment, widowhood, and remaining single. Economic, social, and political conflict led women to join labor, abolitionist, suffrage, socialist, and utopian movements. Religion began to come under the control of women. New organizations and institutions for higher education emerged and admitted women. Industrialism created the typewriter, the electric sewing machine, and other inventions that would eventually free women from the home and tie them to machines. The scientific thinking of the 19th century also affected women's roles. The social Darwinists claimed that physiclal differences in women, such as mammary glands and larger amounts of adipose tissue, made the female more altruistic and better able to care for children and other individuals. Anthropologists and sociologists were predicting that women would eventually return to their natural habitat: home and children. Women used the antebellum belief in female moral influence to lead reform movements and social action groups. Social motherhood permitted women to remain unmarried without being pitied as old maids or castigated for being Lesbians. In contrast to women who rejected domesticity and motherhood, there were other women who became what was later known as the "supermom," women who stretched their energies to superhuman proportions and combined career, family, and community responsibilities.

Misconceptions about "Victorian" America are probably even more prevalent than those about Puritan America. By 1830, the birthrate had begun to decline from an all-time high in 1800. This decline is seen as a result of the availability of birth control literature in the 1830s. In fact, the literature became available after three decades of decreased fertility. Another misconception about 19th-century Americans is that they did not talk about sex or that if they did, it was in extremely vague terms. Actually, ministers, doctors, and quacks were busy writing advice manuals guaranteed to solve all problems. There were notorious brothels and group marriage arrangements. Pornography flourished, as did birth control literature and indictments against the lewd behavior of college students. Public outrage led to the passage of legislation attempting to regulate morality. This legislation was largely ignored.

While it is interesting to note the diversity of literature, laws, and advice manuals, it must be remembered that this "American" view of sexuality was largely being written by white New England males. If a woman did write an advice manual, which was rarely, it was written for young ladies on hygiene and health and did not deal with masturbation and licentiousness because these were largely male problems. By the end of the decade, these latter two topics assumed even more importance in the literature for males and females as the people who were said to need admonition greatly increased, such as Jews, Catholics, immigrants, homosexuals, and the poor.

The difficulties of discussing a topic as extensive as the history of female sexuality in the United States between 1700 and 1978 is evident enough in the vagueness of Lewis's treatment of the 18th and 19th centuries, and they become even more apparent and unmanageable in her attempt to discuss the 20th century as an entity. Also, the history of women does not divide neatly by century, and such a breakdown creates a great deal of fragmentation and omission.

Looking at advice manuals, studies, psychiatrists, and psychologists provides a very narrow view of the history of sexuality in the United States in the 20th century. A far broader conceptual framework needs to be considered, combined with an examination of more extensive and diverse data. In order to provide for a more conceptual approach and to correct for some of the omissions created by a chronological framework, the following questions need to be considered. They are not definitive or terminal; they are a starting point for further research. Generally, for any time period: (1) What are the actual relationships between men and women? (2) What roles do men have in the family for the care and socialization of the children, and what roles do women have outside the home in economics and politics? (3) How are children socialized and role models formed? (4) How much autonomy and power does the woman have in the home and family? (5) What materials are available for study and do they reflect a particular bias or omission?

For the 18th century: (1) Why was premarital sex condoned if the partners were engaged? (2) Is the emphasis on the planter class, which represented 1.8% of the white southern population, legitimate in talking about the "South"? (3) Why did southern women participate in greater frequency in politics and business than New England women? (4) Were geographical differences an important factor in marital and sexual relations?

For the 19th century: (1) How did the furor over sexual roles effect change? (2) Did changing patterns of dress reflect role changes or changes in definitions of male and female? (3) Did changing concepts of marriage affect sexuality and fertility? (4) Why did such a rigid definition of sexual roles evolve? (5) Did socialists and communists and their discussions of the family make an analysis of the role of women harder or easier? (6) Why was it so necessary to suppress and destroy a woman's sexuality by sanctifying motherhood, defining female sexuality as vaginal, performing clitoridectomies to prevent sexual excitement (which was said to cause insanity, hysteria, epilepsy, and other diseases), and accepting Freud's interpretation that woman's low status was given to her by God, who neglected to give her a penis? (7) Did changes from a rural to an urban society make changes in the diet that caused dysmenorrhea and a lower fertility?

The 20th century suggests: (1) Why are contemporary women who advocate equality pictured as radicals or as castrating to men who feel threatened? (2) Why are most methods of contraception aimed at women rather than men? (3) How have changes in role affected the psychic impact of feminism? (4) Why have the issues of the ERA and abortion caused such a furor? (5) Why are numerous questions about role, status, and socialization written and answered by men?

REFERENCES

Demos, J. *A little commonwealth: Family life in Plymouth Colony.* London: Oxford University Press, 1970.

Gordon, M. (Ed.). *The American family in social–historical perspective.* New York: St. Martin's Press, 1978.

Hartman, M. S., and Banner, L. (Eds.). *Clio's consciousness raised: New perspectives on the history of women.* New York: Harper & Row, 1974.

Rabbo, T. K., and Rotberg, R. I. (Eds.). *The family in history: Interdisciplinary essays.* New York: Harper & Row, 1973.

Walters, R. G. *Primers for prudery: Sexual advice to Victorian America.* Englewood Cliffs, N.J.: Prentice-Hall, 1974.

Chapter 3

Physiological Aspects of Female Sexual Development

Conception through Puberty

CORI BAILL AND JOHN MONEY

INTRODUCTION

Although current knowledge of the physiological aspects of female sexual development from conception through puberty is elaborate and complex, it is not complete. The separation of fact from theory is often difficult, but throughout this chapter, every attempt is made to distinguish what is theory from what is fact. Limitations of technology are in part responsible for the uncertainties of today's knowledge. So also are social, cultural, and religious taboos, which hamper full scientific inquiry concerning sexuality.

CONCEPTION

The hormones that govern the fertility cycle of women increase and decrease cyclically, taking approximately one month to complete a full turn. Conception can take place during about three days of this cycle. At that time, the uterine lining is mature, the cervical–vaginal mucus is thin enough to allow migration of the sperm, and a viable ovum (egg) has been released from the ovary into the Fallopian tube. The sperm of the male and the ovum of the female each contribute 23 chromosomes that will unite to form 23 pairs. The sperm meets the

CORI BAILL, B.S., R.N. • Phipps Psychiatric Clinic, The Johns Hopkins Hospital, Baltimore, Maryland.   JOHN MONEY, Ph.D. • Professor of Medical Psychology and Behavioral Sciences and Associate Professor of Pediatrics, The Johns Hopkins University and Hospital, Baltimore, Maryland.

ovum in the Fallopian tube, and they unite. The chromosomes match up in pairs, and a single zygote cell with a full 46 chromosomes is formed. This cell divides and multiplies. By the third day, the zygote implants itself in the mature uterine lining. Programmed by the genetic information coded in the chromosomes, in nine months the zygote cell will have differentiated into all the complex and varied components of the newborn infant.

Phyletically shared attributes of human beings are carried in the chromosomes. All human beings of normal genetic makeup and development have a thumb opposing their fingers, 10 toes, 1 stomach, and so forth. Variations may be genetically coded. Eye, hair, and skin colors are examples. When the human ovum and sperm unite, a unique being is produced from a vast range of possibilities transmitted from the genotypes of the two parents.

Chromosomes are composed of an as-yet-undetermined large number of genes, which themselves are composed of nucleic acids in strands twisted into a double helix. With the exception of the germ cells destined for possible future fertilizations, each cell in the body carries the entire genetic code of 46 chromosomes in 23 pairs, established at the time the ovum and sperm met. The uniqueness of the genetic information contained in each ovum is derived in the following manner: at birth, there are approximately 200,000–500,000 primitive ova (primary oocytes) present in the two ovaries, approximately 400 of which are released during the reproductive years. Two divisions of the oocyte take place to produce a mature ovum containing 23 chromosomes. The first division begins before the woman is born and remains uncompleted until shortly before each occasion of ovulation after she has become an adult. The second division is in progress when ovulation occurs. This division is not completed until after the sperm and ovum meet in the Fallopian tube. There is only one mature ovum created by the two divisions, since after each division a miniature polar body representing one product of the division is expelled.

The processes of sperm and ovum formation are similar, except that during sperm division, no polar bodies are formed. Each division results in two new sperm.

Following conception, the chromosomes are dormant with respect to sexual differentiation until either the 6th or the 12th week of fetal life, depending, respectively, on whether the male partner contributed a Y or an X chromosome. If the father contributed a Y chromosome, at 6 weeks the fetal gonads (left and right) begin to develop as testes. Each Y-bearing sperm and, later, the surface of each Y-bearing cell carry H-Y antigen, which is the stimulus for the gonads to differentiate. In the absence of H-Y antigen, ovaries will arise from the same gonadal tissues, but not until the 12th week of fetal life.

Following this point in sexual differentiation, chromosomes have no known function in the sexual differentiation of internal or external genitalia, nor of an individual's perception and expression of her/his sex, erotically or otherwise. It is a misconception that chromosomes directly determine psychosexuality. They are only the first step; further differentiation depends on the hormones produced by the differentiated gonads (ovaries or testes).

Embryonic Differentiation

After the gonads have differentiated, further morphological bipotentiality of the embryo persists until the third to fourth month of pregnancy, regardless of chromosomal status. The primordia of male and female internal and external genitalia are present in the embryo of either sex. This is illustrated in Figure 1. The internal sexual organs of the female (Fallopian tubes, uterus, upper vagina) arise from the Müllerian ducts; the sexual organs of the male (vas deferens, seminal vesicles, ejaculatory ducts) arise from the Wolffian ducts. In the third month of fetal life, either the Müllerian or the Wolffian ducts proliferate. The set that does not proliferate degenerates.

Male differentiation is dependent on the presence of hormonal secretions from the testes. In a chromosomal male, if testicular hormonal secretion totally fails, then male differentiation of internal genitalia cannot take place, and a proliferation of Müllerian structures occurs, as in a chromosomal female. In other words, female differentiation is dependent only on the absence of testicular hormones. Female differentiation is the basic blueprint. The total absence of ovaries will not deter its occurrence.

Embryologically, differentiation of the external genitalia is the final step in the differentiation of sexual morphology. Whereas the female and male internal genitalia differentiate from separate primordia, the external genitalia arise from the same primordia during the third and fourth months of fetal life. This is illustrated in Figure 2. Initially present in both the male and the female is a genital tubercle above a urogenital slit. On each side of the slit is a urethral fold and, adjacent to each, a labioscrotal swelling. In the female, the labioscrotal swellings remain separate and form the labia majora (outer lips of the vagina); in the male, they fuse in the midline to form the scrotum. The genital tubercle forms into the corpora (erectile tissue) and the glans

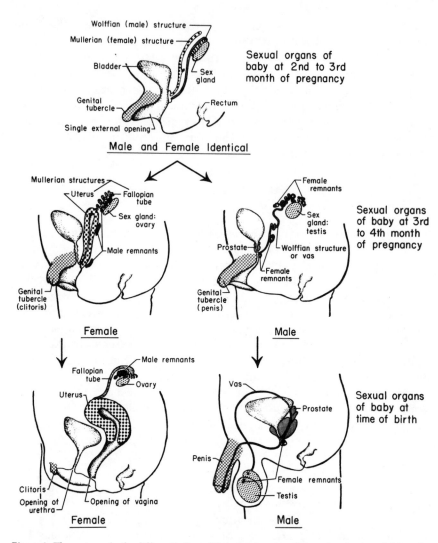

Figure 1. Three stages in the differentiation of the sexual system, internal and external. Note the early parallelism of the Müllerian and Wolffian ducts, with the ultimate vestiges of one and the development of the other.

(head) of either the clitoris or the penis. The urethral folds either form the clitoral hood and labia minora (inner lips of the vagina) or fuse to form the foreskin and the wrap-around skin covering of the penis.

By the fifth month of pregnancy, if all has gone well, the infant's internal and external genitalia are differentiated, and the question "Is it a girl or is it a boy?" can be answered at birth. However, the anat-

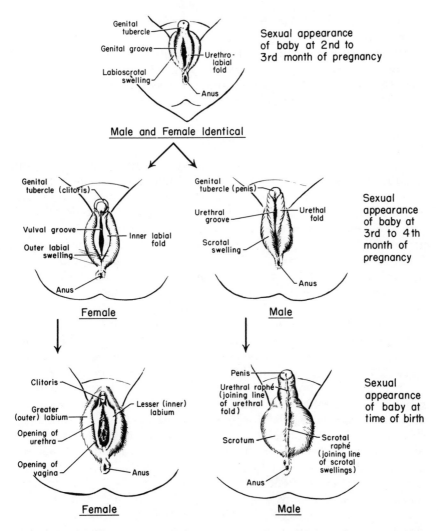

Figure 2. Three stages in the differentiation of the external genital organs. The male and female organs have the same beginnings and are homologous with one another.

omy of the genitals—just like the chromosomal sex discussed earlier—does not ensure and may not correlate with the person's eventual expression of masculinity or femininity.

Modern embryological sexual differentiation can be summarized according to the Adam–Eve principle (Money and Ehrhardt, 1972). The Eve aspect of this principle is that the basic plan of nature is female differentiation and that nothing needs to be added; that is, female differentiation will take place in the absence of either ovaries or testes. If the testes do not develop fully, then the embryo will revert to the basic female plan either totally or partially. The quantity and timing of the hormonal impairment determines the extent of reversion to the female plan. The fact that a male chromosome, antigen, or hormone must be present for male differentiation is the Adam aspect of this principle.

NEONATAL TO PREPUBERTAL YEARS

PREPUBERTAL HORMONES AND BEHAVIOR SEQUEL. The fetally produced hormones that dictate genital formation and the maternally produced hormones that sustain pregnancy affect the central nervous system of the fetus. Primarily, the brain is affected. This occurs prior to birth and hence prior to the main contribution of the external environment to the person's perception and expression of maleness and femaleness. In 1973, Forest, Cathiard, and Bertrand documented that the male infant from birth until three months of age has an elevated concentration of androgen, the predominantly male hormone. By the seventh month after birth, the male's androgen level drops and will remain low until the onset of puberty. The female infant's androgen level does not fluctuate, and once the male's androgen level lowers to its prepubertal norm, the male and female androgen levels are nearly the same from age seven months until the onset of puberty.

The role of the burst of androgen in neonatal males may be to seal in behavioral thresholds. Specific influences of neonatal and fetal hormones on subsequent behavior in humans are not known, though animal experiments that involved the manipulation of the sex hormones by removal of the gonads and hormonal additions and depletions during fetal and neonatal life correlated with changed adult sex-linked behavior. Similar experiments cannot be replicated on the human level, but clinical analogues provide parallel evidence (Money and Ehrhardt, 1972). In lower species, fetal androgenization of the female may reverse gender dimorphic behavior. In humans, such preordained reversal as may occur is no more than a predisposition. Postnatal differentiation permits incorporation of these predispositions into either a male or a female gender identity/role. The role of postpubertal androgen in romantic and erotic behavior remains to be fully elucidated. It may well be that androgen is the libido hormone for both sexes; but it does not dictate whether sexual expression will be homosexual, bisexual, or heterosexual.

Behavioral thresholds vary, determining the strength of stimulus required to elicit a particular behavior. Men and women are capable of the same behavior (except menstruation, lactation, and gestation in

the female, and the capacity to impregnate in the male, to be discussed later), but the behavior may be elicited by greater or lesser exposure to a stimulus. The specific sex-shared, threshold-different traits that have been identified are general kinesis; dominance; assertion and rivalry; roaming and territory mapping; defense against predators; parental caretaking; and possibly erotic arousal in response to visual imagery.

The sum total of evidence is that pre- and neonatal hormones relate to behavioral thresholds in childhood and also at puberty, when hormones again dictate further morphological sexual differentiation. The distinction between the fetal and the maternal hormonal contribution to behavior threshold development also remains unclear.

SEX ROLES. Sex-irreducible, sex-derivative, and sex-coded roles are prepared for in childhood. The sex-irreducible roles pertain to reproduction. They are that women menstruate, gestate, and lactate; men impregnate. These sex roles are not fully established until puberty and are discussed later in this chapter. Some sex-derivative roles, such as wearing a bra, are dependent on pubertal hormones. Sex-coded roles include sex-adjunctive roles, such as that the female prepares meals as well as breast-feeds, and sex-arbitrary roles, such as girls wear more lace than boys. Sex-coded roles are any behaviors encouraged or discouraged according to a child's genital sex. Sex-coded roles are assimilated through learning from birth until puberty. This learning may be categorized as a form of imprinting.

LEARNING OF SEX-CODED ROLES. The process of imprinting was first enunciated by Konrad Lorenz in 1952. It includes learning that conforms to the following four criteria: (1) a responding nervous system and a special set of stimuli must meet; (2) they must meet at a sensitive development period; (3) bonding of signals in the brain at a sensitive period is rapid; and (4) such bonding is tenacious and long-lasting.

The learning of language is an example of imprinting in human beings. Our brains are phyletically capable of language acquisition, but its actualization depends on the interaction of the brain, through the senses, with other members of the species who use language. It is necessary that the infant hear the language at a specific and sensitive period of juvenile life if optimal learning is to take place. Then, the establishment of language is rapid and permanent.

Imprinting regarding gender identity and gender-role differentiation is closely linked with the timing of language acquisition. The baby begins to develop a gender-differentiated self-concept under the stimulus of sex-coded social interaction at approximately the same time that he/she begins to acquire native language. This timing is illustrated in the case of babies born with ambiguous genitalia. Neonatal freedom to decide on a sex of rearing congruent with surgical and hormonal options diminishes with each month of age until it is nearly impossible to reverse a decision after the 18th month. Up until that time, the best option can be chosen, even if it requires a reannouncement of the sex assigned at birth. After 18 months of age, sex reassignment is as potentially disastrous as it would be to an ordinary adult.

The infant's gender identity, incorporated with her/his total self-concept, is practiced and refined in childhood through parental interaction, peer play, and erotic and romantic rehearsals. The labeling of childhood as a sexually latent period is incorrect. If the term *latency* is to be at all applicable, it is restricted to the occurrence of a complete falling-in-love experience, which appears to be a phenomenon that is linked to an internal clock activated at the time of puberty. The child's process of refining, enhancing, and expressing maleness or femaleness takes place through identification and complementation.

A child experiences two sets of stimuli: one, the behavior of females; the other, the behavior of males. A child responds by imitating one set (identification) and by reciprocating the other (complementation). It does not matter if the mother is an engineer and the father a nurse. Arbitrary cultural and historical variations of the masculine and feminine social and vocational roles are assimilated so long as there are boundaries delineating, at a minimum, the arbitrary sex-coded roles from the nonarbitrary, nonnegotiable reproductive and erotic roles of the sexes.

The terms *gender identity* and *gender role,* as related to sexual development, are sometimes loosely and inaccurately defined. Both become fully established after birth, but well before puberty.

> Gender identity is the sameness, unity and persistence of one's individuality as a male or female, especially as it is experienced in self-awareness and behavior. Gender identity is the private experience of gender role, and gender role is the public expression of gender identity. . . . Gender role is everything a person says or does to indicate to others or to the self the degree to which one is male or female. (Money and Ehrhardt, 1972)

The process of gender identity and role differentiation is not irreversibly preordained at conception, nor even at birth. It is a developmental and dynamic process.

Puberty

The initial signal within the body for the onset of puberty in females and males is unknown. However, it is known that the brain activates the flood of hormones, pituitary and hypothalamic, that seal, so to speak, the femininity or masculinity of the juvenile gender identity or role.

The hormonal system of the female, like that of the male, is hierarchial, involving the brain's hypothalamus, which produces releasing factors picked up by the anterior pituitary, to whose products the ovaries in turn respond. In the female, hormones are not secreted in constant, steady amounts, as are those of the male, but fluctuate cyclically.

The differential sexual programming of those pathways of the hypothalamus that will be responsible for cyclically releasing the hormonal secretions of the female occurs in fetal life. Androgen acts at a critical time during male differentiation to abolish cyclicity irreversibly in the male. In the female, an abnormal flux of androgen during the critical time in fetal life will do the same. The Adam–Eve principle is once again illustrated: feminine differentiation requires only the absence of androgen (see above).

The hypothalamus is located deep in the brain, behind the bridge of the nose and adjacent to the pituitary gland. In the female, between the ages of 7 and 11, luteinizing hormone–releasing factor (LH–RF) secretion by the hypothalamus begins to increase the release of pituitary FSH (follicle-stimulating hormone) and later of LH (luteinizing hormone). The range of individual variation is wide. FSH and LH cue the ovaries to secrete estrogen and progesterone, respectively. Small amounts of estrogen are also secreted by the adrenocortical glands, as are small amounts of androgen.

At puberty, estrogen induces the Fallopian tubes and the uterus to increase in size and the vagina to become cornified and able to lubricate. The external genitalia also enlarge. Cells lining the vagina change and become more resistant to trauma and infection. The uterine lining (endometrium) proliferates and develops glands that, if the woman becomes pregnant, aid in the implantation and nutrition of the zygote. The Fallopian tubes, in which ova are transported from the ovaries to the uterus, grow additional cilia. Estrogen also enhances the activity of these fingerlike guides. They beat in a continuous rhythm to guide the ovum through the tubes.

The breasts of boys are indistinguishable from those of girls prior to puberty. It may appear paradoxical in terms of the Adam–Eve principle that breast development depends on the addition of estrogen, whereas androgen inhibits breast growth in males because of the greater ratio of androgen to estrogen. However, if the male receives a sufficient amount of estrogen to override the inhibitory action of androgen, he, too, will develop breasts. If the chromosomal (46, XY) male produces androgen but is unable to utilize it intracellularly, the estrogen normally produced in small amounts by the testes is sufficient to produce total feminization of the body at puberty, including breasts and feminine skeletal, skin, and fat-distribution characteristics.

Pubertal estrogen increases bone growth, which is reflected in a pubertal growth spurt for several months, the peak of which is passed prior to the onset of menstruation (menarche). On the average, women are shorter than men. The sex hormones may, in fact, be implicated. Cartilaginous tissue separating the joints of the long bones becomes calcified (epiphyseal closure) at puberty. Puberty occurs earlier in girls than in boys. Therefore, growth ceases sooner. Estrogen also broadens the pelvis and widens the pelvic outlet to accommodate the birth of an infant.

Skin thickens without losing its softness and smoothness in response to estrogen. The fat underlying the skin increases in the buttocks, the thighs, the breasts, and the face. Estrogen plus progesterone also causes subtle change in protein deposition, metabolism, and electrolyte balance. Their mechanism of action in each cell of the body is not fully known, nor is the full range of their effects. The least-understood influence of the sex hormones relates to romantic, erotic, and mating imagery, thought, and behavior.

In Europe and America, the chronological age for the onset of puberty has been dropping for the last century and a half at the rate of four months every 10 years. Paralleling this trend is an increase in average adult height. The lower age of physiological maturity widens the gap between the physiological and the social and legal milestones of adulthood. Legalities and customs affecting teenagers in their domestic, academic, vocational, and erotic behavior have not paralleled the decrease in age for puberty onset, thus illustrating a disjunction between physiology and society. The obverse may also be true, since it may be improved public health and nutrition that in part are lowering the age of puberty.

One final point: It is a common misconception that there are male and female hormones. The sex hormones—androgen, estrogen, and progesterone—are present in both sexes. Androgen dominates in the male, estrogen and progesterone in the female.

MENSTRUATION

The fact that only women menstruate was, of course, realized long before it was known that the cycle is linked to the cycle of fertility. However, *menstrual cycle* is the term that encompasses the cycle of fertility as well as of menstrual bleeding. The first day of bleeding is considered Day 1 of the entire cycle of menstruation, which lasts for, on the average, 28 days. Bleeding normally occurs for the first few days only. Menstrual bleeding begins when ovarian estrogen is at its lowest level, fertilization is extremely unlikely, and renewal of a conducive internal environment for fertilization and growth of an ovum has yet to begin.

Based on the average 28-day cycle, Days 1–4 encompass the bleeding of menstruation; during Days 4–14, maximal proliferation of the uterine lining takes place; ovulation occurs on Day 14; and during Days 15–28, the postovulatory phase, the uterine lining degenerates, if fertilization did not occur during midcycle. These events are governed by hypothalamic, pituitary, and ovarian hormone secretions. The hormonal control mechanism of the cycle is hypothetically explained as follows.

Menstruation is the shedding of the endometrial lining of the uterus. It occurs when the estrogen and the progesterone secreted by the ovaries during the previous cycle decline. When sufficiently low levels are reached, the hypothalamus produces its gonadotropin-releasing factors, which are also hormones. The cause of low ovarian hormone levels and their effect on the hypothalamus are not fully established. Nor is it certain that there is only one releasing factor from the hypothalamus implicated in triggering the pituitary to secrete gonadotropin, though currently this is thought to be the case. The pituitary responds to releasing factors by secreting follicle-stimulating hormone (FSH) and luteinizing hormone (LH). FSH stimulates the growth of follicles in the ovaries, and LH is necessary for the initiation of estrogen secretion from these follicles.

Estrogen induces the uterine lining to proliferate, and a richly nutritious environment is created for the soon-to-be-released ovum. This is an environment designed to nurture the ovum following fertilization and implantation. The increasing level of estrogen also produces atrophy of potentially developing follicles other than the dominant one, within which resides a maturing ovum. While estrogen concentration rises, LH remains constant and FSH concentration steadily declines. Estrogen is hypothesized to act on the hypothalamus, which induces a decline in FSH production. This is an example of a negative feedback system. The absence of a similar change in LH concentration may reflect a positive feedback of estrogen.

At midcycle, LH concentration rises in response to a rise in estrogen level, which stimulates the pituitary. This LH surge produces the final growth of the follicle and induces ovulation, followed by the formation of a corpus luteum (yellow body) from the ruptured follicle.

Usually, only one human ovum is released per menstrual cycle, thus limiting the chances of multiple human births.

Ovulation marks the end of the proliferative phase of the cycle. The corpus luteum continues to secrete estrogen and now begins to secrete progesterone. Estrogen dominates the proliferative phase. Progesterone dominates the postovulatory phases of the cycle. If gestation does not occur, decreasing levels of progesterone and estrogen negatively feed back to the pituitary, and LH production drops. The corpus luteum begins to atrophy. Concomitantly, progesterone and estrogen production ceases. The uterine lining cannot be maintained. The cycle ends with the sloughing off of the uterine lining and the onset of menstrual bleeding as a new cycle begins.

If fertilization occurs during the cycle, the corpus luteum is kept intact by the hormone chorionic gonadotropin, secreted by the placenta, which is growing at the site of implantation, and the uterine lining is maintained (see below).

Stress, whether it be traumatic, infectious, thermal, or otherwise somatically or behaviorally induced, can drastically interfere with menstrual cyclicity. Thus, ovulation may or may not occur at an expected time.

During normal menstruation, only approximately 35 ml of blood (less than ¼ cup) is lost. When the uterine lining sloughs off, the cervix dilates slightly, facilitating the passage of menstrual material. Sometimes, this dilation produces a cramping sensation, and it would provide a route for infection of the uterus, except that vast numbers of white blood cells are released along with the necrotic material, thus ensuring that the uterus will be highly resistant to infection. The blood usually remains unclotted, or only minimally clotted, owing to the release of fibrinolysin, an anticlotting factor, along with the uterine lining.

Menstruation has been, and, indeed, still is, the subject of much myth and folklore. Prosaically it is no more and no less than the byproduct of the monthly female hormonal cycle when pregnancy does not occur.

SUMMARY

Conception occurs when the sperm and the ovum meet in the Fallopian tube, usually at the midpoint of the 28-day female fertility cycle. The ovum and the sperm each contribute 23 chromosomes that match to form 23 pairs. Chromosomes do not determine psychosexuality. They are, however, the first step. Under the differential influence of H-Y antigen, they dictate that the fetal gonads will differentiate as testes, or without it, ovaries, according to whether the sperm contributed a Y or an X chromosome, respectively. The chromosomes initiate the first step by determining, through the influence of the presence or absence of H-Y antigen, whether the gonads will differentiate as testes or ovaries, respectively. H-Y antigen will be present if the sperm contributed a Y chromosome and absent if an X chromosome was contributed.

The primordia of male and female internal and external genitalia are present in the embryo of either sex. The primordia differentiate during the third and fourth month of fetal life. As epitomized by the Adam–Eve principle, male differentiation is dependent on the presence of the Y chromosome, H-Y antigen, and sufficient androgen; female differentiation requires only that no additions be made.

Prenatal and neonatal androgen concentrations relate to behavior thresholds evidenced in childhood, and later, at puberty. Androgen's full import in gender identity/role development remains to be explored. The child's gender identity/role is acquired at the same time as native language and probably by the same mechanism of learning and imprinting. During childhood, sex-coded roles are assimilated through identification and complementation of gender-differentiated behavior.

At the onset of puberty, the brain activates a flood of hypothalamic and pituitary hormones, which, normally, confirms the juvenile gender identity or role and seals the irreducible sex differences. The irreducible differences are that women menstruate, gestate, and lactate and that men impregnate. The sex-related hormonal system in the female is cyclical and hierarchical.

The menstrual cycle is the average 28-day cycle of fertility. The events of the menstrual cycle are bleeding, proliferation of the uterine lining, ovulation, and the degeneration of the uterine lining when fertilization does not occur. These events are governed by interdependent hypothalamic, pituitary, and ovarian hormonal secretion. The exact mechanism of governance remains unclear.

GLOSSARY

Adrenal cortex: The outer three layers of the adrenal gland, as contrasted with the innermost part, the medulla. The cortex produces steroidal hormones, among them the glucocorticoid, cortisol, and small amounts of sex hormones. The medulla produces adrenaline, a catecholamine. One adrenal gland is located just above each kidney.

Androgen: A sex hormone—testosterone is an example—produced chiefly by the testis but also by the adrenal cortex and, in small amounts, by the ovary. In biochemical structure, there are several different but related steroid hormones that qualify as androgens. They differ in biological strength and effectiveness.

Cervix: The neck of the uterus (womb), which extends into the vagina.

Cilia: More than one cilium. A group of fingerlike cytoplasmic cells that beat rhythmically in one direction, thereby propelling the ovum (egg) from the ovary into the Fallopian tube.

Corpus luteum: (plural, corpora lutea) "Yellow body"; a yellow mass in the ovary formed from the follicle after the ovum is released. It produces progesterone and grows and lasts for several months if pregnancy occurs.

Endometrium: The membrane lining the uterus, which is shed and regenerates in response to the hormone fluctuations governing menstrual cyclicity.

Estrogen: A sex hormone produced chiefly by the ovary but also by the adrenal cortex and, in small amounts, by the testis. So named because in lower animals, it brings the female into estrus (heat). In biochemical structure, there are several different but related steroid hormones that qualify as estrogens. They differ in biological strength and effectiveness.

Follicle (ovarian): The sac formed on the ovary that surrounds the ovum prior to ovulation. After the ovum is released, the ruptured follicle develops into a corpus luteum.

Follicle-stimulating hormone (FSH): Produced by the pituitary gland, stimulating formation of the ovarian follicle on the ovary and the production of estrogen. When the follicle ripens, lutenizing hormone (LH) takes over, and the progesterone-dominated phase of the menstrual cycle ensues.

FSH: See *Follicle-stimulating hormone.*

Genotype: The hereditary components of an organism.

Gonadotropins: Hormones released by the anterior lobe of the pituitary gland that program the activity of the ovary in the female and the testis in the male. FSH and LH are the hormones.

Hormone: A specific chemical product of certain glandular cells; hormones have a specific regulatory effect on cells remote from the site of origin.

Hypothalamus: A portion of the brain of special importance in regulating vital functions, including sex, by means of the release of neurohormonal substances from nerve cells. These substances in turn regulate the nearby pituitary gland.

LH: See *Luteinizing hormone.*

Luteinizing hormone (LH): One of the gonadotropic hormones of the pituitary gland. It induces the release of the ovum from the ovarian follicle and the transformation of the latter into a corpus luteum.

Müllerian (ducts): The structures in the fetus that will, in the female, develop into the uterus and the Fallopian tubes; named for Johannes P. Müller, German physiologist (1801–1858). See also *Wolffian (ducts).*

Phyletic: Of or pertaining to a race. Phyletic components or aspects of behavior in human beings are those shared by all members of the human race, as compared with behavior that is individual and biographically idiosyncratic. Phyletic behavior is the product of both prenatal and postnatal determinants.

Pituitary: An endocrine gland situated deep in the brain in the midline behind the eyes, near the hypothalamus. The hormones of the anterior pituitary regulate many functions of the other endocrine glands of the body.

Progesterone: One of the two sex hormones chiefly characteristic of the female. It is produced by the ovary in the corpus luteum, following ovulation, and also by the placenta during pregnancy.

Releasing factors: Hormones secreted by the hypothalamus that regulate pituitary hormone secretion.

Somatic: Pertaining to the body.

Wolffian (ducts): The embryonic structures that develop into the internal reproductive anatomy of the male; named for Kaspar F. Wolff, German embryologist (1733–1794). See also *Müllerian ducts.*

References

Forest, M. G., Cathiard, A. M., and Bertrand, J. A. Evidence of testicular activity in infancy. *Journal of Clinical Endocrinology and Metabolism,* 1973, *37,* 148–157.

Guyton, A. C. *Textbook of medical physiology.* Philadelphia: W. B. Saunders, 1976.

Hatcher, R. A., Stewart, G. K., Stewart, F., Guest, F., Schwartz, D. W., and Jones, S. A. *Contraceptive technology 1978–1979.* New York: Irvington Publishers, 1978.

Lorenz, K. *King Solomon's ring.* New York: Thomas Y. Crowell, 1952.

Money, J., and Ehrhardt, A. A. *Man and woman, boy and girl. The differentiation and dimorphism of gender identity from conception to maturity.* Baltimore: Johns Hopkins University Press, 1972.

Chapter 4

Physiological Aspects of Female Sexual Development

Gestation, Lactation, Menopause, and Erotic Physiology

Cori Baill and John Money

The scientific inquiry into human sexuality is in many ways incomplete. Political, religious, and cultural taboos contribute to the difficulties of gathering and disseminating information. Unfounded, though popular conceptions of sexuality contribute to sexual repression and oppression. The following discussion of physiological aspects of female sexual development will assist the reader to differentiate better between myth and fact when encountering information about sexuality and to reserve acceptance of data that are not fully substantiated.

Gestation

Gestation, defined in the strictest sense, refers to the development of the embryo from conception to birth. The focus of this section is on aspects of the hormonal mechanisms of pregnancy and their effect on the mother rather than on the fetus. In every culture throughout history, there have been attempts to control fertility. In today's medically and technologically advanced societies, women can elect when and how often to become pregnant or, having conceived, whether or not to

Cori Baill, B.S., R.N. • Phipps Psychiatric Clinic, The Johns Hopkins Hospital, Baltimore, Mayland.   John Money, Ph.D. • Professor of Medical Psychology and Behavioral Sciences, and Associate Professor of Pediatrics, The Johns Hopkins University and Hospital, Baltimore, Maryland.

carry the conceptus to term. The new medical technology affects both individual physiology and societal function. Legalities, customs, and religious views have not caught up with the technological changes.

If fertilization of the ovum takes place during the midpoint of the woman's hormonal cycle, the menstrual cyclicity is interrupted. The corpus luteum remains intact, presumably under the influence of the hormone human chorionic gonadotropin (HCG), which is secreted by the developing placenta, beginning within a week of conception. Once the placenta is fully capable of secreting progesterone and estrogen itself, approximately six to eight weeks into pregnancy, the corpus luteum of the ovary begins gradually to degenerate. These three hormones, HCG, progesterone, and estrogen, dominate pregnancy. However, their precise physiological actions on the mother, on the fetus, and on the placenta are still obscure.

HCG is the hormone measured in pregnancy tests. Originally, rabbits were injected with anti-HCG and later with the urine of the presumptively pregnant woman. If the rabbit died, the woman was pregnant. Modern techniques permit a more sophisticated test that does not require the rabbit. Blood can also be tested for HCG, permitting earlier detection of pregnancy. HCG sustains the corpus luteum and also causes the endometrium to grow and store nutrients. However, uneventful continuance of pregnancy occurs in animals when the corpus luteum is removed surgically. Therefore, either a backup mechanism acts to interrupt cyclicity, or HCG activity is broader in scope than is currently known. For example, HCG may act as a stimulus on the maternal adrenocortical glands. After the fetus and placenta are sufficiently mature to continue the pregnancy without the corpus luteum, HCG continues to be secreted.

During the third trimester of pregnancy, HCG production increases until the last week. It is uncertain what role HCG decrease fulfills, but it is possible that the HCG level is linked to uterine motility and that its decrease during the last week plays a part in the onset of labor.

Progesterone is secreted in moderate amounts by the corpus luteum at the beginning of pregnancy, and it is secreted in large amounts by the placenta for use as a precursor of fetal steroids. The rate of secretion increases as much as 10-fold during pregnancy. The fetus metabolizes about 30 mg of progesterone for every 100 ml of plasma reaching it through the placenta. Progesterone inhibits proliferation of the endometrium, it is important in embryonic nutrition, and it decreases contractibility of the uterus.

In addition to inhibiting the motility of uterine muscle, progesterone relaxes other smooth muscle. Relaxation of the esophageal sphincter of the stomach may cause problems for pregnant women. Acidic gastric secretions splash up into the esophagus, often causing heartburn, a common discomfort in pregnancy. Fatigue, another common discomfort, is a by-product of the mild sedative effect of progesterone. This effect is most pronounced in the first trimester of pregnancy, when progesterone concentration is highest. Morning sickness is not thought to be progesterone-related. Rather, it is thought to be either HCG- or estrogen-related, since the timing of the nausea and vomiting correlates with the peak HCG production and prior to the usual period of adjustment to high concentrations of estrogen. There is another early-occurring phenomenon of pregnancy that may also be related to the etiology of morning sickness. The degenerative products from the rapid implantation of the conceptus into the endometrial lining of the uterus may be implicated. It is known that other degenerative products of occurrences such as burns cause similar symptoms.

Estrogen, unlike progesterone or HCG, is a valuable measure of fetal maturity, since one of its sources in pregnancy is the fetus, and the level falls when fetal death has occurred. Estrogen is produced in daily-increasing amounts that, by the end of pregnancy, reach concentrations as much as 300 times the amount produced in the middle of the normal monthly cycle. Estrogen stimulates uterine muscle growth and vaginal enlargement. It also stimulates breast enlargement and growth of the mammary glands in preparation for breast feeding.

The placenta, in addition to producing hormones, also filters the blood and its nutrients before they reach the fetus. Fetal by-products of metabolism return through the placenta to be eliminated by the mother. During pregnancy, the mother's circulatory, respiratory, metabolic, and urinary systems increase in rate of function as a direct result of hormonal influences and increased maternal weight gain.

Nine months of gestation culminate in labor. No theory of labor fully explains this event. The cervix dilates and thins so that the fetus can be propelled out of the uterus, through the vagina, and into neonatal existence. The pain in labor is due in part to uterine muscle hypoxia during contractions. During the latter part of labor, when the fetus is being delivered, cervical and perineal stretching produces pain, as does the stretching or tearing of the cervix or vagina.

There are several irreversible effects of pregnancy. The cervical opening will appear as a transverse slit as compared with the small rounded opening of a woman who has never been pregnant. Pigmentation changes of pregnancy such as darkening around the nipples and the central line of the abdomen will lighten, but rarely to their pre-pregnancy hue. Stretch marks or striae will remain, though they pale with time. Finally, intramuscular connective tissue increases in the uterus and, owing to its inelasticity, produces in women who have had many pregnancies weaker contractions, increased postpartum bleeding, and cramping.

The uterus itself becomes less than one-half its immediate post-partum weight within one week. In four to six weeks, the uterus may be as small as it had been prior to pregnancy, the cervix closes, and the endometrium regenerates. This process of postpartum uterine in-volution is enhanced if the mother breast-feeds (see below).

Lactation

At the end of puberty, prior to the first pregnancy, the breasts are not yet fully capable of milk production. Additional mammary growth occurs during pregnancy, under the influence of the hormonal changes. Estrogen from the placenta leads to further development of the ductile system; and progesterone promotes lobular and alveolar development, and thus the breasts' secretory capability. A third hor-mone, also produced by the placenta, is human placental lactogen, which governs the milk production. Though its specific role remains unclear, it appears to be similar to prolactin, the pituitary hormone that, among other things, influences lactation.

Theoretically, prolactin is the hormone most essential for milk secretion after the birth of the baby. Information about prolactin is largely inferred from studies of lower animals. During pregnancy, the prolactin secretion by the pituitary is believed to be suppressed by the high concentration of estrogen and progesterone. Immediately follow-ing birth, there is a sudden lowering of the level of both of these hor-mones, and prolactin production by the pituitary increases. For the first one to three days after birth, the breasts secrete colostrum. Colos-trum contains approximately the same amounts of protein and lactose as human milk, though almost no fat. High levels of immunologic an-tibodies, also present in colostrum, help protect the newborn from in-fection until her/his own immune system matures. Prolactin stimulates the synthesis of milk fats, sugars, and other nutrients, so that by Day 3 following delivery, the breasts begin milk production.

The mechanism for pituitary secretion of prolactin involves the hypothalamus, but differently than for follicle-stimulating hormone (FSH) and luteinizing hormone (LH). The hypothalamus produces a prolactin inhibitory factor (PIF) that is continually secreted in nonlac-tating women. Lactation suppresses PIF production.

Milk is continuously secreted into the alveoli of the breasts, where it is temporarily stored until ejection. A second mechanism allows the milk to enter the ductile system. Continual leakage from the nipples is prevented. The "letdown" of milk from the alveoli to the ducts is accomplished by a combined neurogenic and hormonal action, primarily controlled by the hormone oxytocin, which is produced not in the anterior lobe of the pituitary like all the above-mentioned hormones, but in the posterior lobe.

Oxytocin also powerfully and specifically influences uterine muscles to contract, thus helping the uterus of the breast-feeding mother to return to its prepregnancy size in approximately one month. In addition, lactation suppresses estrogen secretion, which enlarges the uterus in the nonlactating mother.

Oxytocin is released by the hypothalamus in response to sucking of the nipple. Sufficient stimulation of breasts in the nonlactating mother may also activate the hypothalamus to act as if the woman were breast feeding, so that milk production can occur in a woman who has not been pregnant. Upon cessation of the stimulation of sucking at the breasts, the prolactin level falls, since prolactin production is also governed in part by the sucking or nipple stimulation. The breasts' ability to synthesize and produce milk is lost within one or two weeks. Milk production may continue for several years if sucking continues, but the rate of secretion usually decreases.

In suppressing estrogen secretion by the ovaries, lactation prevents ovulation from recurring, usually for one to five months. The time period is widely variable from woman to woman. Presumably, the menstrual cycle is not resumed until pituitary prolactin production ceases to interfere with the production of enough pituitary FSH and LH to reinitiate the menstrual cycle. The reinitiation of the cycle can occur without compromising prolactin secretion and therefore need not interfere with lactation.

Human milk differs from cow's milk in several ways. Lactose, or milk sugar, is present in human milk in concentration 50% greater than in cow's milk. By contrast, protein is approximately two to three times greater in cow's milk, and the ash, which contains the minerals, is also two to three times greater. The protein of human milk is easier for the baby to digest, and the quantity of minerals in human milk is sufficient for neonatal development when the mother's nutrition is balanced.

At the peak of a mother's milk production, one day's milk contains approximately 50 g fat, 100 g lactose, and 2–3 g calcium phosphate, as well as trace amounts of other minerals and vitamins. The lactating mother requires about 100 additional calories per day beyond the ideal diet during pregnancy. Foods high in protein and calcium are of particular importance, as is a high fluid intake. Avoidance of medications and nonprescription drugs is wise, as drugs ingested by the mother are excreted through the milk.

Personal hygiene is important, since the warm, moist environment of the breasts is ideal for infection. However, the body does provide its own partial defense against this possibility. The secretory cells that surround the nipples produce an antiseptic secretion. This secretion, in conjunction with warm-water washing and drying before and after feedings, as well as any time that leakage occurs, is usually sufficient to prevent infection.

The hormonal link between the breasts and the uterus is paralleled by the connection between the nervous system of the genitalia and the breasts. This connection is of particular significance when considering the role of the breasts in eroticism. The two roles of the breasts—namely, in lactation and in erotic responsivity—are not necessarily mutually inclusive or interdependent, though they do share common physiological pathways. Breast-feeding alters the breasts' sexual response in at least one way. The size of the virgin breasts, immediately before erotic orgasm, increase one-fifth to one-fourth over unstimulated size. Breasts that have once undergone lactation do not demonstrate this phenomenon, probably because of the alteration in blood supply, and also in fibrous tissue, that occurs during lactation.

MENOPAUSE

Menopause is defined as the cessation of the cyclic menstrual pattern in women. Women experience the changes of menopause for a period of time that ranges from a few months to several years around age 50. The status of information about the onset of menopause is similar to that regarding the onset of puberty or the cyclic timing of menstruation. Much remains hypothetical, including the following explanation of how menopause progresses.

The onset of menopause coincides with the disappearance of all the primordial follicles in the ovaries (Guyton, 1976). Even though the number of follicles far exceeds the number of ova released by the ovary from puberty until menopause, many ova partially mature and then degenerate during each episode of menstruation. Eventually, all the ova have either ovulated or degenerated. When the number of follicles falls to the number found in women from ages 45 to 50, cyclicity becomes irregular and ovulation may fail to occur. Within a few years from the onset of irregularity, all remaining follicles have gone. Estrogen production by the ovaries decreases proportionally, and when estrogen concentration falls below the level necessary to inhibit

FSH and LH secretion by the pituitary, menstrual cyclicity ceases. Thereafter, FSH and LH are produced continuously, not cyclically.

The body responds to this alteration in estrogen level in many ways. The skin loses some of its smooth texture, the internal genitalia gradually atrophy, and lubrication of the vaginal canal becomes more sluggish. Mood changes of extreme individual variability are traditionally associated with the menopause. They are probably attributable to the altered hormonal status, though the interplay between the sex hormones and the pathways of the brain that process mood are poorly understood. One of the most immediately distressing symptoms of menopause is "hot flashes." Their etiology is not well understood. Hot flashes may be related to brief surges of hormone released from the ovaries, which in turn produce short-lived elevations of the body's metabolic rate. Pulsatile catecholamine release in the hypothalamus has also recently been implicated.

POSTMENOPAUSE

The majority of changes in erotic physiology among postmenopausal women studied by Masters and Johnson (1966) were attributable to estrogen-deficient vaginal and uterine atrophy. The breasts underwent little change in erotic response. Masters and Johnson concluded that the postmenopausal women of their group had an anatomical response pattern to sexual stimulation identical to that of younger women. However, the intensity and the duration of response were sometimes reduced. There is no scientific evidence that the hormonal change of menopause acts specifically on a woman's interest in, or expression of, sexuality. Menopause does, however, signify the end of fertility. For some women, this fact may depress the expression of sexuality, whereas it is enhanced for others, since they no longer fear the possibility of pregnancy. Women have a longer life span than men. Older women outnumber men, so that sexual expression is deterred for some. Societal taboos surround geriatric sexuality, though this attitude may alter as the World War II baby generation ages and the aged become a larger segment of America's population.

Without replacement hormones, vaginal and uterine atrophy occur in all women following menopause. The vagina thins, vaginal length shortens, and width decreases. When the woman is sexually stimulated, there is partial loss of vaginal expansion. Vaginal lubrication is slowed and the quantity is decreased. The uterus shrinks in size. Within 5–10 years, the uterus and the cervix become approximately equal in length. The uterus of the premenopausal woman contracts when orgasm occurs. This response is not lost in postmenopausal women. However, probably because of involution, it may cause a sensation of cramping and even severe pain. Other pain, such as vaginal burning or pain with penetration, may result from vaginal dryness, shrinkage, and thinning. There no longer exists a protective cushion between the vagina and the urinary tract.

Problems of painful uterine contractions and problems resulting from vaginal thinning are usually eradicated by estrogen and progesterone replacement. However, this medical practice remains controversial. If at any point after beginning hormonal replacement the woman discontinues it, she will again experience the symptoms and the physiological alterations of menopause and the postmenopausal sequel to estrogen deprivation.

The body's metabolic rate falls during menopause and stabilizes at a lower level after fertility has ceased. Weight gain and a proneness to fatigue may result (see above). Hormonal replacement may not only alleviate these problems but also reverse the effect that hormonal change may have on moods. However, it remains to be established which effects are hormone-related and which are environment-related. Moreover, the replacement hormones may themselves induce undesirable mood effects.

EROTIC PHYSIOLOGY

THE CLITORIS, CLITORAL HOOD, LABIA MINORA, AND LABIA MAJORA. The female's clitoris, clitoral hood, labia minora, and labia majora are homologues of the male's penis, foreskin, penile skin cover, and scrotum, respectively. Though the structure and function of these organs is known, very little is known concerning where and how information from the peripheral nervous system of the eyes, ears, nose, skin, mouth, and other organs is registered and processed in the sexual brain, nor how this information relays to the primary erotic organs, producing sexual arousal and the possibility of orgasm. Prior experience is registered in the brain as memory. The physiology of this process remains to be clarified. Both immediate and long-term memory influence what specifically produces erotic excitement. An example is the sensation of touch, with the hands or any other part of the body. The brain registers the sensation not simply as touch to the skin but also as erotic, sensual, frightening, threatening, comforting, and so on. If a touch is registered as an erotic one, then the clitoris, the clitoral hood, and the labia respond. The clitoris is unique in having no other known function than to receive and respond to sexual stimuli. It responds to sexual stimulation by enlarging as the parasympathetic nervous system stimulates the arteries to dilate and the veins to constrict so that blood congests in the spongy, erectile tissue. This response occurs in all women, though in some the observation cannot be made macroscopically. Clitoral erection typically does not occur with the same rapidity as does penile erection, nor is it the first genital response to erotic stimulation, usually being preceded by vaginal lubrication. As sexual excitement increases, the clitoris appears to retract as the clitoral hood extends. The shaft length is reduced approximately 50% prior to orgasm. Retraction continues until sexual stimulation fades or until orgasm has occurred. Following orgasm, the clitoris returns to its original position in 10–15 seconds or longer, dependent on normal variation.

The normal, unstimulated labia majora meet in the midline and protect the labia minora and the vaginal outlet. In the woman who has not given birth, the labia majora thin in response to sexual stimulation and flatten upward and outward from the vaginal outlet. This is a response to congestion in and around the vagina and/or a neural response. It facilitates penile penetration. The labia minora open up, increase two to three times in diameter, and expand beyond the thinned, flattened labia majora. In the woman who has not been pregnant, blood congestion causes a significant color change, ranging from pink to bright red. Color loss following orgasm is rapid. The labia of a woman who has been pregnant respond differently. The labia majora swell and congest with blood rather than flattening, and the labia minora develop a darker color. The size and shape of the clitoris, the extent of cover by the hood, and the size of the labia all vary from individual to individual. For example, the normal transverse diameter of the clitoral head may range from 2 to 10 mm, a fivefold variation. Regardless of size or proportion, the clitoris, the clitoral hood, and the labia respond to sexual stimulation from any endogenous or exogenous source in a relatively unvarying way, though intensity and duration of response vary.

THE VAGINA. The vagina is the first pelvic organ to respond to sexual stimulation. Lubrication appears on its walls within 10–30 seconds after the onset of any form of effective sexual stimulation. The source of the sum total of lubrication is not yet conclusively established. Glands beneath the labia minora secrete mucus and contribute to vaginal lubrication; but also involved is the sweating of the vaginal wall in response to increased blood volume in the well-developed capillary system encircling the vagina. The upper two-thirds of the vagina expand in responding to sexual stimulation, and its color deepens as a result of vasocongestion. During orgasm, the lower third of the vagina contracts rhythmically. After orgasm, locally congested blood diffuses, so that the entire vagina slowly returns to its collapsed, unstimulated size and shape.

No difference in the peripheral physiology of orgasmic response exists objectively, regardless of stimuli. However, subjectively, the intensity of arousal and orgasm varies widely within the same individual depending on sexual stimuli, whether in fantasy or actuality, with or without a partner, and so on. The individual woman may react more to one type of erotic stimulus than another and may accordingly vary in rapidity of arousal and perception of orgasmic intensity.

The vagina has an additional role as an organ of conception. The acid–base balance in the vagina is delicately held in the 3.5–4.0 pH range (below 7 is acidic, above 7 is alkaline). Lubrication over sufficient periods of time, approximately 30 minutes, will increase the pH toward the neutral range of 7. The sperm in the seminal fluid of the male are maximally mobile in a neutral pH. Seminal fluid, in combination with vaginal lubrication, neutralizes the otherwise acidic environment of the vagina and enhances sperm mobility.

As well as being a coital organ, the vagina is the route for menstrual flow from the uterus, and it forms part of the birth canal. It is extremely elastic in order to distend during childbirth. During pregnancy, the vaginal wall thickens in response to hormonal stimulation, and the blood supply increases, producing a dark bluish coloration. This is one of the signs of pregnancy observed during vaginal examination.

OTHER EROTIC ZONES AND ORGANS. The nongenital parts of the body responsive to erotic stimulus vary widely from individual to individual. For some individuals, the entire skin is an erotic organ, while for others only stimulation of the breasts or the nipples produces arousal. Still others have unresponsive breasts but are responsive elsewhere. Hormonal influences on human arousal are inferred, but poorly understood. The pathways of the brain that perceive stimuli and match them against prior experience to produce erotic arousal have not yet been traced. The mechanism by which fantasy influences the perception of stimuli is unknown, but obviously, it is of great importance in producing arousal. There probably exist critical childhood learning times during which a person develops an individual variation in arousal patterns from a finite set of possibilities. Traumatic prepubertal sexual experiences produce long-lasting effects in some individuals but not in others, perhaps because of their developmental timing.

EROTICISM AND MENSTRUAL CYCLICITY, THE PILL, PHEROMONES, COUPLE SYNCHRONY. Research in the area of the relationship between hormonal menstrual cyclicity and conceptivity is much more advanced than research on the relationship between hormonal menstrual cyclicity and either erotic acceptivity or erotic proceptivity [these terms are applicable to both sexes and were introduced by Frank Beach (1976)]. *Acceptivity* (which includes receptivity) refers to the readiness of the female to accept or receive the approaches of the male, and eventually of her vagina to accept his penis. Proceptivity has two components: the male's attractiveness to the female so that she presents herself and solicits his sexual attention; and the attractiveness of the female to the male, usually by reason of her sexual appearance, sexual smell (pheromonal odor), or, in some instances, her courtship rituals.

Many factors, such as insufficient privacy, may inhibit or interrupt proceptivity and acceptivity. However, the underlying behavioral endocrinology of variability in the occurrence of proceptivity and acceptivity in human beings remains unclear. In subhuman primates, the female's sexual interaction with males is enchained to the hormonal cycle of menses. In human beings, if this does occur, it is much attenuated. Regardless of hormonal levels, the frequency of coitus during the course of one menstrual cycle in young adult couples screened for psychological normality varies widely.

The present state of knowledge concerning menstrual fluctuations of estrogen, progesterone, and androgen (see Chapter 3, the section titled "Menstruation"), and their direct effects on proceptivity and acceptivity (receptivity) in monkeys is updated in an exceptionally well-informed review by Baum, Everitt, Herbert, and Keverne (1977). The review concludes with a statement about human beings:

> The methods currently being used for studying human sexual behavior make it very difficult to distinguish between proceptivity and receptivity and hence to ascribe individual roles to various hormones in the way now possible for monkeys. Rhythmic changes in sexual interaction in humans during the menstrual cycle have been reported, although contradictory reports continue to appear and maximal levels are as commonly found early in the follicular phase as at midcycle. It has been suggested that the human female's attractivity may decline during the luteal phase (as in monkeys) and that this can be counteracted in women taking contraceptive steroids.
>
> The consequences of withdrawing endocrine secretion, or treatment with steroids, have usually been assessed in terms of loss or gain of "libido," although some studies have used other criteria such as incidence of orgasm or "coital satisfaction." It is not clear whether loss of libido indicates change in receptivity, proceptivity, or both. Furthermore, changes in libido may occur secondarily to those in attractivity, as in monkeys.
>
> Ovariectomy is generally agreed not to diminish the human female's libido consistently, and the same conclusions have been reached in studies of menopausal women. Insofar as comparisons are justified, this correlates with findings on ovariectomized monkeys described above. Adrenalectomy, however (which diminishes androgen), has been found to diminish promptly the human female's libido, whereas giving intact women testos-

terone stimulates their sexual interest in many cases. This suggests that
there may be a role for androgens in the human female's sexuality comparable with that experimentally determined for the rhesus monkey, although
exact correspondence await further clinical investigation.

Yet another relatively unexplored aspect of menstrual cyclicity that
may indirectly influence acceptivity and proceptivity is the phenomena of premenstrual tension. Behavioral correlates with premenstrual
tension have been extended to include not only subjectively experienced mood changes but also an increased prevalence of poor judgment, delinquency, violence, accidents, and so forth. However, correlates fail to tell anything about etiology. In some ways, premenstrual
tension has become a fashionable diagnosis, a medical grab bag.
Nonetheless, the premenstrual syndrome does exist in some women.
It is variable in its degree of severity; many women experience it not
at all. It occurs across cultures and classes and so is almost certainly
not an artifact of cultural taboo. Nonetheless, it is not culture-free.
Even in its mildest manifestations, it is multidetermined. One contributing factor may be the increased secretion of progesterone during
the luteal phase of the menstrual cycle and the edema associated there-
with. Therapy for severe premenstrual symptoms is based, like contraception by means of the pill, on the hormonal suppression of ovulation. In the absence of ovulation, there is no postovulatory surge of
progesterone.

There has been much inconsistency in findings on the effect of the
pill on premenstrual symptoms, mood, or sexuality. A large part, if
not all, of the inconsistency may probably be attributed to the fact that
premenstrual symptoms, mood, and sexuality are multidetermined,
and few studies have been designed for multideterminate analysis.
Fortunately, there are some exceptions (Cullberg, 1972). These studies
show little direct correlation between pill use and mood or erotic alteration in women without a prior history of problems. The studies also
show some favorable correlations between pill use and the resolution
of menstrual pain.

Recently, research attention has been directed to the possibility
that proceptivity and receptivity in men may fluctuate in synchrony
with the hormonal cycle of the woman partner. Couples have also
shown synchronous changes in basal body-temperature fluctuations
(Henderson, 1976). This finding resembles that of McClintock (1971),
who found that college women living in the same dormitory established menstrual synchrony.

The most likely hypothesis to explain synchronization is that it is
mediated, possibly subliminally, through the sense of smell by way of
pheromones or odors. In subhuman primates and other mammals, it is
well established that the female, at the time of ovulation, emits a

vaginal odor or pheromone that is an erotic attractant for the male. It is also established that the human female emits an ovulatory pheromone that is chemically the same as that emitted by the rhesus monkey female that is an attractant for the rhesus male. There is as yet no definitive investigation of the role of the vaginal pheromone in human sexuality.

EROTIC APATHY

Hypogyneismus, popularly and often punitively termed *frigidity,* may be subdivided into three categories: an inability to experience erotic–sexual arousal, hyposexuality (incapacity to experience intense sexual response or feeling), and anorgasmy (no orgasm). The inability of a woman to experience psychosexual satisfaction may be neurogenic, vasculogenic, endocrinogenic, and so on. Some causes are classified as psychogenic, which can generally be understood to mean that the physiological etiology is unknown.

The affectionate initiations and responses of a woman to her partner/s are not necessarily reduced by organic disease. Erotic initiation and response, however, are generally dependent on the integrity of the endocrine system and are probably specifically dependent on the integrity of androgen production and utilization. When the endocrine system is assessed as intact, then other known correlates of diminished sexual interest should be evaluated, such as drugs that produce vascular changes and diseases that produce genital pain. When the directly observable possible causes of erotic dysfunction are ruled out, then the problem is most likely a signal that there exists conflict, unhappiness, or fear in the woman or in her relationship with her partner/s. Or, in other words, when the underlying physiological erotic machinery is intact, the problem may be in the affectionate component of the relationship. The problem may be as simple as the fear of pregnancy or as complex as a deep penile phobia. The problem may occur only with one partner or with all, and it may occur during any part of the proceptive or acceptive phase of a sexual interaction.

Regardless of the etiology, erotic apathy is not a normal aspect of female sexuality. Retreating social, cultural, religious, and legal taboos increase the likelihood of full scientific investigation into human sexuality.

SUMMARY

Gestation is hormonally dominated by HCG, progesterone, and estrogen. HCG sustains the corpus luteum and hence plays a part in preventing the endometrial lining of the uterus from shedding, as it would if conception had not occurred during the menstrual cycle. Progesterone, secreted first by the corpus luteum and later by the placenta, governs proliferation of the endometrium, is important in embryonic nutrition, and decreases the contractibility of smooth muscle such as the uterus. Systemic effects of progesterone contribute to the etiology of several common pregnancy discomforts. Estrogen, the precursor of which comes from the fetus during pregnancy, is a useful measure of fetal muturity. Estrogen stimulates uterine muscle growth, vaginal enlargement, and mammary maturation. Lactation is possible only after hormonally induced mammary maturation has occurred. The pituitary hormone, prolactin, is the one most essential for milk secretion. Letdown of the milk from the alveoli to the ducts is controlled by combined neurogenic and hormonal (oxytocin) action. Breast-feeding is not always distinct from the erotic role of the breasts, though the two roles are not directly interdependent.

Menopause is the cessation of the cyclic menstrual pattern in women. The onset of menopause is associated with the disappearance of all primordial ovarian follicles. There is no scientific evidence that the hormonal changes of menopause act specifically on a woman's interest in or expression of sexuality. Hormonal replacement therapy to offset symptoms of menopause such as vaginal atrophy and dryness, hot flashes, and bone porosity is controversial.

The adult's vagina, clitoral hood, and labia respond physiologically to sexual stimulation in a relatively uniform way. The subjective experience of arousal and orgasm varies widely according to individual development. The nongenital parts of the body are also responsive to erotic stimulation. The amount and degree of response are individual.

A person's proceptivity and acceptivity—attraction, solicitation, and reception of a partner—are possibly influenced by physiological events such as menstrual cyclicity, pheromonal odors, and contraceptive pill usage. Findings are inconsistent, possibly because of faulty research designs that do not take into account the multideterminate nature of arousal.

Erotic apathy is not a normal aspect of female sexuality. Psychosexual dissatisfaction may be neurogenic, endocrinogenic, and so forth. Some causes are classified as psychogenic, which can generally be understood to mean that the physiological etiology is unknown.

GLOSSARY

Adrenal cortex: The outer three layers of the adrenal gland, as contrasted with the innermost part, the medulla. The cortex produces steroidal hormones, among them the glucocorticord, cortisol, and small amounts of sex hormones. The medulla produces adrenalin, a catecholamine. One adrenal gland is located just above each kidney.

Androgen: A sex hormone—testosterone is an example—produced chiefly by the testis, but also by the adrenal cortex and, in small amounts, by the ovary. In biochemical structure there are several different but related steroid hormones that qualify as androgens. They differ in biological strength and effectiveness.

Areola: (plural, areolae) The area of pigmented skin immediately surrounding the nipple of the breast.

Cervix: The neck of the uterus (womb) which extends into the vagina.

Cilia: More than one cilium. A group of fingerlike cytoplasmic cells which beat rhythmically in one direction, thereby propelling the ovum (egg) from the ovary into the fallopian tube.

Corpus luteum: (plural, corpora lutea) "Yellow body;" a yellow mass in the ovary formed from the follicle after the ovum is released. It produces progesterone, and grows and lasts for several months if pregnancy occurs.

Endometrium: The membrane lining the uterus which sheds and regenerates in response to the hormone fluctuations governing menstrual cyclicity.

Estrogen: A sex hormone produced chiefly by the ovary, but also by the adrenal cortex, and, in small amount, by the testis. So named because, in lower animals, it brings the female into estrus (heat). In biochemical structure, there are several different but related steroid hormones that qualify as estrogens. They differ in biological strength and effectiveness.

Follicle (ovarian): The sac formed on the ovary which surrounds the ovum prior to ovulation. After the ovum is released, the ruptured follicle develops into a corpus luteum.

Follicle-stimulating hormone (FSH): Produced by the pituitary gland, stimulating formation of the ovarian follicle on the ovary, and the production of estrogen. When the follicle ripens, lutenizing hormone (LH) takes over and the progesterone-dominated phase of the menstrual cycle ensues.

FSH: See *Follicle-stimulating hormone.*

Gonadotropins: Hormones released by the anterior lobe of the pituitary gland which program the activity of the ovary in the female and the testis in the male. FSH and LH are the hormones.

HCG: See *Human chorionic gonadotropin.*

Hormone: A specific chemical product of certain glandular cells; hormones have a specific regulatory effect on cells remote from the site of origin.

Human chorionic gonadatropin (HCG): A hormone excreted in the urine during pregnancy and detected in pregnancy tests. HCG stimulates the ovary to continue production of estrogen and progesterone early in pregnancy.

Human placental lactogen: A hormone which promotes breast growth in pregnancy and afterwards, lactation.

Hyperplasia: An increase in the number of cells in an organ, and thus in the size of an organ.

Hypothalamus: A portion of the brain of special importance in regulating vital functions, including sex, by means of the release of neurohormonal substances from nerve cells. These substances in turn regulate the nearby pituitary gland.

LH: See *Luteinizing hormone.*

Luteinizing hormone (LH): One of the gonadotropin hormones of the pituitary gland. It induces the release of the ovum from the ovarian follicle and transformation of the latter into a corpus luteum.

Müllerian (ducts): The structures in the fetus that will, in the female, develop into the uterus and fallopian tubes; named for Johannes P. Müller, German physiologist (1801–58). See also *Wolffian (ducts).*

Oxytocin: A pituitary hormone which initiates lactation, and also labor.

Pheromone: An odoriferous substance which acts as a chemical messenger between individuals. In mammals, pheromones serve as foe-repellants, boundary markers, child-parent attractants, and sex attractants.

Phyletic: Of or pertaining to a race. Phyletic components or aspects of behavior in human beings are those shared by all members of the human race, as compared with behavior which is individual and biographically idiosyncratic. Phyletic behavior is the product of both prenatal and postnatal determinants.

Pituitary: An endocrine gland situated deep in the brain in the midline behind the eyes, near the hypothalamus. The hormones of the anterior pituitary regulate many functions of the other endocrine glands of the body.

Placenta: An organ developed in the uterus during pregnancy which is the intermediary organ of transfer between mother and fetus. The placenta is also the major endocrine organ of pregnancy.

Progesterone: One of the two sex hormones chiefly characteristic of the female. It is produced by the ovary in the corpus luteum, following ovulation, and also by the placenta during pregnancy.

Prolactin: The milk-stimulating hormone secreted from the pituitary gland. It is the same as luteotropin.

Releasing factors: Hormones secreted by the hypothalamus which regulate pituitary hormone secretion.

Somatic: Pertaining to the body.

Steroids: A specific class of hormones with the same basic organic chemical structure. Aldosterone is an example, as are the sex hormones.

Wolffian (ducts): The embryonic structures which develop into the internal reproductive anatomy of the male; named for Kaspar F. Wolff, German embryologist (1733–94). See also *Müllerian (ducts).*

REFERENCES

Baum, M. J., Everitt, B. J., Herbert, J., and Keverne, E. B. Hormonal basis of proceptivity and receptivity in female primates. *Archives of Sexual Behavior,* 1977, *6,* 173–192.

Beach, F. A. Sexual attractivity, proceptivity, and receptivity in female mammals. *Hormones and Behavior,* 1976, *7,* 105–138.

Cullberg, J. Mood changes and menstrual symptoms with different gestation/estrogen combinations: A double blind comparison with a placebo. *Acta Psychiatrica Scandinavica, 1972, Supplementum* 236.

Fuchs, F., and Klopper, A. *Endocrinology of pregnancy.* New York: Harper & Row, 1971.

Guyton, A. C. *Textbook of medical physiology.* Philadelphia: W. B. Saunders, 1976.

Henderson, M. E. Evidence for a male menstrual temperature cycle and synchrony with the female menstrual cycle. *Australian and New Zealand Journal of Medicine,* 1976, *6.*

Masters, W. H., and Johnson, V. E. *Human sexual response.* Boston: Little, Brown, 1966.

McClintock, M. K. Menstrual synchrony and suppression. *Nature,* 1971, *229,* 244–245.

Nachtigall, L. *The Nachtigall report.* New York: G. P. Putnam's Sons, 1977.

Psychological and Physiological Concepts in Female Sexuality

A Discussion of Physiological Aspects of Female Sexual Development

LYNNE RUBIN

Concepts of sexual physiology are closely related to contemporaneous psychological concepts and even political ideals. Freud described female sexuality in a hierarchy of orgasms, Kinsey provided enlightenment about homosexuality and premarital sex, and Masters and Johnson turned around concepts to describe one type of female orgasm. Thus, woman's erotic life today must be examined in light of the present social environment.

Gestational sexuality is a phase of sexuality that is closely tied to the woman's social environment and the attitude toward pregnancy in her cultural system. There is a dearth of knowledge about libido in pregnancy, but several events take place, the result of which may extend throughout a woman's sexually active years.

Libido in pregnancy can be shown to increase as the woman's pleasure in childbearing stimulates hopeful and pleasant fantasies. In a study by Quirk (1972), it was found that decreased sexual desire in the first trimester resulted from the general malaise or fatigue and the nausea commonly found in early pregnancy. Many other women find increased libido if they feel close to and nurtured by their partners. Some couples are afraid of sexual relations because of fears of harming the mother or the fetus.

The changing body image plays an important part. Many men

LYNNE RUBIN, M.N., Ph.D. • Obstetrics and Gynecologic Nurse Practitioner in Private Practice, Los Angeles, California.

consider the pregnant female's body beautiful. On the other hand, if the man indicates revulsion at the sight of his partner, she will respond with a decreased sexual interest.

Masters and Johnson (1966) found that pregnancy appeared to coincide with many males' beginning extramarital affairs. The reason may be more the stress of the pregnancy on each of the partners than a clear physiological decline in the woman's interest in sex.

In addition, Masters and Johnson noted that sexual appetites increase in the second trimester, possibly because of the increased vascularity surrounding the pelvic area. Notably, uterine contractions often occur with orgasm, and some women may feel these contractions as cramping and aching following sexual stimulation. Masters and Johnson found an effect on the fetus at the time of orgasm. There is a brief decrease in the fetal heart rate. This slowing also occurs during the irregular contractions of pregnancy, that is, Braxton Hicks contractions.

Oxytocin is a powerful stimulus on the uterus during lactation, and it also has a role in erotic arousal. Many women report stimulation while suckling an infant, as well as feeling the sensations of uterine contractions throughout the nursing period. It may be that nursing a baby promotes a woman's awareness of uterine contractions and the consequent pleasurable feelings. This reaction may contribute, along with the increased vascularity of the pelvic organs, to the furthering of a woman's sexual interest.

Various contraceptive agents can cause a change in the erotic behavior of females as dramatic as that caused by menopause or surgical intervention. A contraceptive agent—that is, "the Pill," the diaphragm, the IUD, the condom, foam, or sterilization—should fit the sexual pattern of the person and her partner; otherwise, a less satisfying relationship will ensue. The pill can increase or decrease libido, depending on dosage and the proportions of the two female hormones in the pill. Recent evidence shows that during the end of the pill cycle, when progesterone buildup occurs, libido may be higher than during the first day of taking the pill or early in the cycle (Barnard, Clancy, and Krantz, 1978). In Japan, condoms are a source of erotic enjoyment; it is expected in that culture that sensual pleasures will come from the female's placement of the condom. On one hand, diaphragms may inhibit vaginal sensations for the female or may feel unpleasant to the male partner; on the other hand, if he is encouraged to place the diaphragm in position and to explore her body, an additional positive experience may be provided for the female.

Menopause is a part of sexual development. Kaplan (1978) stated that women become more erotic at menopause and explained this phenomenon by a physiological mechanism. During the menstrual cycle, particularly during the week or so before menses, estrogen and progesterone drop while androgens (male hormones) remain at the same level, that is, unopposed and therefore relatively higher. Androgens are well known to increase libido in both men and women and are relatively higher following menopause.

Psychological factors may also account for this increase in sex drive following menopause. Greater sensitivity, the relaxation of previous sexual taboos, freedom from the possibility of pregnancy, and greater maturity and knowledge may contribute to a better sexual experience. Kaplan pointed out that some older women have more sexual fantasies, masturbate more frequently, and are more interested in sex than when they were younger.

However, the diminishing lubrication during and after menopause may cause severe pain in some women and may consequently dampen sexual desire. Yet, this normal decrease in lubrication may provide the greater friction that the older male needs for adequate erection. It is also true that diminished lubrication delays orgasm, but if the woman's partner is an older man, his orgasm will also be delayed or, possibly, may not occur in every sexual encounter. This change in timing allows for a greater possibility that orgasm will occur for both.

Older women make specific sexual choices as a result of life experience. Older women may be more certain about what they want in a partner. Sexual experiences may have a different significance at this age. Not all postmenopausal women engage in sexual activity. Some may prefer celibacy to indifferent sexual contact. Climacteric women and men are psychologically vulnerable during sexual transitions (Rubin and Rubin, 1977). If the man can't quickly attain or sustain an erection, he may avoid sex because he is afraid of failure. If the woman experiences pain or isn't aroused quickly or, even more importantly, does not *feel* sensuous and beautiful in the sex act, then her adjustment to this new developmental phase may be extremely difficult.

Recently, it has been shown that women, perimenopausal or younger, experience a change in libido, and consequently in the quality of orgasm, following a hysterectomy (Weisberg, 1978). During orgasm, both the vagina and the uterus contract. The ability to sense these contractions varies, and thus, the removal of the uterus has varying effects in different women. In addition, changes in the blood vessel responses may occur because of the cutting or the redirecting of the pelvic blood vessels. Vaginal sensation during sexual activity may be a subjectively different experience, and a decrease in desire may result.

Surgical removal of ovaries may cause a decrease in libido, for the ovaries are a source of androgens as well as estrogens. Since libido depends on androgen levels, estrogen replacement alone does not duplicate a woman's former hormonal environment and changes in sexual response may occur.

It has been the thesis of this discussion that erotic response does not exist by physiology alone and that the study of erotic physiology must include culture, political, and individual, subjective responses. Together, they are responsible for how the physiological arousal response is perceived. Baill and Money acknowledged this fact by pointing out that research designs do not always take into account the multideterminate nature of arousal. Masters and Johnson's finding that the physiological basis of orgasm in the female is clitoral does not explain the subjective response. The qualitatively different experience of orgasm manually induced in the clitoris by masturbation or by the partner as compared with the orgasm induced through the introduction of the penis or other vaginal penetration cannot be explained by Masters and Johnson's findings. It is fallacious to reduce a woman's orgastic range to "clitoral." An orgasm is a total response to a multiplicity of stimuli. Otto and Otto (1972) pointed out that it would be more correct to state that the clitoris plays a role in all orgasms.

Further, women's relationships with their men have changed dramatically in the last few years, and it is to be expected that sexual relationships will also change. Hopefully, these changes will allow a greater tolerance for individual differences in erotic response. The sexual act itself, though filled with variation, will obviously not change, but sexual relationships may. The poet Rainer Marie Rilke (1954) foresaw these changes and offered an optimistic conclusion:

> This advance [of women] will [at first much against the will of the outstripped men] change the love-experience which is now full of error, will alter it from the ground up, reshape it into a relation that is meant to be of one human being to another, no longer of man to woman. And this more human love (that will fulfill itself, infinitely considerate and gentle, and kind and clear in binding and releasing) will resemble that which we are preparing with struggle and toil, the love that consists in this, that two solitudes protect and border and salute each other.

References

Barnard, M. U., Clancy, B. J., and Krantz, K. D. *Human sexuality for health professionals.* Philadelphia: W. B. Saunders, 1978.

Fisher, S. *The female orgasm.* New York: Basic Books, 1973.

Kaplan, H. S. *Sex at menopause.* In L. Rose (Ed.), *The menopause book.* New York: Hawthorne Books, New York, 1978.

Masters, W. H., and Johnson, V. E. *Human sexual response*. Boston: Little, Brown, 1966.

Otto, H., and Otto, R. *Total sex*. New York: Signet, 1972.

Quirk, B. L. *Coitus during pregnancy*, unpublished master's thesis, University of Kansas, 1972.

Reitz, R. *Menopause: A positive approach*. Philadelphia: Chilton Book Co., 1977.

Rilke, R. *Letters to a young poet*. New York: Norton, 1954.

Rubin, R. T., and Rubin, L. E. The psychology of the climacteric. *Encyclopedia Brittanica*. New York: Medical and Health Annual, 1977.

Seaman, B., and Seaman, G. *Women and the crisis in sex hormones*. New York: Rawson Associates, 1977.

Weisberg, M. Sexual–emotional factors in gynecological illnesses. *Human Sexualiaty*, 1978, *12*(10).

Zilbergeld, B. *Male sexuality*. New York: Bantam Books, 1978.

Chapter 5

Some Suggested Revisions Concerning Early Female Development

ELEANOR GALENSON AND HERMAN ROIPHE

⸭EDITOR's NOTE

The tentative and culturally biased early formulations of female sexual development by the founder of psychoanalysis, Sigmund Freud, are well publicized and are often popularly thought to be THE psychoanalytic theory of female development. They are criticized both for confusing the consequences of cultural pressure with innate feminine disposition and for giving scientific validation and enhancement to those cultural pressures. There is, however, more to be said both about Freud and about psychoanalytic theories of feminine development. Freud, for all his patriarchial Viennese Victorian biases and his phallocentrism, took women's sexual life seriously. He learned psychoanalysis from listening to women patients, acknowledged and deplored the repressive forces operating against women's full development, and provided a treatment that supported women's efforts to free themselves from repressive forces (rather than the other current treat-

ELEANOR GALENSON, M.D. • Clinical Professor of Psychiatry, Mount Sinai School of Medicine, New York, New York.   HERMAN ROIPHE, M.D. • Associate Clinical Professor of Psychiatry, Mount Sinai School of Medicine, New York, New York.

The research upon which this paper is based was carried out in the Research Nursery in the Division of Child Psychiatry at the Albert Einstein College of Medicine. We wish to acknowledge the important contributions of the many staff members to this work, particularly Dr. Jan Drucker, who assisted in data analysis, and Ms. Catherine Shapiro, head teacher, who has been responsible for the functioning of the nursery for the past five years. This chapter (excluding the Editor's Note) is a reprint from the *Journal of the American Psychoanalytic Association* (Suppl.) 24(5):29–57, 1976. Permission granted by International Universities Press.

ments by surgical means, which ranged from removing the offending organ, "the hyster" or uterus, to clitoridectomy, to dictatorial and imprisoning "rest cures," to coercive morality).

There is not one, monolithic psychoanalytic view of women's development. As more data have been accumulated by the psychoanalytic method, Freud's beginning positions have been importantly modified. Some of his ideas have proved unfounded and new ideas have been developed. These more current psychoanalytic positions are not yet familiar outside the professional journals. To summarize, feminine development does not begin with the three- or four-year-old girl's disappointment at the discovery of the boy's penis; rather, it begins at birth, with the assignment of sex by the parents and their reaction to the baby as a girl, with the sensations from the baby's genital area and the early important pleasure and pride in her body. Penis envy is only one of many envies that babies have of those who have something they don't have. It is a developmental event turning the girl inward, enhancing her cognitive and speech development, and increasing her interest in her father. However, her identification with her mother remains essential for feminine development and a sense of self-esteem. The desire for motherhood develops from these identifications, not as a compensation for being deprived of a penis. The three papers that follow are written by analysts who have thought about the problems from somewhat different perspectives. Eleanor Galenson and Herman Roiphe have observed toddlers in a controlled nursery setting. Susanna Isaacs Elmhirst draws from her many years of experience as a child-analyst in the tradition of Melanie Klein, as well as from her initial experience as a pediatrician and later, following Winnicott, as the Physician-in-charge at Paddington Green Children's Hospital. Robert Stoller, an authority on gender development, has years of experience in reconstructing and unraveling the influence of childhood on adult patients, many with unusual and deviant adult sexual lives.}

A reevaluation of Freud's ideas concerning early sexuality must take into account new findings from a variety of sources, such as studies of normal children, genetically and hormonally deviant ones, and those who are emotionally disturbed, as well as the changes in psychoanalytic thinking that have taken place under the impact of ego psychology over the past 20 years. We agree with Lichtenstein (1961) that sexuality has been relegated to the position of only one among several variables from the special and exemplary role in development that Freud (1905/1955, 1940) had originally assigned to the sexual drive organization. Lichtenstein, in arguing against this general trend, maintained that sexuality is the most archaic mode, closely related to the primary process and therefore uniquely capable of conveying the emotional truth of personal existence, while only later on do other modes establish, in thought, the conviction that one does in fact exist. In this respect, he followed Freud's views concerning the centrality of sexuality among the other variables of development and held that sexuality both molds and is molded by developing object relations, a position with which we are in agreement. This mutual influence of sexuality and object relations was alluded to in a preliminary and sketchy way in Freud's 1933 paper, where he acknowledged that the early experiences of boys and girls differed, and that the pre-Oedipal relation of the girl with her mother was of a special nature. He described the changing character of the girl's libidinal relations to her mother as

> of many different kinds. Since they persist through all three phases of infantile sexuality, they also take on the characteristic of the different phases and express themselves by oral, sadistic–anal and phallic wishes. These wishes represent active as well as passive impulses. (pp. 119–120)

With the advent of Mahler's infant observational research (Mahler and Gosliner, 1955; Mahler, 1963, 1966, 1968), attention to the area of developing object relations increased enormously, while drive development receded somewhat from both research and clinical interest. In the course of our own research carried out at the Albert Einstein College of Medicine since 1966, we have attempted to encompass both the sector of developing object relations and that of drive organization, focusing upon their interdependence and their reciprocal influence in relation to ego functions. We have been particularly interested in the emergence of the sense of sexual identity during the second year of life.

Review of Pertinent Studies

Before presenting our own data concerning the emergence of genital awareness at 16–19 months, we shall review two other studies of early sexual development, since these point to a critical period in development coinciding with the one we have described. The work of Money and Ehrhardt (1972) is concerned with genetically and hormonally deviant individuals: these authors suggest that it is the sex in which the infant is reared during the first two years of life that plays the major role in the establishment of the sense of gender identity. They have studied several different groups of children. There were genetically male individuals in whom there had been complete absence of all gonadal hormones during the prenatal period and who were therefore born with female-appearing external genitalia. These children developed along female lines if they had been reared as fe-

males during the first 18 months of life. In contrast to this first group
was a group of genetically female children who had been hormonally
androgenized during their prenatal period (without having received
additional androgenization postnatally). These prenatally androgenized
but genetically female girls were also reared as girls. When studied
during their latency years in follow-up, although they showed certain
traits called tomboyishness, which included preference for rough-and-
tumble play and for boys' toys instead of dolls, as well as a disinclina-
tion to have children, their object choice was distinctly heterosexual
and they regarded themselves as female.

Money and Ehrhardt concluded from the study of these two
groups of children that feminine gender identity is primarily dependent upon neither prenatal gonadal hormones nor genetic endowment, but upon the sex of rearing. The presence of tomboyish traits,
however, suggested to them that the presence of prenatal androgens
plays a minor part.

Another group studied by Money and Ehrhardt consisted of genetically male individuals in whom there had been an absence of hormonal androgenization prenatally. Some of these infants were born
with normal or near-normal-appearing female external genitalia and
were reared as females. These children showed feminine preferences
for doll play and for having children of their own later on: 90% of
them said they were content with their female role, and 80% had already established heterosexual relationships when followed up at the
time of early adolescence.

However, those genetically male infants in whom some but not
the normal amount of prenatal androgen hormones had been produced, were born with external genitalia that were anomalous in appearance, neither definitely male nor definitely female. In several of
these infants reared as boys, sex reassignment was attempted after
they had reached the end of the second year of life because of the
surgical impossibility of providing a semblance of adequate male genitalia. These children showed profound psychological disturbance.
Money and Ehrhardt concluded from the study of this group as well
that it is primarily postnatal factors in the human that, in contrast with
lower species, account for much if not most gender identity. They nevertheless believe that it is cognitive development, particularly language, that is responsible for the age-specific critical level of 18
months or so, beyond which successful sex reassignment is impossible. Our own findings are in agreement with the critical age for sex
reassignment, although we do not consider cognitive factors the essential determinants.

The other major research connected with very early sexuality, carried out by Stoller (1968) and his group, emphasizes the decisive influence of early parental rearing during the first few years for the determination of "core gender identity." Stoller has described the importance of the prephallic feminine identification in a small group of transsexual males whose mothers shared a particular type of psychosexual constellation. These transsexual males had apparently reached a critical developmental divide in terms of their sexual identity toward the end of their second year, the same critical period noted by Money and Ehrhardt and in our own research population. However, Stoller did not entirely eliminate the contributions of genital anatomy and physiology, or of endocrine and neurological factors, to the sense of sexual identity, in addition to the effect of the maternal influence.

In regard to female development, Stoller believes there is an early phase of female gender development, followed by a secondary phase, which he feels is the result of the girl's defense against her growing awareness of the genital difference, although no clinical material has as yet been offered in support of this position. A similar point of view was expressed by Horney (1924/1967, 1926/1967), Jones (1927, 1933), Zilboorg (1944), and, more recently, Fliegel (1973), all of whom have disagreed with Freud's emphasis on the phallic phase as the beginning of the gender development of the girl.

In summary, the two most extensive ongoing studies of early sexual development, those of Money and Ehrhardt and of Stoller, have identified a critical period for the establishment of gender identity that occurs by the second half of the second year of life, a critical period that correlates chronologically with our own findings. There is disagreement among us, however, as to the factors responsible for the occurrence of this critical phase of sexual development.

RESEARCH HYPOTHESES AND RESEARCH DESIGN

Roiphe (1968) has proposed an early genital phase, which occurs normally and regularly sometime between 16 and 24 months of age and is characterized by the presence of behavior indicating genital arousal. This would include frequent and intensive manipulation of the genitals and increased curiosity regarding the genitals of others. This early genital phase would be free of any Oedipal resonance but would be closely connected with ongoing consolidation of self and object representations, particularly of the genital area. Roiphe further postulated that although reactions would usually be low-keyed, there would be moderate to severe castration reactions at this time in those children who were exposed to the genital anatomical difference between the sexes and who had sustained, during their first year of life, either some important trauma to the developing body image, such as serious illness and surgical procedures, or had suffered a serious disturbance in the mother–child relationship, because of such factors as prolonged separations or depression in the mother.

Roiphe proposed that these pre-Oedipal castration reactions would consist of a complex of symptoms including negativism, increased dependence on the mother, disturbances in sleep and bowel and bladder functioning, nightmares, fears of being bitten by animals, the fear in boys that the penis would fall off, and, in girls, the question of why they do not have a penis. This early castration anxiety would be indissolubly connected with fears of object loss and self-annihilation unlike the castration reactions of the later Oedipal phase.

Finally, the original hypothesis (Galenson, 1971) was broadened to predict that all areas of functioning, including the emergent symbolism of play and speech, would be influenced and organized by the genital awareness and the reaction to the genital difference; in other words, this era would constitute a true early genital phase, preceding by a year or more the later well-known phallic–Oedipal phase.

During the nine years of our research, we have studied a population of 70 children who are evenly divided between the sexes, mostly coming from a middle-class group; they have been studied from their 10th or 12th month of life through the end of their second year in a naturalistic, informal nursery setting. Ten mother-and-child pairs attend four two-hour sessions each week. Two observers gather developmental information from the mother and observe the child's behavior, recording the data immediately after the observation session. Although individual case studies have already been published, this is our first cross-sectional analysis of our population, a group that is now the subject of a systematic follow-up by colleagues who will be comparing their findings with our own earlier ones.

Every mother lends shape to an "identity theme" in her young infant, as Lichtenstein (1961) has felicitously described it, and it is partly through the feeding relationship that this molding occurs, an experience that appears to be a different one for boys and for girls. Murphy (1962) and Korner (1973) have described differences in maternal handling according to whether the infant is a male or a female.

Furthermore, reports in the psychoanalytic literature have pointed to the difference between the early oral experiences of male and female patients. Greenacre (1950), Kestenberg (1956, 1968), and, more recently, Fraiberg (1972) have described the close relation between oral and vaginal themes in the analytic material from both adult and child female patients. Confirmatory evidence of such combined early oral and genital experience comes from the fact that penile erections occur in boys during nursing (as well as at other times, of course).

Although feeding is certainly a highly significant experience of the first year, it is by no means the only one. As Freud (1933) pointed out, "the mother . . . by her activities over the child's bodily hygiene inevitably stimulated, and perhaps even roused for the first time, pleasurable sensations in her genitals" (p. 120). Kris (1951) elaborated on this point: "The transfer from general affection to the genital zone itself . . . may also arise as a consequence of the general bodily closeness to which, we assume, the child tends to react with sensation in the genital region" (p. 96). We would add that is is likely that the mother's activities are experienced differently by boys and by girls, not only because the genital anatomical structure of each sex provides distinctive sensations, but more particularly because the specific sex of the child provokes special and unique unconscious fantasies in the mother as she handles her infant's genitals. One has only to witness the repetitive and intense genital cleansing practiced by some mothers, in contrast to the almost complete avoidance of the area by others, to be convinced of the impact on the infant of sexual fantasies aroused in the mother.

The mutual influence of drive organization and object relationship just described characterizes all early mother–child interactions. Lichtenstein (1961) described this influence as

> An interaction between two partners where each partner experiences himself as uniquely and specifically capable of serving as the instrument of the other's sensory gratification—such a partnership can be called a partnership of sensual involvement. (p. 207)

And later on:

> . . . there is an innate body responsiveness, a capacity . . . to respond to contact with another person with a specific kind of somatic excitation which is not a drive, because it has no direction, but which is the innate prerequisite for the later development of a drive. . . . This responsiveness we may call sexual because it forms the matrix of later sexual development. (p. 250)

Patterns of sensuous interaction of mother and child—the expression of early drive organization—seem, then, to involve the genital zone from the very beginning of life, not only in the course of the mother's fondling and bodily ministrations and during feeding, but also probably in connection with transmitted pressure and excitation from the adjacent anal and urinary areas, the totality of these sensuous interactions contributing to a substantially different early body image for each sex.

CORRELATION BETWEEN DRIVE DEVELOPMENT AND OBJECT RELATIONS
FROM 6 TO 18 MONTHS OF AGE

The particular importance of the genitals as well as the face, from about six months of age, for the establishment of the sense of identity has been described by Greenacre (1958) as

> The body areas which are then most significant in comparing and contrasting and establishing individual recognition of the body self, and that of others, are the *face* and the *genitals* . . . after six months of age and extending into the second half of the second year. During the latter part of this time, however, and especially during the third year, the gradual increase in genital feelings—clitoral and phallic—gives endogenous sensations and pressures from within a kind of sensory peg which combines locally with the body imagery produced by visual and tactile appreciation of the own genitals and those of the other. (pp. 116–118)

It is specifically this new level of bodily awareness, involving first the anal and urinary zones and then the genitals, that emerges during the practicing subphase of Mahler's separation–individuation process, that is, at about one year of age. Behavioral evidence of these psychological developments has been accumulated during the course of our own research. Whereas the infant of 6 months plays with his toes, fingers, and body in a general exploratory fashion, the 12-month-old examines his body parts in a new way. He compares his own facial features with his mother's by pointing at and touching them, and soon his comparison includes the rest of his body as he proceeds in a regular sequence from facial features to the anal, urinary, and finally the genital area (Galenson and Roiphe, 1974). The emergence of anal awareness is indicated by behaviors such as shifts in the frequency and timing of defecation, attentiveness to the act itself, tugging at the soiled diaper, hiding during defecation, interest in toilets and garbage cans, and the use of anal verbal references. There is also an increased incidence of diaper rashes and diarrhea and/or constipation. With these anal-zone indications come many sequences of play behavior that we have understood as "anal derivative" in nature. These consist of "in and out," filling and emptying, and scattering and smearing behavior, all having structural properties similar to those characteristic of anal-zone functioning (Galenson, 1971).

With the anal awareness, or soon thereafter, the emergence of urinary awareness is signaled by such zonal behavior as attentiveness to the urinary act and such derivative play as interest in faucets and hoses and in pouring liquids. This anal and urinary interest is directed not only at the toddler's own body but at these specific areas and functions in parents, peers, animals, and dolls as well.

In the midst of the progressive anal and urinary awareness, genital behavior of a different quality from the early genital exploratory play emerges for the first time. All 70 children in our research sample (Galenson and Roiphe, 1974) have demonstrated this heightened and qualitatively distinctive genital awareness along with genital derivative behavior, to be described below, beginning sometime between 15 and 19 months of age, confirming Roiphe's original hypothesis (1968). Moreover, in each instance, the genital awareness has emerged in regular and predictable sequence, only after the development of both anal and urinary awareness. This finding agrees with Kleeman's (1976) report of the five infant girls he studied.

CLINICAL ILLUSTRATION. The following excerpts from direct observational data of an infant boy illustrate the type of behavior that indicates the underlying psychological anal, urinary, and then genital differentiation, as well as progressive differentiation in the object sphere.

John, at 12 months of age, explored his mother's eyes, ears, and mouth simultaneously with those areas on his own body and had become interested in his mirror image. As self-object differentiation proceeded, peek-a-boo games with his whole body were his favorites; he pointed and waved bye-bye, and he took his first unaided steps. As evidence of his increasing individuation and body-image emergence, John's interest began to be concentrated more and more in the perineal area; he began to defecate only at night and was now very interested in the toilet and the toidy seat—both of which he used for splashing and playing—and garbage pails intrigued him for the first time. His genital play, which had begun at about 7½ months, continued to be casual and exploratory in nature.

At 13 months, John became interested in his mother's navel and in his own, began to remove his own diapers, was following his mother into the bathroom consistently, and had begun to throw and bang toys and aggressively take them away from other children. At 14 months, an important shift in the object sphere was signaled as John became definitely less clinging to his mother but now sought out his father, anticipating his departure in the morning and his return at night. He succeeded in witnessing his father's urination for the first time, as far as was reported to us. Along with this beginning shift in object ties, there was a definite acceleration of his anal and urinary and genital interests. His stools were softer in consistency, they awakened him in the morning, and he was irritable until he was changed. He pulled at his soiled diaper and at his outer pants in preparation for the change and had also developed a diaper rash. Much anal-derivative play made its appearance soon after: he shredded his pampers and banged and threw toys; the "shape box" became his favorite toy; he messed and smeared his food, searched out garbage pails constantly, discovered and operated light switches devotedly (the element of control was important here), loved push-toys (again the anal expulsive characteristic), and was often found filling the toilet with paper. His object ties assumed anal-phase attributes as he became much more demanding and had angry outbursts, during which he screamed and kicked his mother.

Urinary and genital awareness in the body-image area showed similar intensification. John now began to urinate selectively during diapering and could stop and start his stream while standing in the bathtub. At the same time, he pointed to his own penis and smiled as he manipulated it.

At 15 months, his increasing general autonomy became evident in his "no" behavior and verbalization of that word, but he also began to imitate his father more and more. He now defecated in solitude only, sat on the toidy seat quite voluntarily (but without results), teased, stored and stacked his toys, and still remained very interested in the bathroom. His urination became even more infrequent as he withheld his urine for longer periods, and he labeled his mother's urination "pee-pee"; furthermore, he pointed to his penis and looked down at it as he pulled in his rather protruberant abdomen. It was evident that the anal, urinary, and genital areas were achieving much greater psychic representation, as was the emerging concept of his own identity as a totality. For example, he called himself by his proper name, he had added the word "yes" to his vocabulary, and he was attached to a new transitional object, a teddy bear (his bottle had been his first one).

In the object sphere during the next three months, as an even stronger shift to the father took place, John was increasingly interested in his father, carrying about his shoes and other belongings while he bit and was angry at his mother. As for body-image progression, his own penis became even more interesting to him: he pointed at it through his diaper, pulled at it vigorously, often while it was erect, and in parallel fashion tried to touch his father's urinary stream and penis on many occasions.

This summary description depicts the usual urinary and genital developmental sequence with the concomitant separation–individuation progression, including the beginning shift toward the father that has been observed in most of our normal children.

In contrast to the normal developmental sequence of anal, urinary, and then genital emergence at 16–18 months just described, 29 disturbed children in our therapeutic nursery have shown serious delays not only in their separation–individuation process but also in the emergence of their anal, urinary, and genital awareness (Galenson, 1973). It seems, then, that the achievement of both the practicing and the rapprochement subphases of object relations is correlated with and, in fact, is essential for ongoing drive development, as is illustrated by the delay in progression of anal, urinary, and early genital cathexis and organization, which is evident in these children with serious object-relationship impairment. Drive development is profoundly influenced by the quality of the object relation.

The Line of Development of Genital Drive Organization

It is now generally agreed (Spitz, 1962; Kleeman, 1971, 1975; Galenson and Roiphe, 1974) that the genital play of the first 16 months of life is, under normal circumstances, in the nature of general body exploration and cannot yet be considered true masturbation. The pattern of emergence of this early genital play, as described by Kleeman (1971, 1975) in the five children he reported on, agrees in most respects with our own findings (Galenson and Roiphe, 1974) in the 70 boys and girls we have studied. This early genital play may be summarized as follows: boys and girls show a difference in time of onset and quality of early genital play. Boys begin genital exploration somewhere between 7 and 10 months, whereas girls begin some months later. In girls, the genital play is less focused and less frequent and shows less intentionality than in boys, partially, we believe, in consequence of the more indirect mechanical stimulation by diapers and cleansing experienced by the girl.

Genital behavior in both boys and girls then begins to take on a new quality beginning somewhere between 15 and 17 months. In the 5 girls reported by Kleeman and in the 35 girls in our own sample, genital manipulation was now more focused, the infant was absorbed in the activity, she derived intense pleasure from it, and there were signs of concomitant autonomic excitation, such as skin flushing, perspiration, and rapid respiration. Masturbation was carried out manually as before, but the action was now rapid and repetitive, with vigorous rubbing, pinching, and squeezing, and the fingers being positioned near the mons pubis or on or between the labia. Because the genital area is so small, it is usually impossible to decide whether the vaginal opening is being stimulated at the same time. However, several of our research group mothers have reported that the little girl's finger has actually been introduced into the opening of the vagina itself. In two deviant female infants we have studied (Galenson, 1973), insertion of their pacifiers deeply into the vagina regularly and repetitively was observed in our own nursery.

The usual normal manual masturbation occurs during bathing and diapering, while indirect nonmanual masturbation is achieved mainly through straddling rocking horses, toys, furniture, parents' legs, etc. It is particularly significant that affectionate and erotic gestures toward other people now accompany the genital manipulation for the first time; that is, it appears to be object-directed. In the beginning of this period of new genital awareness, the little girl often looks at or touches her mother with an expression of pleasure and delight as she is touching her own genitals. Gradually, this object-directed affect is replaced by the inner-directed gaze that soon accompanies all her genital self-stimulation.

We consider this new type of genital activity true masturbation, in spite of the absence of a concomitant verbalized fantasy, for various forms of nonverbal yet clearly symbolic behavior accompany the new genital activity, indicating the presence of some accompanying—albeit rudimentary—fantasy state. For example, among the many objects used in direct genital masturbatory contact by many little girls in our study have been nursing bottles, transitional-object blankets, stuffed animals, and dolls. We think it likely that this early fantasy formation includes a partial memory of the earlier maternal contact, since the genital manipulation so often involves these typical "mother-me" objects. Concrete objects are then gradually discarded, and masturbation approaches the adult model, although some people never relinquish them entirely, as has been reported by Greenacre (1969) and by ourselves (Roiphe and Galenson, 1973a; Galenson and Roiphe 1971, 1974).

Genital Drive Organization and the Sense of Femininity

Our view of early female sexual development, as derived from our research findings, includes the following three propositions:

1. As already stated, we believe that sexual drive organization plays a central and exemplary role for the early sense of sexual identity and profoundly influences object relations and ego development.

2. Although Freud in his later papers (1931, 1933) assumed that the pre-Oedipal development in the girl is crucial for certain aspects of her later development, particularly for the shift of love object from mother to father, he vastly underestimated the role of pre-Oedipal psychosexuality.

3. The early castration complex (not as yet connected with the

Oedipal constellation), with its component penis envy, is a pivotal factor for the girl's developing femininity, particularly for the crucial and decisive erotic shift to the father as love object.

Evidence supporting this view of early female development will be presented under the following headings: (1) "The Role of Early Drive Development"; (2) The Discovery of the Sexual Anatomical Difference and Its Impact on Psychosexual Development"; and (3) "Ego Development and the Sense of Sexual Identity."

THE ROLE OF EARLY DRIVE DEVELOPMENT. As already described, the early oral activities with their probable concomitant vaginal stimulation have combined with the stimulation of the mother's affectionate handling and other ministrations to provide the girl with an early sense of the genitals, always in connection with the infant's developing bond to the mother. The early genital exploratory play adds to this vague beginning sense of the genital area. Then, at about 16 months, a qualitatively new type of genital play develops, which we consider true masturbation for the first time. The infant seems now to be newly aware of both the genital area and genital sensations in that she looks at her genitals and alertly attends to her genital manipulations. Furthermore, this zonal behavior is soon followed by a flurry of genital derivative behavior. There are accompanying affective behavioral changes, and ego development now comes under the influence of the genital cathexis. A definite quality of phallic organization appears to both mingle with and finally dominate over the prior anal-urinary organization.

The little girl now not only focuses her attention upon her own ano-urinary-genital area, but from about 16 or 17 months on, she becomes curious about this area and its functions in others as well. As evidence for the widespread influence of the new genital awareness, all the little girls in our study succeeded in being admitted to the bathroom with their fathers at this time, even in the most modest of families, and those who had been present during parental toileting during their earlier months began to be interested in the father's urination for the first time at about 16–17 months. This initial curiosity concerning her father is soon followed by similar attempts to investigate the same area in her mother, her peers, and dolls and animals, if available. Then, the curiosity spreads to other aspects of body differences, such as hair and clothing. Furthermore, in those girls where boy–girl differential verbal labeling had already emerged prior to 17 months of age, distortions in the use of such differential verbal labeling have been noted frequently during the period of their reaction to the genital difference, while use of the word *boy* has often dropped out altogether. A few excerpts from our observational data will give a flavor of the behavioral manifestations of this emerging genital schematization in girls.

Lilly, at 14 months, had been interested in the toilet and its accessories for some time, although toilet training had not yet been attempted. Now she began to pull at her genitals during diapering and bathing. At 17½ months, she wanted to examine her mother's pubic area and asked to see her mother's "penis"; she also inserted her fingers deeply between her own labia and looked up between her widespread legs. She undressed dolls continually and watched other children being diapered.

Peggy had touched her genitals in her bath from the age of 12½ months. At 14 months, she fell asleep with her genitals resting upon her teddy bear, and she fingered between her labia frequently during diapering and bathing, then examining her hand visually. At 15½ months, she rubbed her labia with toilet paper, looking pleased and flushed as she did so. She also examined dolls and became very interested in other children's diapering. A little later, she became self-absorbed and withdrawn during her genital manipulation.

Winnie had been touching her genitals during diapering for some months, but at 19 months she began to smile when she did so and looked up at her mother. She also masturbated while looking at a book.

Jenny was one of our early "rocking-horse" children, but this rocking became an intensely erotic activity with flushing and rapid respiration from 14½ months onward. At 17 months, she began to reach briefly for her genital area manually, although rocking still remained her main form of genital activity. She took possession of her father's pen, hiding it for several days. [This possessiveness and interest in phallic-shaped objects, extremely common in girls during this period, seems to be linked with the emergence of symbols (Galenson and Roiphe, 1971).] At 19½ months, while she was still rocking intensely, she insisted that a little male friend with whom she bathed was a girl and made many male–female errors in verbalization. At 20¾ months, she demanded full possession of all her father's pens.

Mary began to pull at her genitals whenever she was fatigued, beginning at 8 months of age. At 14 months, tentative but now regular genital touching emerged and soon accompanied every diapering. She also began consistently to straddle trains and place dolls between her legs. During a trip with her parents, her masturbation increased, it was now accompanied by a self-absorbed and dreamy look, and she insisted that she, her mother, and her favorite doll all had penises.

Sara began to finger her genitals at 12 months; this activity gradually became more intense and erotic in character, until at 15½ months she was giggling and becoming quite self-absorbed during each episode of genital manipulation.

Discovery of the Sexual Anatomical Difference and Its Impact on Psychosexual Development: Boy–Girl Differences after 18 Months. Boys and girls differ in their later genital development in several respects, although they are initially alike. All 35 boys in our normal sample developed an awareness of the genital difference and began masturbation proper about 15 months, as did the girls, and their sexual curiosity was similar to that of the girls during the early weeks following the initial discovery of the genital difference.

From this point onward, however, there was a clear divergence in development between boys and girls. The boys reflected the effect of the genital emergence in their choice of those toys and play activities that are usually considered typically masculine, such as cars and ball playing, and in the onset of a mild degree of hyperactivity. Furthermore, their masturbation was continuous and fairly vigorous from then on. Only 2 of the 35 boys showed serious disturbances following the emergence of genital awareness, disturbances that seriously distorted their subsequent development. Both boys had suffered marked interference in their maternal relationship during their first year of life, the details of which have been reported elsewhere (Galenson, Blau, Roiphe, and Vogel, 1975; Roiphe and Galenson, 1973a).

In contrast to the low incidence of overt reaction in the boys, all 35 girls in our research sample showed a definite and important reaction to the discovery of the genital difference, and 8 of the 35 developed extensive castration reactions. It should be mentioned here that our sample was not a random one, since we had selected for inclusion in our research group each year at least two children who, because of certain experiences during their first year of life, would be expected to react with disturbance to the emergence of genital awareness in accordance with Roiphe's (1968) original hypothesis. Thus although the castration reactions were definitely more frequent in the girls, this boy–girl ratio is only an approximate one.

The castration reactions in the girls ranged from mildly transient ones, which seemed to have milder prognostic importance, to some profound disruptions involving almost every aspect of behavior. Our data lend support to Freud's (1933) statement that the girl's discovery that she is castrated is a turning point in her growth. However, this discovery of the genital difference, with the fantasy that she is castrated, takes place at an earlier age than Freud indicated, and the advent of the crucial discovery seems to wait upon the emergence of a specific cathexis of the genital area, which in turn follows closely upon the emergence of anal and urinary awareness. The subsequent sense of loss may be profound to only moderate, depending upon many factors, such as the quality of the tie to the mother, earlier bodily experiences, the availability of the father at this time, and the mother's conscious and unconscious attitudes.

We believe that these castration responses to the sexual difference are important organizing influences from this time onward (Roiphe, 1968; Galenson and Roiphe, 1971, 1974; Roiphe and Galenson, 1973b) and that they determine not only the direction of much of the girl's subsequent psychosexual development, but other aspects of her personality as well, in both enhancing and inhibiting directions. For in the wake of the castration reactions, we have seen marked oral-regressive behavior; anal-zone exploration and anal masturbation become markedly intensified; and there is reemergence of the fear of object loss and of anal loss, and a subsequent change in the pattern of genital masturbation in many girls. Manual masturbation is often replaced by indirect masturbation by such means as the rocking horse or thigh pressure, or it is displaced to the anal area or to the umbilicus, while some girls abandon masturbation altogether. Still others continue to masturbate, but no longer seem to derive pleasure from masturbation (Galenson and Roiphe, 1974).

In a previous publication (Galenson and Roiphe, 1971), we described the establishment of a basic depressive mood in connection with a profound pre-Oedipal castration response in an infant girl. Many of the girls with less profound forms of pre-Oedipal castration reaction have shown temporary affective changes, such as quietness and loss of zestfulness and enthusiasm, along with facial expressions of sadness. Since these mood changes have been correlated chronologically with the castration reactions, we have hypothesized that there is a causal connection between these two experiences. Mahler (1966) described similar mood changes in many of the little girls she observed during the same chronological period, although she has emphasized a causal relation between mood changes and the rapprochement phase of object relations.

In contrast to the disturbances already described, many advances in ego development have been noted. It is in connection with these pre-Oedipal castration reactions, for example, that many girls develop a special type of attachment to dolls or other inanimate objects, different from the earlier type of doll play, which appears to serve as "infantile fetishes" in support of the wavering genital schematization (see Roiphe and Galenson, 1973a; Galenson and Roiphe, 1971, 1974). These inanimate objects are involved in the remarkable burgeoning of inner fantasy life, which had emerged in most of the girls in our sample under the impact of the reaction to their recognition of the sexual difference. Furthermore, they began to use crayons, pens, and pencils at this time, earlier than most of the boys in our group, in an early but definite attempt at graphic representation. Many defenses, such as displacement, introjection, and projection, were elaborated as the little girls coped with the fantasy of castration and their renewed fears of object loss and self-annihilation.

The general developmental picture of the 35 boys differed in that all the boys continued to masturbate manually; furthermore, all of them showed some increase in the level of their general motor activity, ranging from a very mild to a quite intense degree. Finally, the boys were not as involved in either fantasy play or graphic representation as were the girls in this same age group.

In summary, most girls in our research sample showed an increased investment in inner fantasy life, expressed in both play and graphic representation; an elaboration of many defenses; and a change in basic mood and in masturbatory patterns; whereas the boys showed a definite tendency toward increased motor activity. The latter might be viewed as defensive in nature, in the service of a denial of the genital difference.

Excerpts from our data will illustrate the many different patterns and types of reaction in the girls of our sample following their discovery of the genital difference.

Lilly, who had been investigating her genital area both visually and manually, began at 18¾ months to inhibit both these activities. At the same time, she became irritable and clinging, her play became less zestful and inventive, and her doll play consisted of labeling all dolls as boys. She called for her father consistently and became distinctly antagonistic toward her mother.

In Peggy, at 15¾ months, all exploration and manipulation of her genitals ceased. She became her mother's well-dressed, neat, subdued, and obedient little girl. Her dolls still remained her prized possessions at 4 years of age, when she was last seen in follow-up.

Winnie had fluctuated in her level of manual masturbatory activity from her 19th month on. At 22 months, while bathing with two little boys, she examined her own genitalia and asked where her penis was. After her baby sister was born, when Winnie was almost 23 months old, her doll play flourished remarkably, whereas her genital play subsided. At 24 months, she persistently tried to open her father's underwear and to grab for his genitals. At 25 months, she started to masturbate again, and at 26 months, she tried to urinate while standing up in imitation of a boy. She had remained an extremely avid doll player when last seen in follow-up, at almost 4 years of age, and her fantasy life was rich and varied.

Jenny, our early passionate horsewoman, was still masturbating this way when last seen in her third year, although there was occasional manual touching as well. She had established ownership of several of her father's pens at the time of the birth of her sister when she was 17 months old, during a period when her anger at her mother had mounted, and she had made many errors in boy–girl labeling of people as well as pictures. By 21 months, she constantly preferred her father in the flesh, or his pens if he were not available. She had also attempted to take possession of her baby sister, with whom she was a very strict and unpleasant disciplinarian.

Finally, Shirley, whose genital manipulation had become intense and was accompanied by definite arousal at 16¾ months, showed extensive preoccupation both with long rods, which she stood upright, and with her Bathinette hose, at the same time as she stared at her baby brother's genitals over and over again. Her formerly very close relation with her mother began to be superseded by a definite wooing of her father; she cried and called for him when he was away and was excited about him when he returned, whereas she refused to allow her mother to read to her or dress her, and she was often sulky. She also developed an abiding preference for two of her dolls at this time and was busily engaged in much make-believe play.

The effect of the castration reaction upon developing object ties has been most striking. Both boys and girls in our sample had developed a special relation with their fathers toward the end of the first year, as part of their increasing separation from the mother. But it was in the midst of their castration reactions that most of the little girls in our group turned to the father in a newly erotic way, seeking the mother's attention only during periods of distress. These little girls seemed to have had a relatively successful experience during their first year. However, in those girls whose earlier relation with the mother had been of poor quality or who had suffered important bodily traumata during their first year, or if they had experienced the birth of a sibling during the second half of the second year, hostile dependence upon the mother was enormously aggravated in the wake of the discovery of the sexual anatomical difference. There is no doubt that these early events in the psychosexual sphere exerted a decisive influence upon the developing libidinal attachment to the father in these little girls, determining whether a definitive erotic shift toward the father took place toward the end of the second year or whether there was a persistence of an intensified and even more ambivalent tie to the mother.

The character of the subsequent Oedipal constellation of the girl will, of course, be influenced in due course. The milder castration reaction would appear to facilitate the girl's turn to the father as her new love object, with a continuing, albeit less intense, attachment to her mother, while the more profound castration reaction would be expected to lead to a predominantly negative Oepidal constellation, with the choice of the mother as the primary but ambivalently loved object.

Our data do not thus far elucidate the question of the site of actual sexual arousal. Intense or exclusive vaginal masturbation has not been reported in any of the girls we have studied, although many have apparently discovered and stimulated the vagina in the course of masturbation involving the labial and clitoral areas. In the two deviant infant girls mentioned previously, extensive and persistent vaginal masturbation with a pacifier was reported by the parents and also observed directly in our own nursery. This vaginal masturbation began at about 12 months of age and continued during the year or so of our contact with these families.

EGO DEVELOPMENT AND THE SENSE OF SEXUAL IDENTITY

Effect upon Symbolic Functioning. We must keep in mind that those male–female verbal labels that appear at 16 or 17 months of age do not represent true concepts but are still bound to concrete attributes; *boy* means "the boy next door" or "the boy in the book named Jim," but not all boys everywhere. It should not be surprising, therefore, to find that these boy–girl labels are quite unstable and that they are either lost altogether for a time or their meaning is confused under the impact of castration reactions (Roiphe and Galenson, 1973a; Galenson and Roiphe, 1971, 1974). This distortion in symbolic functioning persisted over many months in several of the girls we have studied, frequently encompassing the use of masculine pronouns as well.

Not only was verbal symbolism affected, but many aspects of the emerging semisymbolic play that is characteristic of the second half of the second year were profoundly influenced by the developments in the psychosexual area. There was usually a remarkable burgeoning of fantasy life and of graphic representation in the form of early attempts at drawing and writing. The little girls began to use many new defensive measures, such as displacement and introjection and projection, as they very actively coped with the newly aroused anxieties. If the castration reaction was not overwhelming, it was as if a new level of intellectual functioning was achieved. We will mention only a few examples: the avoidance of broken toys, doll play dealing with the genital anatomical differences, the use of phallic-shaped inanimate objects as phallic substitutes, and the attachment to dolls and other inanimate objects as infantile fetishes. These findings have been described elsewhere in detail (Roiphe, 1968; Roiphe and Galenson, 1973b; Galenson and Roiphe, 1971, 1974).

In contrast to the usual reaction, those girls with the more intense castration reactions to the genital emergence suffered a considerable constriction in their fantasy life in that imaginative play of all types became sparse and stereotyped. There was also an interference in their general intellectual curiosity; they explored their world in a much more limited fashion. Their extensive use of such defenses as denial, splitting, displacement to other body areas, total body eroticization, and the use of infantile fetishes led to further disturbances in their development. These children have been described elsewhere (Roiphe and Galenson, 1973a; Galenson and Roiphe, 1971), as have the two boys whose castration reactions came in the wake of unusually severe traumata during their first year of life.

SUMMARY

In our view, Freud's original position that sexual drive organization exerts a special and exemplary role during the various psychosexual stages remains a valid one, although drive organization is in turn consistently and extensively influenced by events in the sphere of object relations. Very early genital-zone experiences during the first 16 months of life contribute to a vague sense of sexual identity and undoubtedly exert an influence over many ego functions. Some genital sensations probably occur consistently in conjunction with feeding, as well as during many other interactions of the mother and her infant.

With ongoing separation and individuation, the genital zone emerges as a distinct and differentiated source of endogenous pleasure sometime between 16 and 19 months of age, exerting a new crucial influence upon the sense of sexual identity, object relations, basic mood, and many aspects of ego functioning, such as the elaboration of fantasy and graphic representation in girls and the increased use of the motor apparatus in boys—the latter probably in the service of denial. This era constitutes an early genital phase, preceding that of the Oedipal period, and the later Oedipal constellation is inevitably shaped by the pre-Oedipal developments we have described.

The discovery of the sexual difference and the new genital sensations of the early genital phase should not be regarded merely as several of many variables that influence the growing sense of identity; they are unique, exemplary, and of equal importance with the oral and anal aspects of psychosexual development that have preceded them.

Furthermore, the pre-Oedipal castration reaction rapidly reactivates and becomes fused with earlier fears of both object and anal loss, and it is therefore particularly threatening to the child's still unstable sense of self and object.

In other publications, we have presented data from direct observational research indicating that the little girl's early relation with her mother, as well as her early bodily experiences, is important in determining the effect upon her when she discovers the sexual anatomical difference at about 16–18 months of age. At this juncture, depending upon the nature of her earlier experiences, as well as the availability of the father, she may either turn more definitively to the father or remain even more ambivalently attached to the mother, a choice having fateful consequences for the Oedipal constellation shortly to emerge.

We have described the little girl's reactions to the discovery of the sexual difference: they include complex pre-Oedipal castration reactions and penis envy, basic mood changes, and the development of many defensive measures. There may, in addition, be a partial or complete renunciation of direct masturbation. We believe that Freud's original position was partially correct in that penis envy and the feminine castration complex do exert crucial influences upon feminine development. However, these occur earlier than he had anticipated, they are closely intertwined with fears of object and anal loss, and they shape an already developing, although vague, sense of femininity, stemming from early bodily and affective experiences with both parents. Furthermore, the castration reactions vary in intensity from child to child to a marked degree, and they profoundly influence ego development, in both enhancing and inhibiting directions, depending upon specific individual factors. From this period on, there are marked differences between boys and girls in many sectors of their psychological development.

References

Fliegel, Z. O. Feminine psychosexual development in Freudian theory. *Psychoanalytical Quarterly,* 1973, 42, 385–409.

Fraiberg, S. Some characteristics of genital arousal and discharge in latency girls. *The Psychoanalytic Study of the Child,* 27, 439–475. New York: Quadrangle Books, 1972.

Freud, S. Three essays on the theory of sexuality. *Standard edition,* 1905, 7, 125–243. London: Hogarth Press, 1955.

Freud, S. Female sexuality. *Standard edition,* 1931, 21, 225–243. London: Hogarth Press, 1961.

Freud, S. Femininity. *Standard edition,* 1933, 22, 112–135. London: Hogarth Press, 1964.

Freud, S. An outline of psychoanalysis. *Standard edition,* 1940, 23, 141–207. London: Hogarth Press, 1964.

Galenson, E. A consideration of the nature of thought in childhood play. In J. B. Mc-

Devitt and C. F. Settlage (Eds.), *Separation–individuation: Essays in honor of Margaret S. Mahler.* New York: International Universities Press, 1971, pp. 41–49.

Galenson, E. Psychopathology of the very young child (unpublished), 1973.

Galenson, E., Blau, S., Roiphe, H., and Vogel, S. Disturbance in sexual identity beginning at 18 months of age. *International Review Psycho-Analysis,* 1975a, 2, 389–397.

Galenson, E., Drucker, J., Miller, R., and Shapiro, C. Detection and treatment of early childhood psychosis (unpublished), 1975b.

Galenson, E., and Miller, R. The choice of symbols. *Journal of the American Academy of Child Psychiatry,* 1976, 5(1).

Galenson, E., and Roiphe, H. The impact of early sexual discovery on mood, defensive organization, and symbolization. *The Psychoanalytic Study of the Child,* 1971, 26, 195–216. New York: Quadrangle Books.

Galenson, E., and Roiphe, H. The emergence of genital awareness during the second year of life. In R. C. Friedman, R. M. Richart, and R. L. Van de Wiele (Eds.), *Sex differences in behavior.* New York: Wiley, 1974, pp. 223–231.

Greenacre, P. 1950, Special problems of early female sexual development. In *Trauma, growth and personality.* New York: International Universities Press, 1969, pp. 237–258.

Greenacre, P. 1958, Early physical determinants in the development of the sense of identity. In *Emotional growth.* New York: International Universities Press, 1971, pp. 113–127.

Greenacre, P. 1969, The fetish and the transitional object. In *Emotional growth.* New York: International Universities Press, 1971, pp. 315–334.

Horney, K. On the genesis of the castration complex in women. In H. Kelman (Ed.), *Feminine psychology.* New York: Norton, 1967, pp. 37–53.

Horney, K. The flight from womanhood. In H. Kelman (Ed.), *Feminine psychology.* New York: Norton, 1967, pp. 54–70.

Horney, K. The phallic phase. *International Journal of Psycho-Analysis,* 1933, 14, 1–33.

Jones, E. The early development of female sexuality. *International Journal of Psycho-Analysis,* 1927, 8, 459–472.

Jones, E. The phallic phase. *International Journal of Psycho-Analysis,* 1933, 14, 1–33.

Kestenberg, J. Vicissitudes of female sexuality. *Journal of the American Psychoanalytic Association,* 1956, 4, 453–476.

Kestenberg, J. Outside and inside, male and female. *Journal of the American Psychoanalytic Association,* 1968, 16, 456–520.

Kleeman, J. The establishment of core gender identity in normal girls. *Archives of Sexual Behavior,* 1971, 1, 117–129.

Kleeman, J. Genital self-stimulation in infant and toddler girls. In I. Marcus and J. Francis (Eds.), *Masturbation: From infancy to senescence.* New York: International Universities Press, 1975, pp. 77–106.

Kleeman, J. Freud's views on early female sexuality in the light of direct child observation. *Journal of the American Psychoanalytic Association,* 1976, 24(5), 3–27.

Korner, A. F. Sex differences in new borns with special reference to differences in the organization of oral behavior. *Journal of Child Psychology and Psychiatry,* 1973, 14, 19–29.

Kris, E. Some comments and observations on early autoerotic activities. In *Selected papers.* New Haven, Conn.: Yale University Press, 1975, pp. 89–113.

Lichtenstein, H. Identity and sexuality: A study of their interrelationship in man. *Journal of the American Psychoanalytic Association,* 1961, 9, 197–260.

Mahler, M. S. Thoughts about development and individuation. *The Psychoanalytic Study of the Child,* 1963, 18, 307–324. New York: International Universities Press.

Mahler, M. S. Notes on the development of basic moods: The depressive affect. In R. M.

Loewenstein, L. Newman, M. Schur, and A. J. Solnit (Eds.), *Psychoanalysis—A general psychology.* New York: International Universities Press, 1966, pp. 156–168.

Mahler, M. S. *On Human symbiosis and the vicissitudes of individuation.* New York: International Universities Press, 1968.

Mahler, M. S. and Gosliner, B. T. On symbiotic child psychosis: Genetic, dynamic, and restitutive aspect. *The Psychoanalytic Study of the Child,* 1955, *10,* 195–212. New York: International Universities Press.

Money, J., and Ehrhardt, A. A. *Man and woman, boy and girl.* Baltimore and London: Johns Hopkins University Press, 1972.

Murphy, L. *The widening world of childhood.* New York: Basic Books, 1962.

Roiphe, H. On an early genital phase; With an addendum on genesis. *The Psychoanalytic Study of the Child,* 1968, *23,* 348–365. New York: International Universities Press.

Roiphe, H. A narcissistic disorder in the process of development (unpublished).

Roiphe, H., and Galenson, E. The infantile fetish. *The Psychoanalytic Study of the Child,* 1973a, *28,* 147–166. New Haven and London: Yale University Press.

Roiphe, H., and Galenson, E. Object loss and early sexual development. *Psychoanalytical Quarterly,* 1973b, *42,* 73–90.

Spitz, R. A. Autoerotism re-examined. *The Psychoanalytic Study of the Child,* 1962, *17,* 283–315. New York; International Universities Press.

Stoller, R. J. *Sex and gender.* Science House: New York, 1968.

Zilboorg, G. Masculine and feminine. *Psychiatry,* 1944, *1,* 257–296.

Chapter 6

The Early Stages of Female Psychosexual Development

A Kleinian View

SUSANNA ISAACS ELMHIRST

There is no such thing as an official Kleinian position and therefore no such creature as a Kleinian spokesperson. My qualifications for accepting the task of writing this chapter are that I am a child psychiatrist, and a former pediatrician, trained in the Kleinian technique of analyzing children and adults, a method I have been using in psychoanalytic practice for nearly 20 years.

It is now over 50 years since Melanie Klein developed a technique of child psychoanalysis applicable to children from about the age of two onward. She did this by a direct and logical development of Freud's discovery of free association and the transference as keys to the unconscious mind. Klein went on to modify the use made of the material produced by adults in analysis. Analysis of children and adults using the Kleinian adaptations of Freud's technique has already yielded a lot of information about female development in its sexual and in all other spheres.

Misunderstanding of the Kleinian technique and difficulties in applying it have contributed to the Freudian–Kleinian controversy, an unscientific struggle that would be farcical if it were not so sad. The pity is that anti-Kleinian prejudice within the profession has denied the scientific basis for disagreement with some of Freud's opinions and has thus fostered female hostility to Freud and to the psychoanalytic contribution to human psychology as a whole.

SUSANNA ISAACS ELMHIRST, M.D., F.R.C.P. • Associate Clinical Professor of Child Psychiatry, University of Southern California Medical School, Los Angeles, California.

The original antagonism to Melanie Klein's work was not primarily based on the ways in which her views of female development
differed from Freud's. Nor did it have much at all to do with the fact
that she was a woman. Freud was not prejudiced against women as
psychoanalysts; indeed, he was very troubled about the future of psychoanalysis in America because of the medical model to which it was
committed, which also meant a masculine model since so few women
went into medicine then. Ernest Jones devoted a whole chapter of his
biography to Freud's views on this and related problems.

Freud once wrote, "we are now obliged to recognize that the little
girl is a little man." I do not see that we are obliged to agree; nor do I
see that we need to turn against all that Freud discovered because he
was sometimes mistaken. His greatest contribution was a method of
studying the fundamental importance of childhood emotional experience to adult life, and that method has only been extended, by the
Kleinian approach, to include infantile emotional experiences.

The shock and horror with which Melanie Klein's work was
greeted mainly resulted because she found that babies and very young
children have very intense, and often violently aggressive and terrify-
ing, feelings and fantasies. This assertion ran counter to the idealized
picture that people have, consciously and/or unconsciously, of themselves as the perfect baby; the good, peaceful, loving baby either in
union with a perfect mother or persecuted and deformed by a very
bad one.

From time to time, Freud gave evidence of having perceived the
strength of the hostility and fear even an infant is capable of feeling.
Freud's connecting fears of being poisoned by milk or food with the
experience of weaning has been amply supported by clinical child
analysis. Freud thought of an infant passing meconium during delivery as revealing fear; Melanie Klein added that the baby is trying to
evacuate fear, and W. R. Bion (1962) added that the infant is also attempting to communicate fear in the hope of help. Another example is
that the life and death instincts as described by Freud have turned out
to be manifest from infancy onward in the emotional struggle between
feelings of envy and those of gratitude. One implication of Klein's discovery of the complexity and intensity of infantile emotional life was
that it was necessary to reconsider the real role of the mother in
human mental development. Freud certainly did not consistently mis-
understand or underestimate women's role in human development either. He wrote of "a lovely dream," a patient's dream, in *The Interpretation of Dreams* (1900), the book he considered his most important. In
thinking over the patient's associations to this dream, in which there
were references to an apple tree and an inn, Freud wrote (and had in-

terpreted to the patient at the time, though not necessarily in the same words):

> . . . there cannot be the faintest doubt what the apple-tree and the apples stood for. Moreover, lovely breasts had been among the charms which had attracted the dreamer to his actress. The context of the analysis gave us every ground for supposing that the dream went back to an impression in childhood. If so, it must have referred to the wet-nurse of the dreamer, who was then almost 30 years old. For an infant the breasts of his wet-nurse are nothing more nor less than an inn.

This interpretation could, of course, be taken as insulting to women and as devaluing the vital, active role of the breast. But there is no reason that one has to take it in that vein. I see Freud as being unable, despite his already near-miraculous self-analysis, to get down to the roots of his conflicting feelings about his own adored and respected mother. With much greater help, many find themselves in the same position nowadays, or they are equally unaware without knowing the depth of their own ignorance. Despite the apparent dogmatism of some of Freud's statements, especially when misquoted, he knew how much remained to be discovered. "If you want to know more about femininity, enquire from your own experience of life, or turn to the poets, or wait until science can give you deeper and more coherent information," wrote Freud in 1932. But it cannot be denied that Freud did indeed use the word *passive*, not *receptive*, as synonymous with *feminine*. However, I see no evidence that he went along with others who translated that term into infantile terms, as Helene Deutsch (1944) did when writing of a "passive–oral function." No one could seriously continue to use that phrase if he had put his finger in a tiny baby's mouth, or at least it would take a great degree of denial to fail to perceive the force with which the baby sucks or to fail to link the sucking with affectual experience.

It certainly does not take a psychoanalyst to observe the objective facts of the behavior of infants and young children, so I am perturbed by the new term *psychoanalytic direct observation*, with its suggestion that only psychoanalysts can be objective observers, open to the existence of the unconscious. Even more serious is the implication that observations by psychoanalysts can supplant, not just supplement, those made in psychoanalysis. The term *psychoanalysis* has a specific meaning. Whether used with adults or children, it is a method of studying the workings of the unconscious mind in a way that enables the patient to enlarge his mental awareness of himself and his relationships to others. Only under certain constant conditions, which are not available in everyday situations, can psychoanalysts perceive manifestations of the unconscious with any reasonable degree of accuracy.

Therefore, it is only under such specific circumstances that psychoanalysts can interpret and assess their patients' responses to interpretation. In other words, psychoanalysts put their view of their observations into words for the patients, who are then studied for how their reactions confirm, refute, and alter the analysts' suggested explanations. The aim is a convincing and usable increase of both analyst's and patient's knowledge of the workings of the patient's mind.

Of course, a psychoanalytic theory must encompass and must be compatible with objectively observable facts. Observation of a mother and infant in the privacy of their own home has proved invaluable in the training of psychoanalysts and psychotherapists in England because of the vivid conviction gained of the emotional interaction between mother and baby. It also gives evidence of the link between a growing, increasingly satisfying relationship and the growth of the mind. But often, the direct observer cannot even glimpse the ways in which the psychic mechanisms of splitting, projection, denial, and repression are being used and, indeed, often lead to the denial of their existence. Observations made in grossly abnormal circumstances, such as residential nurseries or even the smaller groups of very young children now popular, are observations of infants exposed to excessive stimulation and thus are not comparable to those of a mother and infant in their own house or in more carefully controlled and limited experimental conditions. In all forms of observation, more serious consideration needs to be given to maternal anxiety and its influence on the infant. Such a consideration will involve gaining further understanding of the effect on mothers of being scrutinized, filmed, recorded, and generally "looked into" as well as the effect of the interaction of anxiety in infant and adult.

As originally defined and used by Freud, the word *ambivalence* meant that type of intense conflict between loving and hating feelings seen in obsessional neurotics. In that sense, it may be true to speak of "unambivalent" or "postambivalent" phases in emotional development, so that strictly speaking, the love and hate of a very young infant may not be ambivalent in that they are not at that stage felt to be directed toward the same person or "object." However, the extension of analytic investigation to the areas of infantile experience does not support the concept of an early phase of postnatal life when the baby has no hostile feelings; infants do not know anything of a "conflict-free area of the ego."

Of great importance to the theme of this chapter is the way in which *ambivalence* has now come to be used as synonymous with any mixed feelings of love and hate toward the same person. If the word is taken in that way, it is seriously misleading to postulate a "postambivalent" phase of development, with its implication that such a state is desirable and attainable. When analysts have such an aim for their own work, they will also, consciously or unconsciously, maintain that mothers could and should normally rear children to the "postambivalent" state of adulthood. From my point of view, that approach is an invitation to cripple children and their parents by encouraging pathological ways of avoiding the mental pain that is at times the inevitable consequence of being a normal human, with mixed feelings of love and hate toward those to whom one is closest.

Overexpectations of mothers, and consequent blame of them, compounded by maternal guilt and ways of trying to avoid it, have gone to extremes in this country. An idealization of Anna Freud and Donald Winnicott and a professionally fostered horror of Melanie Klein have helped to bring about a situation in which many women fear, and loathe, motherhood, with a good deal of justification. This is both sad and worrying.

One of the fundamental discoveries of the Kleinian group has been that unconscious mental activity is as continuous throughout life as the beating of the heart. There are innate, instinctual patterns of physical response, and they are accompanied by—and in earliest infancy, are often experienced as synonymous with—unconscious fantasies. There is no action or inaction that is not accompanied by fantasy. In other words, all human responses include unconscious imaginative activity. An example from everyday experience is the hungry baby who, if allowed to cry too long, will reject or fight off the breast or bottle when it finally appears. The Kleinian view is that the infant's frustrated, angry fantasies have rendered the breast bad in its imagination, and the external object is accordingly responded to as an attacker.

In the early stages of life, fantasy and behavior are indistinguishable; at birth, there is no differentiation of mind and body. Yet, babies are human beings, not paper bags to be filled with what their parents feel they should contain, nor lumps of clay to be molded in accordance with some plan. Innately, they are obviously physically different, and they differ emotionally, too. Babies *in utero* behave and develop according to a basic plan, but even there, where there is limited scope for individuality, they are recognizably individuals. So, of course, such differences show even more clearly after birth. In my opinion, there is so far no scientifically convincing evidence of babies' mental and emotional development being in any way innately dependent on their sex in the first few months after birth. Girl babies and boy babies respond physically and emotionally in those early months as babies, and their contribution affects the quality of maternal care.

The mother's responses to a baby's behavior and to its genetic endowment, including its sex, are of immense importance and very hard to study without disturbing the relationship. It can be very helpful for mothers to know that much of the variation babies show in their adaptation to the extraordinary state of being so dependent results from variation in their innate ability to tolerate feelings of frustration and gratification.

Once a baby is born, relationships with people are found to be essential to its very being. Babies die if they are provided with purely material care; they starve in the face of what may be physically as much as or more than a healthy infant needs. The observations of Rene Spitz (1945) demonstrated this phenomenon with harrowing conviction. Lesser degrees of emotional uninvolvement or maladaptation of the environment result in infantile illness or distorted development. Donald Winnicott (1949) has expressed his view of the importance of infancy to the whole of mental life in the phrase "psychosis is an environmental deficiency disease of infancy" (p. 247). But in his deliberate association of the problem with vitamins, he laid a false burden on mothers by the implication that it is as simple to satisfy an infant's emotional needs as it is to administer a daily dose of vitamins.

The inevitable helplessness and dependence of infancy frighten and enrage babies and provoke great greed and envy. What an infant does with these feelings depends on their intensity and on the infant's tolerance of them. But to some extent, all babies use the psychological mechanism of projection; they have to, as a form of communication.

By *projection*, I mean a mental maneuver whereby the person rids himself or herself of an unwanted response or experience by projecting it to the outside. When a baby yells, it is projecting its incomprehensible, unbearable distress into the mother, whose basic function it is to respond creatively and return a satisfying experience to the baby in the form, say, of a feed or a smile or a song. This form of communication is based on the very young infant's experiece of feelings as concrete, as things to be evacuated if they are unpleasant. A mother's normal, satisfying response is responded to by the baby with appreciation and with love, as well as in other ways. Pleasing communications such as a smile or a voice are apparently at first experienced partly as concrete, as good things put or taken into a mind and barely, if at all, differentiated from the baby's body. But differentiation of the concrete from the abstract begins with birth itself and is the basis of an inner, mental world. Very interesting work, well described and discussed by Mary Boston (1975), is going on now in the nonanalytic—but not antianalytic—psychological field; in this work, importance of the mother's voice to the infant is incontrovertibly demonstrated. A baby in a normal—what Donald Winnicott called a "good enough"—environment can distinguish the mother's voice from the father's, and both from a stranger's, by the time it is at least four weeks old. Therefore, by this early age, the infant has achieved mental images of the mother and the father that are pleasing, that stimulate hope of further nonphysical satisfaction, and that are not mutually exclusive. Yet, a healthy baby responds to a smile not only with a smile and interest but with its whole body, also expressing sensual gratification and sometimes, but by no means always, a wish to move on from talking to touching. Babies, like adults, do not live by bread alone.

The physical growth of an infant is normally accompanied by a growing ability to perceive what helps it to feel safe and enriched and thus increasingly less helpless. The baby begins to love those who provide the necessary physical and emotional care. The mother or the main mother substitute is the initial, and the most intense, object of this love. If it is any comfort to fathers who envy mothers their central position in a baby's development, or to mothers who envy their baby-minders in the same sort of way, the primary caretaker is the most hated and feared, as well as the most intensely loved, object in the infant's world. When a normal baby is around the age of four months, mothers notice a change that they describe spontaneously in phrases such as "He has become a person"; "She gets really upset, not angry but upset, and she cries tears"; "He won't go to anyone he doesn't know now"; "She seems afraid of losing me." This behavior appears to coincide with a stage of development deduced from psychoanalytic observations in which the baby begins to realize that some of its angry and painful feelings arise within itself, that they are not put into it from outside. Along with this realization comes the baby's awareness that its hostile feelings are directed, inside and out, toward those whom it loves and needs most. The sense of having harmed what we analysts call its *good object* leads to a dawning capacity for sadness and concern and to the emotional precursor of the creative and constructive activities of later life. In the baby's inner world, the damage done in imagination is repaired; the loved mother is returned to her former goodness and is then felt to exist as an inner image more strongly in favor of the infant's growth and separateness. The importance of this capacity to repair one's inner images of loved persons cannot be overestimated. In the process, the external object is established in the infant's inner world as a symbol, an abstract image. Speech depends on the existence of abstract symbols and so does the capacity of normal creative thought. With the capacity to form symbols, the creative life of the mind is under way.

There is no such thing as a static situation in the mind, ever, but especially not in babies. The urgency of this active state and the baby's need to be in frequent communication with a person who is aware of it and able to grow with the baby places a huge demand on those who do the work of rearing it. Having been a baby is, in one sense, an experience common to us all. But having tolerated and accepted infancy in all its aspects—let alone having come to enjoy an interest in all these aspects—is by no means the lot of all parents. Nor is it easy to predict who will be able to grow and learn with a baby and who will turn out to be crippled emotionally by his own split-off, formerly unrecognized, unsymbolized infant experiences, which he is still unable to digest mentally.

Babies and young children are in vital, continuous need of help in differentiating subjective from objective reality. Many of their fantasies are loving, but many are frustrated, angry, or jealous. To babies or young children, what is going on in the inner world of the imagination is felt also to be going on in the world outside, so that when the sense of being excluded from a grown-up world provokes hostility, the infant *needs* that outer world to be actively cooperative and productive, as a sign that the infant is not as all-powerfully destructive as it feels itself to be.

Babies and young children also need their parents to survive and thrive as proof that their good feelings are effective; just as a child feels that disaster is the consequence of its aggressive feelings, so will the child feel that growth and happiness in the world of the family results from its own love and helpfulness. Of course, the child is still left with the task of discovering the extent of its real constructive powers as well as of its destructive potential. When asked to what he attributed his success in life, Oliver Wendell Holmes put it down to having discovered at an early age that he was not God.

The baby's dependence on its mother for its very life and her gratification of its basic needs give rise to fantasies of the mother as the container and source of all good experiences, physical and mental. Narcissistic notions of the infant itself as the source of all pleasure and satisfaction are sometimes consolatory, what Freud called "hallucinatory wish fulfillment," and are temporarily essential to the survival of all infants. Everyday examples are finger, thumb, or tongue sucking. However, such satisfactions are not as purely benign psychically as some would suppose. If an unduly narcissistic solution to the sufferings of infancy is sought, whether because of excessive frustration or undue innate omnipotent envy, the underlying greed and the contemptuous rivalry with the maternal object give rise to many fears and abnormal defenses against them. Babies with a tormenting internal state of affairs need more, not less, consistent and sensitive attention from the environment. But those babies who appear unusually content may, in fact, have psychically split off their awareness of emotional pain and fear.

The details of the baby's fantasies depend on the stage of its instinctual development. In the oral stage, love is equated with the giving and getting of food and sounds, the eyes also often appearing in dreams and fantasies as mouths receiving and bestowing love. Similarly, oral aggressive fantasies are of sucking out, biting, tearing to bits, and spitting. A little child in treatment once drew "a loaf-of-bread house" and spoke of tearing to bits what she could not devour of her "lovely Mummy."

A 17th-century member of the Medici family was described by a contemporary in these terms: "Leopoldo always kept a book in his pocket to chew on whenever he had a moment to spare, like a little boy with a piece of bread." A nice example from three centuries ago of the relationship between mouth and mind.

In the oral stage, an infant's attempts to counter the desperate helplessness that is associated with its dependence center on imaginatively acquiring the breast or its contents, with or without the accompaniment of regurgitation, finger sucking, mouthing toys, and so on. In a consultation, an eight-year-old discussed her sense that liquid came out of her thumb when she sucked it; she knew it couldn't do so, and yet she had a delusional, and thus frightening but also delicious, sense of self-sufficiency. She was a highly intelligent, well-functioning child in other areas, struggling with split-off, unresolved infantile ways of trying to handle anxiety.

From the beginning of life, anal activity is evidently accompanied by varying emotions, painful and pleasurable. The baby's fantasies about its bowel contents and their powers predominate in the anal stage of development, say, from 9 to 18 months of age. However, oral fantasies are never absent and never superseded, nor are those of the anal stage. Babies of both sexes idealize and exaggerate the delights the mother is felt to be enjoying while they are frustrated. Among the satisfactions that the mother is felt to contain within herself, and to deprive the baby of, are penises and babies. These types of fantasy are common to patients of both sexes, including young children. They are partly based on innate preconceptions of the instinctual phases, and thus, in due course, they include spontaneous unconscious awareness of the existence of the penis and the baby.

These objects are at first experienced as parts of the mother, who is thus the prototype of the combined parental image. On the other hand, the breast and nipple, like the mother with the penis inside her, are also seen as the original couple in mutually advantageous, loving, productive intercourse. Buses or boats are very commonly used by children in psychoanalysis to symbolize the mother with living objects inside her. These inhabitants of the mother are at times seen as rivals, as with the two-year-old twins who insisted that they had not shared the uterus with their singleton sister or each other but had "grown one in each breast." However, insofar as the penis and the baby come to be seen as separate from the mother they are also seen as enriching and gratifying her. Therefore, the baby's rivalry with the father's penis or with the baby inside the mother can be both *for* the mother's attention and for the role of benefactor *to* her.

An infant's helplessness and desires are so inordinate that frustration is an inevitable part of babyhood. Even Winnicott (1949/1957) once wrote that "there is absolutely no need to try to make him (your baby) angry, for the simple reason that there are plenty of ways in which you cannot help making him angry whether you like it or not" (p. 43). The frustration gives rise to aggressive feelings and distress, which are often dealt with by a mixture of greedy and intrusive attacks in fantasy that lead the infant to experience its mother as damaged and damaging. A normal response to such fears and frustrations, in both sexes, is to turn to the father. At first, the infant has fantasies of oral incorporation of, and sucking on, the penis. This turning to the father often results, in both sexes, in a relationship with him that is less fraught with fear and ambivalence than that with the mother, apparently because the baby's dependence on the father is not so great. The good feelings toward the strong, gratifying father are thus less threatened by the infant's hostility. They are also commonly protected by the projection of hostile impulses into the mental image of the mother, which she is then felt concretely to contain. This psychological maneuver is also used in an attempt to protect the baby from painfully conflicting feelings. But when this maneuver is used to excess, the resulting internal, unconscious image of a dangerous mother results in her being experienced as forbidding or interfering with the developing relationship with the father. In due course, this process leads to difficulties when the highly idealized father inevitably frustrates the baby, too, and it dare not turn back to the mother.

Clear differences in the psychosexual development of girls and boys begin to manifest themselves around the last quarter of the first year of life, when the genital phase is incipient. Evidence available to anyone, as compared to that obtained from psychoanalyses, particularly those in which the Kleinian technique is used, can be seen in the spontaneous development of children's play, with boys showing an increasing preference for thrusting, pushing toys and girls a greater absorption with the insides of toys and with their contents. There is also much as-yet-unpublished information accumulated from individual observations of mothers and babies in their own homes. As regards nursery-school- and kindergarten-age children, the books of Susan Isaacs (1930, 1933) on intellectual and social development are classic and still relevant.

In girls, the wish to have a penis is only partly the inevitable consequence of the infant wish to have every object and attribute possessed by those whom it admires and trusts. Possession of the penis is also desired as a way of getting gratification from the loved mother, an important source of rivalry with the father. But there is also the extremely important aspect of coveting the penis as a source of the gratifying experiences that it is felt to bestow on the mother. This process, of course, also leads to rivalry with the mother for the good food, feelings, and babies the father is felt to provide her with from his penis. The oral desire actively to suck the penis is normally largely transferred to the vagina, but like other early sexual components, it continues in adult life to lead up to genital sexuality, rather than replacing genitality as in the perversions.

Many anal fantasies in girls center on the idea of the bowel and its contents taking over both parental roles, with the feces often representing the father's penis as well as the babies inside the mother. When these fantasies are very grandiose and envious, both parents are felt to contain, and to be overwhelmed by, the greedy and spoiling parts of the infant. A female's common way of attempting to preserve some good internal object relationship then consists of idealizing the penis as a source of babies and denigrating sexuality, or vice versa.

The baby boy also makes fantasied greedy and envious attacks on his mother, whose breast with the nipple and whose body with the penis inside it represent the combined parental image. So young children of both sexes have to deal somehow with the fact that they do not have breasts and cannot make babies and thus often feel incomplete and inadequate in comparison to the feeding and sexual mother. This feeling can be experienced as proof of an attack by the attacked and revengeful mother on her infant rival. Similarly, rivalry with the father, including rivalry for his genital, can lead to fear of retaliation. However, when a small boy fears castration as a revengeful response, he has the consolation of being able to see and feel that his genital is still there, a penis and testicles that, though smaller and different than father's, are evidently made on the same model. It is not at all uncommon for small boys to run out of a therapy session to urinate, as a cover for reassuring themselves that their penis is intact. Preoccupation with the intactness of penis and testicles is often found in analysis to have a component of displaced fear about having no breasts.

But where can a little girl run to for such reassurance from her fears of revenge for similar yet different fantasies of attack? It is with her inside that she becomes preoccupied, and yet about this, she can get very little direct or spontaneous reassurance.

Girls have to wait a long time for direct confirmation of their innate sense of having a productive inside, potentially like that of the mother. One little girl patient of mine had no conscious awareness of her internal genitalia but had many dreams of a lush, velvety, generous inner place or room that was at times very clearly differentiated from the anus. Yet at the age of six or seven, she sometimes felt very strongly about her apparently permanent, plain, outwardly undecorated physical state.

"I have nothing," she said, "nothing outside and nothing inside." She felt empty or full of bad stuff, and her parents' conscious idealization of her gave no lasting consolation. Then, one day, she discovered that

> Anyway I had an extra face:
> Two nipples for eyes,
> An umbilicus for a nose,
> The crease between my legs as a mouth.

A 3⅓-year-old asthmatic girl once said to her mother, "Johnny's got a titty on his bum and I want one." Her mother told the psychiatric social worker that she had not at first understood and that when she realized what was being demanded of her, "All I could think of to say was, I wish I could help." Actually, she did help, by allowing the child freedom to fantasize, by allowing the child freedom to verbalize, and by acknowledging her own lack of omnipotence.

There is, of course, an endless amount of work to be done, psychoanalytically, sociologically, educationally, on the relationship between cultural and other factors affecting female psychosexual development. Nevertheless, I think that the long period in childhood when a girl has no spontaneous avenue of physical reassurance about the existence or intactness of the organs vital for childbearing or sexuality does have a fundamental effect. So I think it will emerge that the small girl's, and the woman's, frequent preoccupation with external appearances and attire is often part of a search for reassurance about what they feel to be their inadequate state. So, also, do I think that it will come to be seen as evidence of a normal female need that girls are more dependent on environmental approval and reassurance than are boys. It does appear to me that at times of great emotional importance, when potential for progress is great but when, of course, failure is inherently possible, women are more in need of the kindly, reassuring attention of their mothers or other women than men are in need of that of their fathers or other men. I am thinking of the menarche, marriage, pregnancy, and child-rearing in particular.

Normally, children seek privacy for their masturbation from a very early age, apparently because they sense its personal nature and also because it is inevitably accompanied by conscious and unconscious aggressive fantasies about the parents they love and trust, with the result that they feel spontaneous shame and fear of reprimand. It is inevitable that small children should at times feel excluded from their parents' private adult activities. Such a sense of exclusion is, in fact, increased by some of the well-meaning attempts to avoid it, for children feel their small size and helplessness acutely. I have found in my practice of clinical child psychiatry, as well as in child analyses, that frequent confrontation with adult genitalia and sleeping in the parental bedroom or in the bed of one or the other parent are titillating and frustrating, often enragingly so. These responses are often unconscious and dealt with in abnormal ways. For example, Herbert Rosenfeld (1964) has found evidence that many adult sufferers from severe hypochondriacal illness have in childhood shared a bed with an adult, usually the mother. Excessive secrecy or modesty are not indicated, but neither is a denial of differences between adults and children. On the other hand, under normal circumstances, young children get a good deal of satisfaction and reassurance from some visual and tactile exploration of each other's genitalia, despite the provocation of some penis envy in girls or castration fears in boys. But situations in which children engage in a great deal of personal or mutual masturbation are disturbing and are signs of emotional difficulty.

From well before they can intellectually apprehend motherhood or be consciously aware of the genital structure of others, little girls show an interest in the insides of objects, in containers and in babies, dolls, and animals to put into them. This activity contrasts with a small boy's spontaneous interest in pushing, thrusting, exploratory play. But young children of both sexes are much helped by being given freedom to play according to their varying inclinations and to talk about their feelings and ideas without inhibition. Something that can be talked about is at least potentially thinkable. The paucity of words and the reluctance to use those there are to describe and differentiate the little girl's external genitalia only compound the problem of their mystery.

A mother who calls everything between the umbilicus and the

knees "the wee-wee department" is presumably too muddled and fearful herself to be more explicit.

A mother who believes that "babies are made from menstrual blood" or that they "come from the hospital" cannot help her daughter sort out fact from fantasy.

These examples are both from women clinically known to me, but their difficulty in verbalization may not present nearly such a serious intrusion on their daughter's sexual development as does possessiveness, or loathing and fear, of their daughters' bodies when they are babies. Babies and very young children are especially sensitive to nonverbal communication, so that they are bound to be affected by their mothers' fears and hatreds, perhaps particularly if the feelings are unconscious to the mother. An extreme example from my clinical experience was the mother whose baby cried a lot at the breast. It took weeks before the poor woman was referred for psychiatric help, when she was able to verbalize a conscious delusion that her baby was a tiger. The more subtle yet also intense influences of a mother who weans her baby for fear of its teeth or cannot touch its genital region because of loathing or terror are clearly important, but hard to study. The mother who cannot distinguish sensuality from sexuality in her handling of her baby is intruding on its spontaneous differentiation of the two. A mother who expresses her possessiveness, be it greedy or fearful, by administering enemas to her infant is in my experience far more disturbingly intrusive than one who is inarticulate or uneducated about verbal nomenclature.

A daughter's dependence on external reassurance faces a mother with the task of coming to terms with her envy of her own daughter. The daughter will be moving forward to opportunities that her mother will never have again and hopefully into many areas that were not available to the mother's own generation. One female patient was rather thrilled, albeit apprehensively so, when she started menstruating at the age of 11. She rather excitedly told her mother, whose crushing response was "What do you expect me to do, put the flags out?"

Another young adolescent was brought for enuresis. She was the youngest of three girls, and it emerged that the mother had developed delusional disgust at her "baby's" adolescent bodily changes. The girl's enuresis stopped when she was allowed, and was able, to weep at the very real external loss of a formerly "good-enough" mother. The mother was, in my view, suffering from a regression to her own early, envious, and formerly unconscious imaginings about her *own* mother's mature female shape and sexual and maternal capabilities, an eruption consequent on her last child's moving on and placing her psychically in the position of a left-out little girl "with nothing."

Similar problems arise in connection with a father's attitude toward the physical and emotional reality of his children, and his daughter is much in need of outward approval and appreciation that does not foster her rivalry with and fear of him or her mother.

I was once consulted about and by a highly verbal 2½-year-old girl who began to have night terrors, of which she had no memory on waking. They began when her father went abroad to work for a few months. In the course of the consultation, the little girl was relieved enough to tell me, in a sudden burst of confidence, how "a jacket comes out of the closet, a jacket and shoes, an empty jacket and shoes." It turned out that she was remembering her nightmares. Father's empty clothes came and terrified her, as though they were an emptied skin that would devour or suck her dry. I hope some of the implications of this example are obvious, but I will elaborate on some of them.

Biologically, it is still evidently true that babies need two parents of different sexes, in that a sperm and an ovum must unite; that is the fundamental act of procreation. Parthenogenesis is not yet possible for humans, and if it does become so, the resulting psychological problems will be horrendous, for humans are not rabbits or pigs, despite the satirical parallels of *Nardik* and *1984*.

In my opinion it is also psychologically necessary, if not in quite the same absolute way, for a baby to have two parents of different sexes to live with. My clinical experience confirms the expectation, based in psychological theory, that this is so. I will try to explain why.

Three-ness is inherent in the life of the mind, as it is in the body. All interactions, all relationships, have an outcome. Creative relationships are those in which the union between objects or ideas produces something new and valuable. Inevitably, these unions are between unlike entities; two identical ideas or bodies do not unite to produce an original one, despite the fact that a patient of mine had a dream of a mother who had a daughter identical to her, who had a daughter identical to *her,* ad infinitum. Bion's way (1962) of describing the innate roots of this mental state of affairs is that we are all born with innate preconceptions that, when they meet with realizations, form concepts. For example, a baby sucks if you put a nipple or your finger or whatever in its mouth. The mouth is a container, the nipple the contained, and the result—a satisfying feed or sensation—leads to a mental concept, the basis of a good internal part-object. This, of course, is a dynamic view of the mental accompaniment to an innate, spontaneous physical response. It is evidently active at the root of normal sexuality, but in very early life, it is not perceived as directly related to genitality. However, it is interesting that in situations of great frustration, whether arising from external deprivation or arising from an infant's incapacity to permit good internal experiences, premature and concrete genitalization of mental processes occurs. For the disturbed baby who develops a schizophrenic disorder in adult life, everything is sexualized, and concretely so, although the development of genitality in the creative sense is interfered with. Crude, overtly sexual drawings in the prepubertal period are often a sign of past and future trouble of this kind.

Although three-ness is inherent in the life of the mind, there need to be external relationships of a similar nature in the young child's world. Children need appropriate gratification if they are not to be unduly provoked and thus confronted with excessively hostile or frightening fantasies. Deprivation and the emotional responses to it also intensify the continuing problem that young children have in distinguishing internal from external reality, fantasy from fact.

Appropriate gratification is not gained solely by the existence and maturation of two parents of opposite sexes. The inner consequence of mixed feelings toward both parents is inevitably some degree of grief and sadness at the fantasied damage to loved objects. The normal way out of such states of mind, which are akin to normal mourning, is by a process of mental re-creation of the damaged objects, a process technically known as *reparation*. This difficult emotional task involves the individual in an acceptance of his or her own hostile impulses and an acknowledgment, conscious and/or unconscious, of their impact on internal objects. Failure to complete this task results in identifications with damaged, abnormal objects rather than with a parental couple experienced as capable of creative life together. There are two familiar distorted identifications to which women are particularly prone. One involves the woman's becoming identical with the fantasied image of "Mother-turned-into-a-baby," with all that image implies about a dependent relationship to men. The other consists in identification with a masochistic mother partnered by a sadistic swine of a father. In both cases, whether the man is experienced as an infantilizing mother or an aggressive father, the paternal images are experienced as the aggressors and are thus the ones who should suffer guilt and remorse.

The acting out of variations on these Oedipal themes plays an important part in the sexual and marital relationships of women with character disorders. The problem of frigidity is a complex one, by no means fully understood, but, clearly, identification of the vagina with a biting, sadistic mouth will lead to fears for the penis, while projection of infant sadism *into* the penis will lead to its being experienced as dangerous. These problems are by no means mutually exclusive. I do not mean to imply that all the psychopathology of sexual relationships lies in women, or vice versa.

Among many unanswered puzzles in the developmental differences in boys and girls are why boys suffer so much more often from enuresis and encopresis than do girls, why females are so much more prone to heterosexual dysfunction in adult life, and why males are more often transsexuals. Certainly, a boy *has* to achieve some degree of reconciliation with his primary object, his mother, if he is to satisfy the normal instinctual urges that drive him, in genitality, back to a female object. No such reconciliation is imposed on a girl, in that by being mothered and impregnated by a man she may experience herself as identical with, and never having been separated from, her mother, and so she may not have achieved an adequate degree of symbolization of the mother. Be that as it may, a better understanding of the feminine need for reassurance from the outside world leads, in my opinion, to the recognition of girls' especial need for appropriate educational opportunities. Girls are often, traditionally, educated in practical housewifery and crafts that provide some of the reassurance lacking from their own child's bodies. But the use of the girl's mind in symbolic creation, in intellectual and artistic pursuits, is often neglected, explicitly and implicitly. Yet, the reassurance and joy to be found in the creative union of intellect and imgination are devalued as much by those who overvalue physical unions as by those who undervalue the woman's contribution as "only a homemaker." Furthermore, no service is done to either sex by an exaggeration of the simplicity of the small boy's sexual or intellectual situation; recognizably equipped like his father he is indeed, but by no means is he thereby protected from the helpless sense of permanent smallness and inadequacy that is the source of so much childhood suffering and so much distortion of adult psychosexual life.

There is not space here to go into the details of abnormal sexual development in girls or the impact on children of parental sexual abnormality. I hope that some of the implications of my views on the interaction of external reality and the inner world of the imagination, and the importance of that interaction, will enable the reader to draw his or her own conclusions and to read and study further. Despite some current social tendencies, a mutually respectful and loving relationship can be developed between a mother and a father and between parents and a child. That such a relationship is not always achieved does not mean that it is not desirable and indeed necessary. Knowing what is needed, even if it is unattainable, is psychologically a much more promising and productive state of mind than denying and denigrating the need, for thus treated, the unsatisfied need is unconsciously perceived as a persecuting internal object, which interferes with growth and development.

There is a story of an American university where a notice was put up saying: "From tomorrow, there will be a tradition in this university that nobody walks on the grass."

If one can succeed in gradually developing a family tradition of not walking on the growing grass of anyone's personality, child's or parent's, many of the problems of human relationships can be faced and overcome. But any notion of instant tradition-making or any idea that emotional insensitivity is normal will gravely interfere with such an aim. So too will anything that interferes with a mother in emotional difficulties seeking appropriate psychiatric help. Many professionals retain an infantile belief that mothers can switch love on, or hate and fear off, by conscious effort alone. Thus, they are unaware of the problem presented to a woman who finds herself feeling, let alone expressing, fear or loathing, disgust or greed, envy or jealousy to her own baby. The sense of guilt and painful responsibility can be made unbearable, and concern for the baby may be abandoned altogether by such a mother, if she is approached with attitudes of reproach or idealization.

I once worked with a woman who had consulted her family doctor because she feared she would hurt her baby. His response was "People don't do that sort of thing." On the other hand, there appears to be a tendency to approach marriages and families in difficulty as though people can't be emotionally hurt by what is "usual" or what is becoming accepted by a society. One potential for progress in our society is that, at least theoretically, people do not have to be parents if they do not want to. For those brave enough to do so, there are many rewards among the responsibilities, even though the delights of parenthood can never attain the Cornucopia ideal set by babies for their parents and for themselves.

REFERENCES

Bion, W. R. *Learning from experience*. London: Heinemann, 1962.

Boston, M. Recent research in developmental psychology. *Journal of Child Psychotherapy*, 1975, 4(1), 15–33.

Casseguet-Smirgel, J. *New psychoanalytic views*. Ann Arbor: University of Michigan Press, 1970.

Deutsch, H. *The Psychology of Women*. New York: Grune & Stratton, 1944.

Freud, S. The interpretation of dreams. *Standard Edition*, Vols. 4, 5, 1900.

Freud, S. The question of lay analysis. *Standard Edition*, Vol. 20, 1926, p. 177.

Freud, S. Femininity. *Standard Edition*, Vol. 22, 1932, p. 112.

Isaacs, S. *Intellectual growth in young children.* London: Routledge & Kegan Paul Ltd., 1930.

Isaacs, S. *Social development in young children.* London: Routledge & Kegan Paul Ltd., 1933.

Isaacs Elmhirst, S. *A Kleinian approach to Psychoanalysis* (3 taped lectures). Psychotherapy Tape Library, 59 Fourth Avenue, New York City.

Journal of the American Psychoanalytic Association. Supplement: Female psychology, 1976, 24(5).

Klein, M. The effects of early anxiety situations on the sexual development of the boy. *The writings of Melanie Klein.* London: Hogarth Press, 1975.

Klein, M. The effects of early anxiety situations on the sexual development of the girl. *The writings of Melanie Klein,* Vol. 1. London: Hogarth Press, 1975.

Klein, M. Envy and gratitude (1957). *The writings of Melanie Klein,* Vol. 3. London: Hogarth Press, 1975, pp. 176–235.

Klein, M. Our adult world and its roots in infancy (1959). *The writings of Melanie Klein,* Vol. 3. London: Hogarth Press, 1975, pp. 247–263.

Mitchell, J. *Psychoanalysis and feminism.* New York: Pantheon Books, 1974.

Rosenfeld, H. The psychopathology of hypochondriasis. *Psychotic states: A Psychoanalytical approach.* London: Hogarth Press, 1965.

Segal, H. *Introduction to the work of Melanie Klein.* London: Hogarth Press, 1964 (rev. 1973).

Spitz, R. Hospitalism. *The Psycho-Analytic Study of the Child,* 1945, 1, 53–74.

Winnicott, D. W. Mind and its relation to the psyche-soma. *Collected Papers.* London: Tavistock Publications, 1949.

Winnicott, D. W. Why do babies cry. *The child and the family.* London: Tavistock Publications, 1949/1957.

Chapter 7

Femininity

ROBERT J. STOLLER

INTRODUCTION

There being, I think, no such thing as femininity, one is in a bit of a fix if he or she wants to discuss the subject. Still, it and masculinity are hard to ignore since we all believe in them, and so it may be useful to sort psychoanalytic ideas on this subject once again, adding a few hypotheses. In doing this, I shall challenge my own hypotheses by discussing the development of marked femininity in males as well as in females (for it is reasonable to suggest that similar behavior has similar causes, even in different sexes) and also the development of marked masculinity in females.

A few thoughts on vocabulary will orient us.

First, let us take up and be done with the awareness that femininity (or masculinity) does not exist, so that we can continue to talk about it. People do not *have* femininity; there is no such entity or substance. Rather, there is a myriad of behaviors springing from innumerable identifications, fantasies, and beliefs, the algebraic sum of which is called femininity, none being necessarily—in all places and at all times—distinctively characteristic.

An instance. Deutsch (1944), following Freud, defined femininity by these parameters: narcissism, masochism, and passivity. Undoubtedly, years ago, those women whom Western societies felt to be feminine exuded, from bounteous flesh, movements and communications that the authorities felt exemplified these categories—and the memory still lingers in many circles. Yet, the closer one looks, the more amorphous, undefined, and unmeasured narcissism, masochism, and pas-

---

ROBERT J. STOLLER, M.D. • Professor of Psychiatry, University of California School of Medicine, Los Angeles, California.

sivity become. And even with consensus—"Of course, women are narcissistic"—can that quality be linked more to them than to men? Is masochism not part of masculinity (as in combat bravery)? Is child-bearing passive? In which phase? For which organs?

Granting it does not exist, what is femininity? It is natural appearing, unselfconscious, ordinary, normative behavior (of which an essential part is fantasy) typical of and expected of girls and women and not of boys and men. Although this definition sounds naive, I now define it as whatever a person, family, group, or society considers femininity. Outsiders should impose their judgments with the greatest caution. For instance, what one culture or era considered feminine, another does not; long hair is feminine only if its possessor believes that his or her long hair is feminine; a shaved male face is feminine only if the shaver feels that his shaving serves femininity; easy public crying is feminine only if one feels feminine in crying publicly; if a feminine woman believes that orgasms are unfeminine, then orgasms are unfeminine. Femininity, then, is not what *is* but what people *say is*, an opinion. A caution: the observer, such as a researcher, should not impute the motives, intent, or psychological state of those he observes by measuring their public appearance only; an obvious example is the hypermasculinity that some men affect to cover fears of latent femininity (which may also be labeled unmanliness by him).

Second, let me differentiate femaleness from femininity, sex from gender. Femaleness is a purely biologic state, defined by chromosomes (XX), external genitals (vulva and vagina), gonads (ovaries), internal sexual apparatus (e.g., uterus, tubes, broad ligament), hormonal state (dominated by estrogens and progesterone), secondary sex characteristics (breasts, subcutaneous fat distribution, pelvic measurements, carrying angles of the arms, absent body and facial hair), and certain submicroscopic diencephalic differences as compared to males. Femininity, on the other hand, does not *per se* imply anything about biology; it refers only to a psychological state and its resultant behavior. This is not to say that there is no relationship between sex and gender; rather, I maintain that in humans, biologic forces contributing to masculinity in males or femininity in females are usually overpowered by the psychological—postnatal experiences.

BIOLOGIC FACTORS

A brief review of what is now fairly common knowledge should suffice. All mammalian cells, including those of humans, require the addition of androgens (male hormones) for tissues to become male. This process of androgenization starts early in the fetus. In normal males, a mechanism controlled by a gene on the Y chromosome causes the development and the migration of the cells that will become the protomale gonad; androgen production then starts up in a few cells, which modifies contiguous cells, causing them also to make androgen. This process, at its appropriate pace, effects the unfolding of the anatomic structures and the physiological functions that define a male. Without these processes (plus another, perhaps also controlled by a Y chromosome gene, that suppresses female reproductive structure), normal femaleness results. More important to our present purpose, the circulating androgen produces changes in the midbrain that contribute to behavior typical of the males of each species.

Animal experiments confirm these rules. Regardless of chromosomal sex or the expected correct sexual development, all animals—male or female—given enough androgen at the necessary time behave like males, and, conversely, all experimental animals deprived of androgens during fetal life behave like females. Confirmatory data in humans must, of course, come from "natural experiments." Here are a few.

If an otherwise biologically normal female suffers *in utero* from hyperadrenalism, with its production of excessive androgen, not only will the infant have androgenized genitals, but also, as these girls grow, they become more tomboyish and are higher in "athletic energy expenditure" than a control series of girls (Money and Ehrhardt, 1972).

There is a condition—androgen insensitivity syndrome—in which chromosomal males (XY) are unable to respond to androgen, although they have it in normal amount. The result is not only the anatomic appearance of femaleness but also a femininity more pronounced than that of a control series of girls (Money and Ehrhardt, 1972).

In Turner's syndrome (XO), the expected second sex chromosome does not appear. In the absence of the Y chromosome and its influence on the production of androgen, these girls, too, have an external appearance of femaleness and are also more feminine than a control group (Money and Ehrhardt, 1972).

The normal human male, then, is born prenatally primed to become masculine and the female to become feminine. But except in rare "experiments," such as those cited, there is no evidence in humans that the biologic dominates the postnatal development of masculinity and femininity (Stoller, 1976); external events—psychological issues—do.

GENDER IDENTITY

Gender identity is the algebraic sum of the mix of masculinity and femininity found in an individual. I do not know when it begins to form (one cannot get into an infant's mind), but, between ages one and two, we see behavior that can be judged masculine or feminine. We have reason to believe that by age three or so, one's sense of being a male or a female (or, in the rare case when the genitals are hermaphroditic, of being neither a male nor a female or of being both) is permanently laid down (Money and Ehrhardt, 1972; Stoller, 1968). I have called this *core gender identity* (a term not synonymous with *gender identity*). It should be evident that if one is to be feminine, it is an advantage to be convinced without question that one is female: a fundament of femininity in women is their fixed sense of femaleness. That sense is created from the following:

1. The biologic anlagen (summarized above).
2. Sex assignment: at birth, an infant is unequivocally assigned to the female sex on the basis of female-appearing external genitals.
3. Parental attitudes: the innumerable behaviors and attitudes of parents and others, with which they transmit to the infant their conviction that she is female.
4. Body ego: the infant, as the months pass, becomes aware of the dimensions of and the sensations produced by various body parts, gradually forming a picture of herself as an anatomic assemblage. Genitals are a powerful factor in this awareness because of their sensations and because they are the focus of special attention by parents.

As time passes, life gets complicated and gender identity expands. No longer is it just a sense of femaleness or maleness; infants move into childhood, and along with their increased awareness of an outside world (especially, at first, of the mother), conflict between the infant and the outside world starts to impinge, along with the capacity to manufacture and contain intrapsychic conflict. The above-listed "forces" are transmuted into attitudes, conflicts, defense mechanisms, identifications, fantasies, and stable modes of confronting oneself or the world (character structure). With this advance, gender development enters phases long the domain of psychoanalysis. Observations extrapolated from the adult patient to childhood, observations of children, and appropriate theory for shaping these observations have filled the analytic literature and need only be touched on here. We are especially familiar with these data and concepts in descriptions of pre-Oedipal and Oedipal development and conflict, penis envy, castration anxiety, and the resolutions of these issues into more mature forms of masculinity and femininity.

PRIMARY FEMININITY

Being in agreement with analytic work, from Freud on, that describes the dynamics of later femininity, and having nothing to add—neither data nor ideas—I shall concentrate on the earliest stage, to be called *primary femininity*. This concept was argued by others—primarily Horney (1924, 1926), Jones (1927, 1933), and Zilboorg (1944), who were disagreeing with some of Freud's fundamental beliefs on the origins of behavior. In brief, Freud's position was that maleness is superior (the penis being the prized organ) and masculinity the original and preferred state for both sexes; one's sense of femaleness and of femininity is built on the pained awareness (with resultant humiliation, anger, denial, or resignation) that one does not have—perhaps was even robbed of—a penis, that most ideal structure.

A girl is doubly cursed, for she must also, Freud said, contend with a primary homosexuality: since her first love object is her mother, a female, she starts life as a homosexual. She then must perform a great feat in order to oppose her most profound desire: she must give up her mother, give up her hope to become a male, and get herself to want—to be excited by and to love—a male, the first representative being her father. Femininity, then, was to Freud a secondary, bedraggled, defensive state, built from pain, renunciation, and the capacity to accept what one did not really want. No wonder women are such wrecks. No wonder *passivity* and *masochism* are synonyms for *femininity*.

In disagreeing, Horney, Jones, and Zilboorg, pointed up different data, especially their belief that in earliest childhood, a girl has no reason to question the adequacy of her genitals, certainly not before being confronted with penises. I do not see how one of Freud's persuasion argues against these contentions except by proposing that females have an inherited memory of penises and a capacity to suffer envy when the inherited memory bangs at their awareness. In addition, Freud's logic is weak. I think he felt this too; consider his phrasing in this quotation: "At some time or other the little girl makes the discovery of her organic inferiority" (1931/1961, p. 232). He seems to have known, and then dropped from consciousness, a belief in a primary femininity.

I prefer to start with the concept of core gender identity. If it stands for accurate observations, then a powerful place of permanently established behavior, an identity, is fixed in place in the first few years of life. This identity results from primarily nontraumatic, nonconflictual forces, especially the shaping of character traits by the positive and negative reinforcement that expresses parents', especially mothers', attitudes. If one wants the appearance of femininity in a baby, all one need do is encourage and encourage and encourage. Examples are everywhere; proof does not require complex research. Carried on the diathesis that normal femaleness provides, shaping creates, I think, a powerful, immovable sense of femaleness with fantasies and behavior appropriate to what one's parents think is feminine.

I am in disagreement with those who believe that all personality development (except for that to be foisted off on biology) is the result of intrapsychic conflict (i.e., conflict between one part of oneself and another part). I think, rather, that huge masses of permanent character "structure," including some identified as femininity and masculinity, are laid down in the first years of life from nonconflictual influences, especially parents' attitudes and ways of dealing with their children.

But shaping results especially in appearances; giving more dimension requires that the girl move these attitudes somehow into her fantasy life and use them to help her solve the traumas, frustrations, and conflicts that must arise. At first, parents and then others teach a girl what is expected of her regarding clothes, choice of vocabulary, ways of sitting and walking, subjects of interest, games to be played, companions to associate with, styles of erotic behavior, themes for daydreaming—an unending flow of suggestions, commands, disapprovals, and enthusiasms. This process seems so obvious that I do not understand why it is not part of analytic descriptions of the development of femininity.

LATER FEMININITY

Early in life—earlier than Freud had thought, but only, I believe, after aspects of primary femininity are laid down—the more complex, painful, conflict-laden creating of oneself begins. As early as around a year and a half there is evidence of penis envy in girls (Roiphe and Galenson, 1972), struggle with a mother who is no longer simply an object of love, awareness of the father's presence and attractiveness (Abelin, 1975), and a turn toward the Oedipal conflict and resolution that Freud described. The primary homosexuality is a barrier to be surmounted and femininity a style to be cultivated if one is to catch the father's admiring attention. Now the girl is in as much trouble and life is every bit as complicated as it is for the boy. But this new, complex, painful, exciting, demanding, and creative phase is not the beginning—as Freud said, in the face of all observations of earlier feminine behavior—but rather a later femininity woven into the more fundamental, primary femininity. The mix of the two is the basis for the adult woman's sexual, reproductive, productive, and social life.

The girl can have had emplaced an uncomplicated primary femininity, which leads to the *appearance* of femininity, but then, in the traumas, frustrations, and conflicts of later pre-Oedipal and Oedipal development, she can end with her femininity in shambles (e.g., a belief that she is worthless because she is female, anger and humiliation regarding aspects of her female anatomy or physiology, a damaged capacity for erotic pleasure, defiant masculine behavior, and an incapacity for nonhostile relationships with any males). My hunch is that women with hysterical personalities represent this course of maldevelopment; they present a fine display, but it is literally skin deep. Reflecting and underlining society's most superficial though emphatic definitions of femininity, they cannot make it in the richer and more complicated experiences confronted by women in our society.

Case Example

Belle was classic. She was, unfortunately, born in the wrong century; like that of other women we label *hysterical personality,* her style got less credit than it would have in Victorian times. Nowadays—in her environment, at least—sugar-plum masochism makes one as much a pest as a princess.

She was always on display, fully or subliminally concerned about whether each garment had been chosen properly and was showing her off well: hair, face, figure, movements. Too often, she was sure some detail was awry, signaling her presumptuous and foolish pride. Erotic experiences were always a performance. She was chronically sexually aroused, spending each day on stage, performing in her sadomasochistic, exhibitionistic role.

The other side of the coin was her fear that no one would look, would care, that is, of abandonment. And this fear was all too nonerotic. It drove her to call attention to herself at any price; if the sex show failed, she fell back on irritating others lest she be unnoticed. It was tiring. Acting so much, she usually felt awkward. False behavior demanded its price in chronic guilt, loneliness, loss of hope, a sense of falseness, and constant exaggeration to rectify the feeling that no one would believe her unless she was operatic.

Yet, for all this, she seemed stylish, feminine, lively, and comfortable in her body until she lay on the couch. Then—at least, during storms of exhibitionism—the flailing, histrionic, wriggling, miserable display was enacted. A peak performance went like this: instead of lying down, she sat on the couch, but before that, she signaled what was afoot by wearing a soft, silky, light, delicate skirt that flowed at her slightest movement. In time, she might sit or lie, but in either case, I would gradually become aware that first her knees and then an

inch or more of thigh twinkled at me. At the same time, as if uncon-
nected to her legs, she chattered away. The subject could be anything,
potentially important or inconsequential; it made no difference, for
she was reducing the thought content to mincemeat. Sooner or later in
the hour (sooner when I got wiser), I recalled that the previous hour
had been filled with masochism—for instance, with her insistence I
could no longer stand her. At first, whipped to a frenzy with these
fantasies, she would return the next hour, calm, quiet, talking briskly
and lightheartedly as her skirt slowly and casually floated up her
thighs. It was a neat show.

Though the price may be high if one's parents are disturbed
enough, most of us in infancy are objects at times of their proud and
narcissistic pleasure in us. We find ourselves on view, clothed or
nude, admired for nothing more than that we exist in an anatomic
form that thrills one or both of them; heady stuff, though not enough
on which to build a personality. For the grand exhibitors, that may be
the best they have. To some degree, this was true of Belle. Her
mother, a histrionic child-woman, was preoccupied with her own
physical beauty and, shoving it under her daughter's nose, saw her
child as mostly an extension of her own body, a female deserving attention and credit only for having come out anatomically the same as
herself. If a mother is into the femininity number, and if she encourages it in her daughter, then her daughter will develop the appearances our culture defines as femininity: primary femininity. (That a
mother may both encourage behaviors she considers feminine and
discourage others or that she may both encourage her daughter to
appear feminine and at the same time put the child down for being a
potential rival are examples of the many complexities in this process.
These parental maneuvers all show up, I expect, in their child's adult
behavior. You can see that I am not alleging that primary femininity
takes only one form, for example, like Belle's hyperfeminine style.
Each woman's, I presume, is distinctive. A woman can also be sure
that she is forever female but be taught by her mother from infancy on
that being female is a degraded state.)

The theme of being lovely yet simultaneously disgusting was constantly present in Belle's relationship with me, reflected in an endless
number of memories meant to prove this a true representation of herself. And so as one of her analytic rights, she went on and on about
her disgustingness: she was sweating on the couch; she was not in a
ladylike position; her hair was ugly; a wrinkle was starting on her
face; she knew she smelled even if she could not smell it herself; her
outfit today was a mess; her sexual feelings were dirty and unbearable
to me; her associations were not neat, clever, and organized as are
good patients'.

Thus, two contradictory fantasy systems were at work. In one, derived from being her mother's doll, she was lovely, while the other, the result of her mother's and father's lack of attachment to Belle, confirmed that she was unacceptable. This business was then played out on a stage in which she assigned people in the real world the roles that she could prove they always filled, since she interpreted whatever they did as "really" meaning whatever she needed the meaning to be.

Belle was driven by a preoccupation with being lovely. What caught my attention was that *lovely* was not, for her, an adjective describing behavior that revealed a sense of herself but was a noun, a specific "substance" within that was drawn on when necessary and could be depleted with too many withdrawals or with age; her "lovely" was a commodity. On rising in the morning, she had to put on her "lovely"; she could only hope, as the day unfolded, that if she had "lovely," then she was lovely. She was really sure that she had it only when sensing that others saw it.

Her mother had lots of "lovely," had had it since childhood, had never earned it, and could not lose it no matter what happened in the way of physical or mental deterioration. This was a source of the greatest envy to Belle, who felt that she had to work constantly to keep up her own depletable reserves. Being her mother's daughter entitled her to a certain amount of "lovely"; she had been assigned it at birth by three generations of women in the family (the "family" was her mother's family; her father's was not acknowledged)—a family in which for generations almost no acceptable men had resided. Her father wore the labels of *fool* and *useless;* he left when she was six. She lived in an ambience that forever spoke of the superiority of femaleness. Although this attitude was a defensive creation of the earlier generations, for Belle, endlessly soaking in this tradition, it became part of her, as natural as breathing, not an effortful resolution for trauma. (Later, however, she came to use it defensively.)

What contributed to "lovely"? First, at birth, she was unequivocally assigned to the female sex. This was a piece of good luck, since all the women in the family openly liked femaleness; it was purely and simply to Belle's credit. Her mother was happy to have borne a daughter. (Belle was lucky to have been female; an infant male would have been at jeopardy simply because he was male.) Because she had an ineffectual father and no brothers, no maleness was present at first to contradict the evidence of female value. That became a lifelong theme: her femaleness was fine.

Beneath her histrionic displays, it was easy to feel her conviction that the parts of her body that were anatomically and physiologically female were solid, dependable anchors, making the prognosis for treatment better than in those women whose primary femininity contains no pride in femaleness. This admired biology was ever-present, a literal central core of her body that was safe and unalterable. She never, after a fit of masochism, fell into a state of complete despair, for the sense of femaleness was always a home to which she could return if frightened or unhappy. Unfortunately, since earliest childhood, the women of her family would not let it go at that; the stories they inculcated in the child had complications beyond simple self-esteem: your mother is a strange one, and since you are her daughter, you will also be strange; the worth in being female is not to be considered the same as that of being a woman; if you ever get married, you will not marry normally; you are truly a female, and that is fine, but some females, like your mother, are more luscious than you.

Competition with her mother was significant only in the arenas of femaleness and femininity; and her mother was too tough to beat: "Mother often bragged about her periods, telling me that her menopause would come at a later age than mine." "My mother wanted to own, to control, my insides, but she didn't want to take responsibility." A dream: "A PBX [telephone] switchboard. Because of a strike, I was supposed to help out. Lights were going on all over the board and I couldn't do anything. When I tried to plug in, I either just couldn't get in or else in place of a hole there was just a blind indentation" (a nice way to describe an exciting, unhuman mother one cannot plug into). The next day, another dream: "There were two nuns and my mother playing, and none of them knew how to play [i.e., mother's two breasts are, like nuns', without milk; the breasts are nones, no good for mothering]. No one [none, nun] paid attention to me or acknowledged me. They didn't remember who I am. Then I was eating medicine off a bell [breast-shaped] . . . Ma Bell. That's in the telephone company's ad. Yesterday's dream" (of the PBX wherein she cannot plug into mother connects with today's addition that I, the doctor, make treatment like "eating medicine off a bell," starving her need for love as her mother did long ago). Dream: "I'm in a low room. My mother is moving out. There are many plugs in one socket. It's overloaded and unsafe. Then they're all unplugged except one." Associations to uteri and hysterectomies. Belle is connected to her mother only by the prized femaleness—and that is not a firm enough contact. In brief, then, she got a solid start into femininity in the encouragement she received for being female, but too many unpleasant messages were also transmitted on the same subject.

If, therefore, everyone surrounding a girl is thrilled when she does something "lovely" or when she looks "lovely," she will repeat that behavior, and in time, when not discouraged, it becomes automatic. (I do not know what inner processes occur that make the behavior change from a single act to one that the child builds in as a part of the permanent repertoire any more than I know how "identification" works.) Just when and how appearances change from imitation to identity is hard to conceptualize, though not very hard for the practiced eye to discern.

Learning the outward forms of femininity does not go on only early in life; obviously, it persists indefinitely, with reinforcements coming more and more from outside the family. We also do not need a simpleminded picture. In real life, innocuous words like *reinforce, reward, discourage,* or *punish* are complicated events: rewards are mixed with options, cautions, threats, and punishments. For instance, the act of spanking a child may contain multiple messages of reward and punishment, advice and warning, predictions and observations: a father preoccupied with his own erotic feelings toward his daughter may announce them and encourage hers when beating her for being, as he accuses, oversexed; perhaps you will agree that *all* his messages get through, including his secrets.

One pays a high price for the privilege of being a living doll. Here is part of a dream: "You had a picture of me. It was me as a cute, chubby child, a very little girl, with ribbons and dolls; but all the stuff just hanging down disorganized. The picture was supposed to represent your attitude about me, which was that I am very lovable and that that was the only part of me that you wanted to think about." Reruns of Shirley Temple movies had had a big pull in her childhood; the most delicious parts were the waif scenes. Too bad her only happy endings were in the movies. A main task of treatment, therefore, was to see what more substantial qualities were present in addition to her acts: Was her "lovely" only a front or was it all there was? I fear those analysts who agree with Freud's version (at least as he wrote of it; it seems that in his actual relationships with women, the theory did not always hold sway): femininity is jerry-built, erected after—and only if—the girl accepts that she is not the boy she wanted to be and learns to settle for second best. If, God forbid, an analyst's private beliefs are the same as this theory, the outcome in treatment would be unfortunate.

When a woman shows us one of these awful facades, we must look to see if she has nonetheless hidden away qualities more substantial than those of a doll; our evaluation, for better or worse, is influenced not only by our theory and training but by our personalities. To get through the bad spells, it does not hurt to be optimistic. One day, before she had found her fuller sense of self, Belle was arguing her case: "I'm lovable because, when I look at my driver's license, I see a picture of a woman that's me. It doesn't look like me; but that's all right because anybody who saw her would think, 'How lovable she is.' '' For a therapist of my ilk, it pays at such times not to fall into despair. On the other hand, if we can determine that that is all there is and have confidence in our capacity to evaluate accurately, then the form of treatment used should not be analysis, which cannot create what does not already exist.

And one must be patient to bear the repetitions of emptiness. Another dream: "I was kissing a lovable baby. Its skin was lacelike. It actually looked like the holes that are punched in piano rolls. It was to disappear in time; nothing would be left."

I suppose the biggest advantage of "lovely" is that it makes one tempting. If she could only manage it—if only smells are a bouquet, skin stays smooth and unblemished, hair gossamer, figure firm yet soft, conversation a tinkling delight—then this whole precious morsel will be swallowed by someone good enough to keep her forever safely, softly, silently inside.

She came in one day dressed deliciously—an impression designed to be clearly different from other appearances and underlined by her wearing a new dress—kneeled on the couch in order to go on display, and proceeded through a number of associations, including dream elements having to do with eating and a shade of red that is the color of "inside organs." She was so edible that I wondered to her if the couch was not functioning as a table on which she was serving herself up. The suggestion gave her an acute erotic attack, for which she had been ripe; from the start of the hour, her clothes and position indicated that, although not yet conscious, the affect was close by. (Incidentally, after much reading on the metapsychology of affects, I still do not see how one can question the existence of unconscious affects.) In addition to responding erotically, she said, "I don't feel right now as if I'm going to be exploited, but I *do* feel like I am a meal that's going to be eaten up." The kneeling position, she said, offered her up as "a bounteous, Renoir woman."

Her mother endlessly filled Belle with stories of romantic and sexual exploits with mother the irresistible heroine. But Belle had another version, latent, about the nature of sex: she had heard from a girlfriend, around age eight, the anatomical facts of intercourse, news that stirred both primary and later feminine identity themes. She first said no, telling her friend that boys would never do such a thing; even if they tried, it was too astonishing and awful an act for a woman to permit. At any rate, she said, *she* would not allow it, but when her friend insisted it really happened, the child knew it was true (touching earlier, long-unconscious knowledge) and became frightened. Fear was the affect that remained through childhood, and it was still there, she said during the analytic hour, mixed with the good feelings that came later. But when one is small there is the threat to one's body, especially its insides, and just as severe is the shame: "Someone pushes inside of you, and you are supposed to come to like it! But I knew that would be impossible. I knew of no way that I could ever get rid of those bad feelings, and there was nothing about what sex seemed like that could ever make it pleasant, much less exciting. It was not just the penis in there but other things I did not know, perhaps dirtiness, certainly more even than that." That intimate part of boys' bodies was going to be inside her, her valued, vulnerable vagina, with which she was already becoming familiar: it had been described. It was an allowed subject of conversation, a part not only female but, for her family, feminine. It had been represented to her as not only precious but also delicate and unsure.

"The kids [young girls] know it's a rape and not pleasure. I knew as soon as I heard that it was nothing like when you're tickling your clitoris. And almost the worst part of it was that they had the right to do that because they marry you. It makes no difference about your body and whether it belongs to you or not. It doesn't belong to you. Marriage gives them the right, and you're supposed to love it and think that it feels marvelous. After that, the little boys just never looked the same to me. Before, they just looked like little boys who were boys, no better than I was, just grubby or nice little creatures. But now it made no difference if they were grubby or nice, good-looking or not, rich or poor or whatever. That was all aside from the point." She knew they knew she knew that they had the fundamental right legally, biologically, and from God to do that to her interior and that she had no right to prevent it. What made it all the more fantastic was the universe of adult women who obviously indulged, who had managed to traverse this rite of passage, and who, probably genuinely, got fine, if not incredible, sensations from the act (she read a lot).

"In order to survive, I had to teach myself that I liked it." Here her body helped out.[1] She found, soon enough, that the sensations from clitoral tickling spread inside, created erotic tension, one aspect of which was a need to have that inside stimulated, and pressed her, despite her limited knowledge in childhood about the act of intercourse, to invent scripts to account for and cater to these sensations.

---

[1] Of course, in the sense now being used, her body was no more than an extension of her mind (as in the concept *body ego*). We still would want to know why the erotic sensations arising in her body, as childhood progressed into puberty, were acknowledged to be intensely pleasurable; that is more a function of "mind" than an inevitable, unalterable response of the body.

Obviously, the development of this erotic capacity went a long way to solving the question of how one could bear to take that alien organ in.

To repeat: a woman's sense of integrity (meaning completeness, intactness) is based in part on her parents' attitudes toward her anatomy, not just on penis envy or on the belief she is castrated. That core of gender identity, once established, is impervious to damage from neurosis and even psychosis. Then, the girl must deal with such pressures as the discovery of male genitals, envy of the functions male genitals enjoy, and the related but not identical powers and responsibilities that males are granted by society. Belle struggled with these issues, doing the best she could; an adequate account of her Oedipal struggles, of the lacerating abandonments to which she was subjected by each of her parents, or of the symptoms and the distorted character structures she created to save herself are crucial to understanding her femininity but too complex to be dealt with here, where our purpose is limited mostly to understanding her "lovely"—the primary femininity. My version of these struggles says that her sense of femaleness was intact and served as a bulwark against traumata and conflicts that tended to spoil later aspects of her femininity. Contrary to Freud, I do not see either the sense of femaleness or femininity as just constructions built on a fundamental despair at not being male. The evidence, I think, is clear: there are many women, in many cultures, who, from the beginning of life on, neither question nor hate being female but like that state and would not give it up. (I am embarrassed to fuss about something so obvious.)

In Freud's theory of masculinity and femininity, castration is a central feature; the male fears that it can happen, the female mourns that it did. That idea should be enlarged. Men fear not just the body wound to those precious parts; even more, the genitals represent their identity as males and as masculine. Castration, then, would mean that they were cut off from their being, from their selves. But by castration, Freud meant the same thing for both sexes: male organs. I think that formulation is incomplete. Each sex also suffers its own distinct threat. Just as the loss of a penis means, for a man, the loss of a penis, so— whatever else it could be—the loss of a breast is the loss of a breast, the loss of an ovary is the loss of an ovary, and the loss of a uterus is the loss of a uterus.

Yet, there is good enough evidence of penis envy in females, and breasts and uterus can be used as organs for attacking, humiliating, overpowering, and revenging oneself. My argument (unproven but strongly believed) is that beneath these elaborate ideas is, in most females, an earlier-established and permanently fixed conviction of and acceptance of femaleness, just as one accepts—without sense of inferiority—having two arms, not four.

One day, when she was being (she said) stubborn, Belle reported a dream: "My leg was amputated and was being replaced by a man's leg, but the operation wasn't working. It started to turn black around the knee cap, which meant it was going bad." In another part of the dream, a teenage girl "was having surgery on her ovary. There was some question whether it had to be removed, and yet it was dangerous to put surgical instruments inside her. The doctors didn't know much about what the condition was. I preferred they would just look in and then close her up without really operating. But they wanted to rip it out, without even knowing what they were doing." She wondered if this had to do with analysis. She had read that analysts think women believe themselves castrated males, and, she said, she feared that I would give her an interpretation that said she really wanted a penis. The dream, among other things, was a warning that that kind of interpretation would not take but would turn gangrenous.[2]

The key words in this discussion have been *female* and *femininity*, their meanings worked out in relation to Belle's "lovely." She never doubted, at any level of awareness I found, the intactness of her femaleness, and when anatomic bisexuality appeared in her thoughts, it represented punishment. Nonetheless, her "lovely" was not an uncontaminated psychic structure; it also had defensive aspects in its construction and was used defensively. Her preoccupation with her appearance and her sadomasochism were examples. There is no question that sometimes she laid it on pretty thick and did so in order to convince herself that being a woman was as good as being a man, but she did this at times when she was envious or enraged at a man because she felt humiliated. One can envy an attribute of another without wanting to be that other in entirety; she wanted men's power, but she was not looking for a penis. I do not believe that her pride in her femaleness was just reaction formation against wishes to be a male.

Appearances can mask their opposite; it is easy, with exhibitionistic women, to talk of "the body as a phallus." Certainly, men and women have such experiences, but, at times, that explanation may be an incomplete, if not a glib, interpretation of a woman's displaying her body in revealing clothes. Perhaps because of the regression that comes with age, I have finally decided that if it looks like steak, sizzles like steak, smells marvelously like steak, and tastes like steak, I shall think it believes itself to be a steak. And if she says she is a delectable female and expresses pride in her female attributes; if she always looks feminine and never masculine; if she dreams incessantly

---

[2] It had other meanings for her equal in importance to the above one but away from the theme dissected in this paper. For instance, she was warning me not to analyze further lest I (she) discover the conflict she had that questioned her core conviction of being female and feminine.

of being pregnant or giving birth, of babies and children; cupboards, cooking, and ovens; mothers with their children; making, buying, and trying on clothes; menstrual periods; vestibules; flowers, grassy lawns; mirrors, carpets, shops, curtains, kitchens, household appliances; lace, linen, silk, cotton; textures, patterns, colors, sizes, functions, styles; fields, earth, soil to be fertilized or planted; and if she is excited exclusively by men, I shall think she believes herself a female and a woman, not just a castrated male.

FEMININITY IN MALES

If part of femininity is the result of postnatal influences, of learning, then it is possible that femininity in males has some of the same origins as femininity in females. That seems the case, especially in regard to primary femininity. The most feminine of (biologically intact) males—those who are so at present, have been so throughout their lives without episodes of masculine behavior, and have been so since the first appearance of any gender behavior—make up a clear-cut group (true transsexuals) insofar as similarity of clinical picture, dynamics, and causative forces is concerned. Without discussing this condition at length—it has been examined more completely elsewhere (Stoller, 1968, 1976)—let me point to only two factors contributing to this femininity. The first is that from birth on, these boys are kept in the most intimately close relationship with their mothers that such a mother can devise. She tries to spare this son any painful experiences. In addition, the powerful impulse toward intimacy is motivated by the mother's sense that this baby, whom she considers her ideal of all creatures on earth, is the cure for a lifelong sense of worthlessness and hopelessness that she endured until his birth. Not only does she create this blissful symbiosis, but she fights to maintain it as the years of infancy pass into childhood. And because the boy's father is passive and absent from his family most of the time, there is no male presence either to interrupt the pathological symbiosis or to serve as a model for the boy's masculinity.

Skipping the data that might make the hypothesis plausible, let me simply state it: the more profound the closeness between a mother and her infant, male or female, and the longer that symbiosis persists, the more feminine will the child be. If this were the case with an infant girl, the resulting femininity would be unnoticed. The less intimate and prolonged the symbiosis with a male or female infant, the less likely that femininity will appear. This latter thought, however, suggests that a remnant of oneness with the mother is present in males, forming a protofeminine core against which most men must work ("symbiosis anxiety"; see Stoller, 1974); some of what we call masculinity may be a defensive "structure" raised against the desire to merge again with mother and with her femaleness.

Then, in very feminine boys, once feminine behavior begins to appear, as early as a year or so, the mothers encourage every form it takes and discourage behavior that they consider masculine. In these two mechanisms that augment femininity—the primitive merging with the mother's body in the symbiosis and the reward and punishment shaping of behavior—we find at work forces that create gender identity without trauma, frustration, or intrapsychic conflict. It may be, then, that a primary femininity comparable to that in females is present in very feminine males. But, as noted elsewhere (Stoller, 1976), when one gets to know such people beyond the superficial engagements of research questionnaires and evaluation interviews, one does not see the more complicated and rich femininity produced by the family dynamics and conflicts we call the *Oedipal conflict*. The femininity of these transsexuals, although genuine and natural-looking, does not contain, for instance, mothering impulses or the capacity to remain in an extended, loving, hating, or envious relationship with males.

Anna Freud (1976) is helpful:

> In our categorization of infantile disorders, we have learned to distinguish between two types, intermingled though they are with each other. One belongs to the infantile neurosis and its forerunners, its earliest appearances caused by conflicts between drive activity and environmental forces, its later stages due to purely internal conflicts between contrasting tendencies within the personality structure, both accompanied by fear, anxiety, guilt, inhibition, loss of pleasure or function and by symptom formation. Experience has proved that psychoanalysis is the method of choice for treating these disorders since interpretation of the repressed, of transference and resistances enables the child's ego to undo the damage it has done to itself by adopting pathological conflict solutions and to replace these faulty structures by more adaptive ones.
>
> The second type of disturbance is of a different nature. It arises during the child's early period of growth and maturation and has to be ascribed to direct interference with the course of normal development. Instead of being born with the average expectable physical and mental equipment, reared in an average environment and developing its internal structure at the usual rate, a child can be subjected to deviations in any or all of these respects and consequently develop deviant, atypical or borderline features. There is no question here of the child's ego having done harm to itself; on the contrary, harm has been inflicted on it by circumstances entirely beyond its control.
>
> Developmental pathology, no less than the neurotic one, is open to psychoanalytic exploration, explanation and understanding. In spite of this, it does not answer to psychoanalytic therapy in the same manner.

> Even the most correct uncovering of past and forgotten circumstances and events (such as physical or mental handicap, neglect, rejection, lack of security and maternal care, precocious or delayed ego or superego functioning) does not blot out their impact on the shaping of the child's personality or eradicate their roots, i.e. does not act as a radical therapy. At best, it helps the child to cope better with the after-effects of what has happened to him. (pp. 258–259)

In thinking about the earliest stages of behavior, including gender identity, I feel that we must go beyond the awareness that, as Miss Freud noted, there are pathological states that are fixed and unchanging from earliest life on, to recognize that the same is true for all kinds of ordinary development, development for which the word *pathological* is inaccurate.

MARKED MASCULINITY IN FEMALES

If we persist in our "experiment" to test hypotheses relating to femininity, we should also examine markedly masculine (biologically normal) females to see if effects opposite to those found with femininity are present. They are. Leaving out a more complete description of the findings in these patients, I shall emphasize here only the two underlined in our review of marked femininity in males: the measure of mother–infant intimacy and the encouragement of either masculine or feminine behavior. In the histories of these transsexual females, one finds a severe disruption of the mother–infant relationship, with the mothers, for one reason or another (e.g., depression or physical illness), unable to function enough to create a symbiotic relationship. Second, the girls have a strong relationship with their fathers, in which they are encouraged to identify with them and in which any behavior judged as masculine is rewarded (Stoller, 1976). Again, then, it would seem that a primary gender identity—in this case, masculinity—opposite to that appropriate to the sex is created. If the hypothesis is that primary femininity is enhanced by closeness to the mother and by encouraging feminine behavior, then there should be less femininity if there is less closeness and if feminine behavior is not encouraged. Transsexual females confirm the hypothesis.

CONCLUSIONS

Here, then, is an outline for the development of femininity. Given the biologic anlagen, which in humans are rarely strong enough to overpower the effects of rearing, one can find, granting overlap, two phases of feminine development, each of which results from different

influences. The first is called *primary femininity;* it is especially manifested in an unshakable sense of femaleness (in females, of being un-
questionably anatomically female; in the true transsexual male, of
being female despite one's anatomy) and in a feminine appearance
that conforms with society's clichés for femininity, especially the result of shaping by parental, peer, and wider social influences. The second phase, not so much connected with appearance, is especially the
result of trauma, frustration, intrapsychic conflict, and conflict resolution. It is mostly intrapsychic and is discovered more in fantasies than
in external behavior.

The two phases and their underlying mechanisms are best observed in early childhood; in later life, they are so interwoven that
separating them is more an exercise in theory than in observation.

These, then, are hypotheses about femininity; perhaps other
workers with a more disciplined research intent will want to test
them.

REFERENCES

Abelin, E. L. Some further observations and comments on the earliest role of the father. *International Journal of Psycho-Analysis,* 1975, *56,* 293–302.

Deutsch, H. *The psychology of women.* New York: Grune & Stratton, 1944.

Freud, A. Changes in psychoanalytic practice and experience. *International Journal of Psycho-Analysis,* 1976, *57,* 257–260.

Freud, S. (1931). Female sexuality. *Standard edition,* 1961, *21,* 225–243.

Horney, K. On the genesis of castration complex in women. *International Journal of Psycho-Analysis,* 1924, *5,* 50–65.

Horney, K. The flight from womanhood. *International Journal of Psycho-Analysis,* 1926, *7,* 324–329.

Jones, E. The early development of female sexuality. *International Journal of Psycho-Analysis,* 1927, *8,* 459–472.

Jones, E. The phallic phase. *International Journal of Psycho-Analysis,* 1933, *14,* 1–33.

Money, J., and Ehrhardt, A. A. *Man and woman boy and girl.* Baltimore: Johns Hopkins University Press, 1972.

Roiphe, H., and Galenson, E. Early genital activity and the castration complex. *Psychoanalytic Quarterly,* 1972, *42,* 334–347.

Stoller, R. J. *Sex and gender,* Vol. 1. New York: Science House, 1968.

Stoller, R. J. Symbiosis anxiety and the development of masculinity. *Archives of General Psychiatry,* 1974, *30,* 164–172.

Stoller, R. J. *Sex and gender,* Vol. 2. New York: Jason Aronson, 1976.

Zilboorg, G. Masculine and feminine. *Psychiatry,* 1944, *7,* 257–296.

Chapter 8

Masturbation in Women

VIRGINIA LAWSON CLOWER

This paper attempts to delineate the role of masturbation in female sexual development and function. There is little on this topic in the literature of any discipline. Long after medical and religious taboos against masturbation in human males gave way to more enlightened scientific and humanistic attitudes, masturbation in the female was felt to be somehow not right. The prevailing point of view seemed to be that psychologically healthy girls and women do not practice genital self-stimulation as a rule. Like so many other aspects of female sexual development, the entire subject has been obscure and myth-ridden.

Work with children makes it clear that the earliest impetus for touching the genitals comes from a wish to repeat the gratification felt when a loving mother cares for the infant's body. This is true for both boys and girls. Genital play in the first two years does not give rise to great visible excitement nor lead to any climax that can be called orgasm. It is in the service of self-exploration and defining the boundaries of self, rather than for any focused, volitional pleasure-seeking.

At about 2½–3, there is a change in the interest of the child in its genital area. The sex organs are manipulated intentionally, and self-stimulation persists until satiation is achieved. Masturbation in young children is stimulation of the genital zone with the qualities of self-absorption, consciously intended self-arousal, and mounting excitement, and seeking pleasure predominates over exploring and acquiring knowledge.

VIRGINIA LAWSON CLOWER, M.D. • Training and Supervising Analyst, Adult and Child Psychoanalysis, New Orleans Psychoanalytic Institute, New Orleans, Louisiana.

The unabridged version of this paper appears in *Masturbation from Infancy to Senescence,* Irwin Marcus and John Francis (Eds.). New York: International Universities Press, 1975.

Freud believed that the discovery that they lack a penis makes girls feel disgusted with the clitoris and induces them to abandon self-stimulation. The suppression of masturbation in latency-age girls has been discussed repeatedly and has been attributed to the inferiority of the clitoris compared with the larger, more accessible, more responsive penis of the boy. To this frustrating organic inadequacy has been ascribed the inevitable penis envy, the lower sexual drive, and the emergence of the feminine characteristics of masochism and receptivity.

While it is true that some girls entering latency give up masturbation entirely, it is not true in every case.

It is important that girls in latency continue some masturbatory activity as a means of discharging sexual and aggressive impulses. It is also important that the girl maintain awareness of the existence of her external genitalia and a perception of the nature and the limits of the gratification available from clitoral stimulation. This is a vital step in progress toward final renunciation of any wishes for a penis and readiness to experience and integrate the internal genitalia when they become functional in puberty. Far from being normal, permanent rejection of the clitoris comes from excessive penis envy and is found as one cause of total frigidity (Harley, 1961a, 1961b).

Latency-age girls masturbate differently from boys of the same age. Typically, girls continue to stimulate the clitoris, the labia, and the introitus by indirect means, with less focused digital manipulation of the clitoris. Rhythmic physical exercise, from playing games to sliding down ropes and bannisters, bicycle riding, and horseback riding, afford tactile stimulation; thigh and pelvic muscles exert pressure on the perineum, creating strong sexual excitement, sometimes to orgasmic climax.

Often girls themselves do not identify their activity as masturbatory. Latency games like jumping rope, playing dodgeball, and folk dancing are characterized by rhythmic movement, counting, or chanting to peaks of stimulation followed by temporary exhaustion and lethargy. Some girls less disposed to vigorous group play bicycle, skate, or swing rhythmically for hours.

The fantasies accompanying healthy girlish pastimes are not easily elicited, even in psychoanalysis. What can be gleaned from doll play, storytelling, and allusive conversation indicates a mixture of fantasies. Some are narcissistic and autoerotic, accompanied by diffused pleasure from indirect stimulation of the genital area. In these fantasies, the girl is usually alone, experiencing her body as its own source of pleasure. She imagines herself floating, flying, dancing solo, skating like a feather. If she is inclined toward passivity, one component of the satisfaction may come from the fantasy of being carried along by the activity and the feeling. More often, either as a defense against ego-threatening passive wishes, or because of more active drives toward mastery, the pleasure comes from the manipulation of the body in skillful ways and control of the source and the degree of physical sensation.

Clinical findings show how guilt over sexual and aggressive wishes may interfere with focused genital stimulation and with masturbatory gratification. Suppression of specific genital manipulation may lead to familiar displacements: playing with the nose or the ears, twirling the hair, foot shaking, and rubbing, nibbling, or mouthing the fingers. These activities are accompanied by nonspecific spreading excitement but probably not by localized genital sensation or by sexual fantasy.

Latency-age girls who have strong superego prohibitions against pleasure itself, especially those who have not relinquished the primitive oral- and anal-sadistic wishes toward the mother, have exceedingly painful conflict over masturbatory urges. Avoidance of masturbation itself can spread to limitation of physical activity and even of fantasy that could serve to discharge sexual and aggressive tensions. Attempts to ward off masturbation may result in symptom formation or in behavioral disturbance manifested as a general restlessness, as in the girl who elicits from her parents and teachers the description "she can't sit still and doesn't know what to do with herself."

Our concern at this time is not with the question of whether or not normal girls at this age masturbate—they do—but with the meaning of the activity and what an understanding of it can tell us about the development of the individual girl and about feminine sexuality as a whole.

Fraiberg (1971) has described genital sensations in two latency-age girls in analysis. Her cases both showed transient anesthesias of the genitalia, which became "silent" for variable periods of time. This process was accompanied by a similar deadness of affect, which seemed to be the counterpart of the genital silence. Both girls described a sense of incompleteness in masturbation; both localized sensations in the genital area, not specifically the vagina. It was not clear, however, what each girl experienced as her vagina or how this word was represented mentally to her.

We need many more published clinical examples, since the number of cases available to any one child therapist is limited. Not only are cases few, but such material is very elusive in clinical work. Girls do not often speak freely of their experience with masturbation. Most of the material we have on masturbation in latency-age girls is gained from inference and the interpretation of clinical work with children seen by intuitively gifted and experienced child therapists.

Another source of information is from recollections of adult women. These are particularly unsatisfactory because they are distorted by retrospective falsification, unavoidable when the patient is a physiologically mature, sexually oriented adult woman. It seems to be virtually impossible for a woman who has once experienced coitus and has integrated her vagina into her body image to regress so completely that she reexperiences earlier sexual feelings and fantasies untinged by a capacity for participation of the internal genitalia and the need for vaginal penetration in the sexual act.

Before puberty, the female's perception of her genital apparatus is vague. Attempts to look at her own vulva are awkward and uninformative. Inspection of other girls, as in the "doctor game," discloses at best some small, ill-defined structures and openings. Nowhere does she find a part comparable to the male penis, which is compact, visible, clearly functional, and easily manipulated, so that the sex organ becomes a familiar source of pleasure for a boy.

Some investigators have found instances of vaginal excitability and of fantasies interpreted as coming from vaginal sensation in this age group or earlier. Other evidence indicates that before the influence of gonadotropins at the beginning of adolescence, the internal genital organs have no mental representation and play no part in masturbatory activity or fantasy. Exceptions occur with vaginal irritation from infection or parasites and with premature vaginal entry because of sexual abuse, accidental injury, or medical procedures. Urethral irritation is also stimulating to the adjacent vaginal tissues and may encourage rubbing of the external genitals and tentative exploration of the introitus or the distal part of the vagina itself.

Prepuberty, characterized by progressive increase in estrogen production and early development of breasts and body hair, brings unlocalized inner sensations that promote anxiety. The girl's sexual interests at this time center on her growing, changing body. Pregenital conflicts, penis envy, and the Oedipus complex are reawakened. Clitoral masturbation may increase sporadically with vivid fantasies that express blatant wishes to have a sexual organ that will "do more," that is, provide a better discharge for instinctual tension. In some girls, manipulation of the clitoris may stop altogether for a time. The limitations of genital satisfaction are compensated for by idealizing the entire body, including the smoothness and the intactness of the genital area, and by increasing interest in the growing breasts, with their excitable erectile nipples.

From about age 10, the secretion of gonadotropic hormones is detected sporadically by urinalysis, implying the sporadic production of estrogen. The endometrium develops proliferation phases corresponding to ovarian estrogen cycles. The first menstruation appears when swings in estrogen levels become pronounced enough to bring on vascular crisis in the endometrium. Later, estrogen production is periodically sufficient to stimulate the release of luetinizing hormone from the pituitary, initiating ovulation and the luteal phase of the menstrual cycle.

Benedek (1952) and Kestenberg (1967–1968) have postulated a correlation between phases of the menstrual cycle and psychic manifestations. The mature menstrual cycle consists of a relatively long period of growth and differentiation and a shorter period of regression. This cycle is most prominent in the endometrium, as manifested by menstrual bleeding, but cyclic changes also occur in the vaginal mucosa.

Kestenberg noted that while the menarche has been understood as one of the literally bloody experiences (menstruation, defloration, childbirth) that are components in normal female development, it has not been so well recognized that menstruation affords the means whereby the previously invisible, unfelt, and nonfunctioning uterus and vagina are experienced and incorporated into the body image. The girl's discovery of lacking a penis has been called *the* traumatic episode in feminine development. Resentment of males and refusal to accept a painful bloody hole have been thought an inevitable consequence, necessitating "normal female masochism" to make female sexuality endurable, let alone enjoyable.

But as Kestenberg (1961) pointed out, pain can sharpen and define body boundaries. In the normal course of development, menarche brings a focal point around which body image and genital function can be organized. However mixed with fearful fantasy and physical discomfort it may be, menstruation, with its regularity, source of flow, limited time, and learned ways of caring for the body, is a stabilizing experience.

Masturbation continues in early adolescence and even increases, as the clitoris grows in size and the glans is more sensitive. There is cyclic capacity and desire for vaginal receptivity, but the lingering fear of penetration and the anxiety about intense orgastic sensation and loss of identity usually inhibit vaginal excitation and limit tactile stimulation to clitoris and introitus.

Freud (1905/1953) postulated a preliminary phase at puberty in which clitoral sexuality is repressed (*clitoral* being equated with "active, thrusting, masculine") before vaginal (equated with "passive, receptive, feminine") dominance can be established. He felt, however, that the clitoris still retained a function even after the transfer from clitoris to vagina, that is, the function of transmitting excitation to the vaginal zone "just as shavings can be kindled in order to set a log of harder wood on fire" (p. 221).

Clitoral masturbation is not normally abandoned when passive–receptive feminine wishes for vaginal penetration are established. In fact, neither physiological research nor clinical work supports the identification of clitoral masturbation exclusively with activity or masculinity; the clitoris remains the female's responsive and accessible erogenous zone, and clitoral masturbation expresses both active and passive, sexual and aggressive aims in adolescence. My own clinical observation bears out that of Harley (1961a), who said that the extension of clitoral to vaginal responsiveness is gradual and may well be dependent on the actual experience of intercourse for its completion.

When ovulatory cycles are established, the adolescent girl has uterine contractions, vaginal sensation, and repeated discharge of blood and tissue from within her body. She associates these with what she understands of penetration and childbirth. Fear of being torn inhibits direct genital stimulation, and she defensively maintains the masturbatory techniques established in latency. However, the excitement may be intense enough to produce vaginal exudate, itself exciting and alarming, and to lead to orgasm, which brings anxious feelings of losing control.

Masturbation at this stage serves to discharge sexual excitement, and at the same time, it initiates fantasies of penetration and acts as a source of genital stimulation that promotes the inclusion of the internal genitalia in the female body image. Individual patterns of masturbatory behavior do not change much from latency to adolescence in girls who have no more than the usual phase-specific conflicts. However, the psychological basis for the behavior shifts, and there is a gradual changeover from clitoral masturbation because this is the only genital organ available for discharge in latency to clitoral masturbation as a defense against sensation from the internal genitalia and the wish–fear of vaginal penetration in early puberty, and finally—by late adolescence—to clitoral masturbation as the trigger and the focal point of spreading genital excitement, which heralds and augments the readiness for coitus. The fantasies of adolescence reflect the movement of the libido from self-stimulation of the genitals and other erogenous zones for narcissistic gratification, to heterosexual experimentation in fantasy, and, finally, to sex play and exploration with partners.

Boys are more likely than girls to engage in transitory homosexual episodes in early puberty because their genital urges are more peremptory. Girls at this age are dreamy and have elaborate fantasies of being wooed and carried away by an idealized lover. Dating, going steady, breaking off, and then reengaging with a nonincestuous object are no longer play at being grown up, like an Oedipal child, but a reasonable facsimile of the real thing. Masturbation fantasies in adolescent girls are not so concerned with the sex act *per se* (as is usual with boys) as with the whole romantic complex of love, marriage, and motherhood.

Masturbation in adolescence has a vital new dimension; it is the activity of a person with mature genitals. It permits a trial of the new sexual resource in fantasies of adult intercourse, and at the same time, it satisfies unconscious pregenital wishes. Repeated experience of the body with its growing capacity for sexual gratification and the feeling that the body belongs to the self help complete the dissolution of symbiotic infantile ties and supports autonomy. Clinical work has demonstrated that long-delayed or absent masturbation in adolescence may signify the incomplete of pregenital conflict and results in defects in the body image and inability to tolerate and master sensation arising inside the self.

The need to masturbate and conscious conflict about it are less severe in girls than in boys, explained in part by the psychology of menstruation. The menses force periodic reworking of the body image and acceptance of the uterus and the vagina as feminine organs. Cycles are established in individual patterns. The length of time between periods, the kind and degree of discomfort, the amount of bleeding, and the necessary steps in caring for personal hygiene vary from girl to girl. The total experience marks her as a woman and thus like other women, including her mother, but at the same time not exactly like anyone else. The girl who has menstrual periods on a timetable and of a character very different from those of her mother, sisters, and friends is asserting her sexual individuality and reinforcing it in a much more subtle but no less significant way than the boy who masturbates frequently and frantically.

Adolescent girls developing normally are quite aware of genital sensation. They have urges to masturbate and do, using various techniques and elaborate erotic fantasies to reach climax. Unless they are in undue conflict about sex, they do not talk to adults about their masturbation or directly about fantasies. They are precariously balanced between progressive and regressive pulls, and the phase-specific need to keep optimal distance from adults interferes with intimate discussions of sex.

The adolescent girl needs to masturbate enough to reinforce her awareness of her genitality, especially to experience vaginal lubrication and excitement spreading from the clitoris. She must not masturbate so much that her sexual gratification is fixed on her own body and that fantasies of being able to satisfy herself are promoted at the expense of accepting the need for vaginal penetration in coitus.

Until quite recently, psychoanalysts were discussing female sexuality almost exclusively in terms of the consequences of the anatomical differences between the sexes and the fate of penis envy. Most of them followed Freud in believing that penis envy is a stage in normal development, primarily determined biologically. A few, like Karen Horney, Melanie Klein, and Ernest Jones, thought that penis envy was secondary and essentially defensive as a flight from the perils of femininity. Both groups derived their understanding from clinical work with patients; neither group had any information on the sexual behavior of the population as a whole or, from studies in basic anatomy and physiology, on sexual response and orgasm. Longitudinal observations of normal girls and endocrine studies correlating hormone changes with behavior were even less available.

In 1953, Kinsey and his co-workers published *Sexual Behavior in the Human Female*. The report was based on histories of 5940 white females living in the United States, aged from 12 to 90. Kinsey reported that 62% of the 2800 women from whom he had information about self-stimulation had masturbated at some time, that many had been engaged in true masturbatory (pleasure-seeking) behavior at an early age, and that 58% reached orgasm at times, many invariably. He found that neither age, educational level, nor religious background was very important in determining whether or not a woman masturbated. Another group, 44% of the nonmasturbators, stated they had not masturbated because they considered it morally wrong. Kinsey's figures show that of the 2800 women from whom he had information about self-stimulation, about 2200 masturbated at some time, or wanted to. Kinsey thought the majority of those without other means of sexual satisfaction who never masturbated had little sexual appetite. I suspect that this group included a number who masturbated like latency girls without direct genital stimulation, never identifying the experience as sexual.

The report brought out the fact that the incidence of masturbation fell somewhat after marriage when regular coitus became available, but it did not disappear. Some women did not begin to masturbate (or were not aware of it—my note) until after they had coitus. Others masturbated after unsatisfactory coitus, still others when their sexual partners were unavailable.

The techniques of masturbation described in the Kinsey report are well known to clinicians. Most frequent is digital manipulation of the clitoris and/or the labia minora. The labia majora are less often the focus of stimulation, and then usually by some pressure that is felt in the entire genital area. Of techniques other than those involving direct or indirect genital stimulation, manipulation of the nipples was cited in about 11% of those who masturbate. Breast stimulation alone was rarely effective in producing orgasm, and simultaneous manipulation of the genitals was usually employed. Another 11% used a variety of techniques, including stimulating the vulva by rubbing against furniture, applying streams of water to the clitoris and the labia, and holding vibrators on the vulva. Least common was the use of douches, enemas or other anal stimulation, and urethral insertions.

Some 20% per cent of those who masturbate reported inserting fingers, rarely other objects, into the vagina during masturbation. The authors questioned this incidence because they noted that most women did not distinguish between the vestibule of the vagina and the vagina itself. In many instances, fingers were inserted only far enough past the introitus to anchor the hand while it rubbed the external genitals.

Kinsey did find, however, that many women derive erotic gratification from deep vaginal penetration in coitus. Furthermore, he noted that probably a majority of women feel that deep penetration provides a type of erotic satisfaction different from that secured by stimulation of the labia or the clitoris alone. He speculated that some women *might* have nerve endings in the vaginal walls but added that the gratification from deep penetration may be the result of psychological associations with vaginal penetration and coitus, and therefore not explained entirely by physiology.

The Kinsey report took issue in lively fashion with the Freudian theory that masturbation in women concentrates erotic responsiveness in the external genitalia and interferes with vaginal response. The data bore evidence that the nature of premarital sexual experience was not as important for a woman as whether she did or did not achieve orgasm. The report stated (1953):

> We have seen very few cases of females who had encountered any difficulty in transferring their masturbatory experience to coitus, although we have seen some hundreds of cases of females who were unable to accomplish the anatomic impossibility of "transferring their clitoral reactions to vaginal responses." (p. 171)

Whereas the Kinsey work is a classic in sociological investigation, the work of Masters and Johnson is pioneering research in the anatomy and physiology of sexual response in the human male and female. *Human Sexual Response* was published in 1966. Information set forth in the book has been elaborated in a number of papers from the Masters and Johnson project and in *Human Sexual Inadequacy* (1970).

These studies have inspired a fresh interest in reexamination of the concepts of female sexuality and an impetus toward the integration of data from many disciplines. One ambitious undertaking was Sherfey's (1966) paper, which focused attention on the biological roots of psychosexual experience.

From Masters and Johnson, we now have the information about female sexual anatomy and physiology needed to supplement our knowledge of sexual behavior and fantasy. Outstanding among their contributions is the elucidation of the respective roles of clitoris and vagina in female sexual function. Masters and Johnson demonstrated a dual function for the vagina: it provides the primary physical apparatus for heterosexual experience and simultaneously acts as a part of the apparatus for conception. They stated (1966):

> To appreciate vaginal anatomy and physiology is to comprehend the fundamentals of the human female's primary means of sexual expression. In essence, the vaginal barrel responds to effective sexual stimulation by involuntary preparation for penile penetration. Just as penile erection is a direct physiologic expression of a psychologic demand to mount, so expansion and lubrication of the vaginal barrel provide direct physiologic indication of an obvious psychologic mounting invitation. (p. 68)

And:

> It should be stated parenthetically that vaginal (natural or artificial) response to sexual stimulation develops in a basic pattern regardless of whether the stimuli originally are primarily somatogenic or psychogenic in origin. (p.69)

The first physiological evidence of female sexual response is the appearance of vaginal lubrication. Within 10–30 seconds after effective sexual stimulation is initiated, droplets of mucoid material appear throughout the rugae of the normal vagina, and the sexually responding woman is ready for coitus. This response is followed by a lengthening of the vaginal barrel and a distention of the inner two-thirds. In this excitement phase, there may be irregular patterns of expansion and contraction. At the same time, the cervix and the body of the uterus retract backward and upward into the false pelvis.

In the second, or plateau, phase of sexual excitement, the entire outer third of the vaginal barrel becomes distended with venous blood, the labia minora are engorged, and vaginal lubrication reaches its peak. Masters and Johnson termed the area of plateau-phase vasocongestion the "orgasmic platform."

The intensity of the vaginal response mechanisms always parallels the degree of sexual excitement felt by the individual. This excitement culminates in an abrupt physiological reaction confined to the orgasmic platform. The localized area of vasoconcentration contracts strongly in a rhythmic pattern that varies from woman to woman and from one orgasmic experience to another in the same woman. Then follows a gradual resolution, with retrogressive changes, usually requiring 10–15 minutes for completion.

The vagina functions also as an organ of reproduction. The excitement-phase expansion of the vagina forms a receptacle for a pool of seminal ejaculate, and the orgasmic platform produces a stopperlike effect in the outer one-third of the vagina to retain semen. If orgasm does not ensue, the orgasmic platform may not be lost for 20–30 minutes, and the exposure of the cervical os to the seminal pool is thus increased. There is a physiological basis for the view of Helene Deutsch, who has long contended that the vagina is primarily an organ of reproduction. Masters and Johnson show how true this view is, but they also provide a demonstration of the vagina's total function in sexual expression.

The clitoris of a mature woman retains its function as both a receptor and a transformer of sensual stimuli. Masters and Johnson pointed out that in the clitoris, the human female has an organ system that is totally limited in physiological function to initiating or elevating levels of sexual tension. No such organ exists within the anatomic structure of the male, a lack that may help to account for the confusion in conceptualizing the role of the clitoris in female sexual response. The fact that anatomically the clitoris is a true homologue of the penis and that it has long been considered the "female phallus" has obscured understanding of its functional role. The penis is the male organ providing for urinary release and the deposit of seminal fluid, in addition to operating as a means for the discharge of sexual tensions in the male. The clitoris serves only as an erotic focus for sexual stimulation. This capacity is a biological given, manifest in the pre-Oedipal girl, never entirely lost in normal latency, reinforced in adolescence, and retained in mature women as an integrated part of the genital apparatus.

Masters and Johnson have demonstrated that either psychogenic or somatogenic stimulation produces characteristic physiological changes in both clitoris and vagina, the first response being vaginal lubrication. The clitoral response appears with mounting excitement, seen as turgor in the glans and experienced as a feeling of warmth and pressure in the lower pelvis (possibly vasoconcentration), with varying degrees of local irritation, swelling, and need for release (possibly glans enlargement). Masters and Johnson's description of the role of clitoral response was echoed by a clinician's note (Gillespie, 1969) to the effect that clitoral excitation may lead to the wish to be penetrated and may express "the desire to be penetrated and so stimulated both vaginally and clitorally—the outcome to be expected in normal female psychosexual development" (p. 497).

Masters and Johnson emphasized the fact that there may be great variation in the duration and the intensity of orgasmic experience in individuals, and they made repeated references to the psychogenic element inherent in any approach to sexual stimulation of the female. But they stated unequivocally that when any woman experiences an orgasmic response to effective stimulation, both vagina and clitoris react in consistent physiological patterns. Clitoral and vaginal orgasms are not separate biological entities.

Adult women, unless they are severely inhibited by cultural taboo, religion, or neurosis, all masturbate on occasion, and recourse to sexual gratification by self-stimulation does not invariably indicate pathology. An analysis of what individual women actually feel and fantasize in masturbation yields insight into their level of psychosexual development, their defenses, and their object relations.

For a number of years, I have been observing and discussing masturbation in females of all ages with all kinds of problems. They have been patients in the diagnostic study and treatment of medical illness; patients on gynecological, obstetrical, and surgical services; and infant girls and their mothers in a well-baby clinic. Some have been children, adolescents, or adult women hospitalized for psychiatric care. Others were in evaluation or psychotherapy as outpatients. A large number have been girls and/or their mothers seen in child guidance clinics, wives with marital problems, and students seeking counsel. Much insight has come from intensive psychotherapy and analyses of females from the age of 4 to the middle 60s, and more was contributed from the supervision of psychotherapy and psychoanalysis. Direct observation of girls in families and in nursery school has answered some questions and raised more.

None of this observation has been research in the sense of systematic, organized investigation, but it has produced impressions to be tested against comprehensive data from facts learned in research on behavior, physiology, and psychoanalysis.

Masturbation in adult women may be chiefly "normal"—meaning that it serves stable ego functions, supports nonincestuous object relations, and evidences progressive trends in growth and capacity for adaptation—or chiefly "pathological"—meaning that it serves pathological defenses, maintains in fantasy conflict-laden infantile relationships, and evidences regressive trends in the ego and insufficient capacity for adaptation.

Normal masturbation, when a satisfying sexual relationship with a love object is not available, can provide some aspects of the gratification found in coitus. Young adult women who are physiologically and psychologically ready for coitus but who have not made an object choice may masturbate as a substitute and as preparation for coital experience. Masturbation in the case of young adults may be a more mature kind of sexual expression than casual sexual intercourse. If there has been vaginal penetration in lovemaking, the fantasies are of coitus with a real or an idealized object. If sexual experience has not included penetration, the fantasies are of whatever is understood or imagined of coitus.

Women who are in stable heterosexual alliances may resort to masturbation when their partners are absent. Some women who are deprived of coital relationship suffer greatly not just because they lack genital satisfaction. The mature feminine wish for coitus comes from many levels, and the need for sexual connection to assuage separation anxiety, to reaffirm sexual integrity and identity, and to express the ability to love and be loved is exacerbated when self-esteem is low. Masturbation with a fantasy of loving relationship can be restitutive here. If the separation is not unduly prolonged and does not coincide with other stress, some women do not masturbate, not necessarily because they are any less desirous or less sexually responsive; apparently, the object relationship is supportive enough to make the sexual deprivation tolerable without substitute gratification.

It is not unusual for mature women to masturbate when coitus is unsatisfying because of intermittent or permanent sexual inadequacy of the partner. Unrelieved sexual arousal makes many women uncomfortable and irritable. When coital connection is infrequent or cannot be sustained by the male, the female may be left with a buildup of vasocongestion in the pelvis and turgor in the vaginal walls and the clitoral glans, making her feel tense and heavy physically as well as emotionally disappointed. Masturbation to orgasm in these instances may be a positive factor in maintaining the relationship if it relieves frustration and anger at the male. If the relationship is otherwise a good one, the fantasy with masturbation is frequently of intercourse with the lover, who performs capably. If there is a lot of anger, the partner in imagination may be another man who is fantasized as a good lover.

The characteristic shared by all kinds of normal masturbation in adult women is that the fantasies are of coitus with a male love object.

It has been my observation that some sexually responsive women in satisfactory heterosexual object relations are not so intent upon orgasm in itself, though they welcome coitus. This type of woman may seldom resort to masturbation even in the absence of regular climax; for her sexual gratification seems less important then other aspects of a good relationship. Such women may be like those described as being satisfied in lovemaking without orgasmic climax, feeling a slow relaxation that is completely pleasurable (Deutsch, 1925/1948). In Deutsch's opinion, the majority of mature feminine women are in this category. She did not say whether the women she described ever resorted to masturbation, or if they had a different kind of orgasm with self-stimulation. These may be women of the type that Sarlin (1970) referred to as having achieved adequate object relations without orgastic capacity. He stated, "Frequently such women manifest a generous, kind maternalism toward mate as well as child; but this is a far different state of affairs than a truly mutual, heterosexual object-love relationship" (p. 295).

Pathological masturbation is readily identified in clinical practice. It may appear as a substitute for coitus where the physiological capacity and need for orgasm are established, but the ability to sustain an object relationship with a man is undeveloped. Some women with this characteristic get involved in homosexual relationships and practice both self-stimulation and mutual masturbation. Some are so fearful of intimacy of any kind that they cannot tolerate physical closeness with either sex. The well-known examples of psychotic women observed masturbating to climax that seems to include the vagina may fall into this category (see Greenacre, 1950).

Women with a severe disturbance in their capacity for object relations are not amenable to classical psychoanalysis because they are likely to have psychotic transference to analysts of either sex, and they develop no true therapeutic alliance and have little observing ego. However, their fantasies are often given spontaneously and unguardedly. In my experience with hospitalized psychotic women, I found fantasies, usually polymorphous, with no clear perception of which organ was involved in the masturbatory experience. Severely regressed women sometimes vomit, urinate, or defecate at the same time as they exhibit sexual excitement. Some patients verbalize sadomasochistic fantasies or hallucinations of being beaten at climax.

In less disturbed women whose reality testing and capacity for object relations are intact, an analysis of masturbation fantasies can delineate areas of failure in psychosexual development and regression that give rise to some of the most familiar sexual problems in women. One intelligent and attractive young woman undertook analysis because she longed to be married and have children but seemed unable to attract a suitable object. In the course of analysis, she revealed compulsive masturbation, which went on nightly for hours, in which she pounded her vulva against a pillow, having repeated orgasms felt as a brief twitching of the clitoris but with no satiation. The frenetic activity would cease only when she was exhausted or when shame and humiliation made her stop. She had been the only girl in a large family of boys, the favorite of both parents. The onset of menstruation was a bitter blow to her fantasy that she was one of the boys, but she gradually accepted the feminine role in social relations. She enjoyed attention from men and felt sexual excitement in limited physical contact, as in dancing, kissing, and having her breasts touched. The masturbation, she recalled, began in adolescence. Her fantasies were of watching brutal assaults on a woman who was forced to stimulate the genitalia of another woman and a man with her mouth. The patient experienced both the masochistic degradation of the abused woman and the sadistic pleasure of the attackers as she masturbated. Deeper analysis of the fantasy revealed that this patient had completely repressed awareness of her internal genitalia. She had no concept of a vagina and could not imagine where the penis would go in intercourse.

Analysis of sexual activity in adult women demonstrates that a great deal of what may pass for a normal, mature heterosexual relationship is quite immature and, in fact, masturbatory at the level of adolescence or earlier. The sex act may take place with a lover, but the fantasies are of looking and being looked at; of thinly disguised Oedipal objects; of romantic encounters with old boyfriends, paternalistic bosses, and attractive neighbors. If the woman has much unresolved fear and resistance to being penetrated, the fantasies may be quite sadomasochistic, with images of rough treatment, rape, or injury. There may be an orgasmic experience that is dutifully reported to the analyst, but careful attention discloses that it is the same kind felt when the woman stimulates the external genitalia. The experience excludes the sexual partner as a real object. Rarely is there tender feeling, a wish to share pleasure, or association to the relationship with the man as a person in the sex act.

Certain borderline women with a tenuous hold on reality and a fear of ego regression cannot surrender in the transient loss of ego boundaries that is the source of elation in the sexual climax. Yet, many of these women report great sexual interest and activity and describe profound orgasmic climax. Deeper understanding of the experience reveals it as pseudocoital and psychologically more autoerotic than some specifically masturbatory activity that involves a love object in fantasy.

The impressive research of Masters and Johnson proves conclusively that, physiologically, orgasm is orgasm, but their studies make no attempt to evaluate what women with the satisfying experience of climax in coitus know well: orgasm in masturbation and orgasm in coitus are not felt as the same. The importance to the individual is not what is occurring physiologically but how it is perceived, mentally represented, and interpreted.

It is unfortunate that we have no psychoanalytic data from the women who participated in the Masters and Johnson study to compare with what women say they wish for, imagine, and feel in sexual congress. Information from patients is likely to be vague and incomplete. Even lengthy and detailed description spontaneously offered is difficult to evaluate. The dimming of contact with external reality and the blurring of self and object boundaries interfere with the observing ego in an intense experience. Many intelligent and otherwise well-informed women remain hazy in their grasp of sexual anatomy. One hears such statements as "He touched my vagina" or "My vagina hurt," when the context makes it clear that some part of the external genitalia or the urethra is being described.

Glenn and Kaplan (1968) discussed the problem that women have in describing sexual feeling and reported that there is a marked variation in the location of the experience of orgasm. The area in which it is finally felt need not be the same as the area of maximal stimulation. They concluded that the type and the location of orgasm experienced depends on the cathexis of mental representations of specific areas, the nature of the fantasies associated with the feelings, and the degree to which sensation may be repressed.

There is general agreement that normal women prefer heterosexual intercourse with coital orgasm to any other form of sexual gratification, but there is no consensus about why this is true. Kinsey's data show that masturbation or mutual stimulation in homosexual intercourse more often produced orgasm; Masters and Johnson have demonstrated no differences in the physiology of orgasm brought on by any effective stimulation. Clinicians are more familiar with the vicissitudes of accepting the feminine receptive sexual role than they are with the fantasies of untroubled women. Masturbation fantasies in patients concern fear of penetration, penis envy, anxiety that dirty or voracious insides may damage the sexual partner, fear of losing ego boundaries, and other fears that shed more light on interference with vaginal participation in coitus than on the wish for it.

Coitus with intravaginal ejaculation is essential for reproduction, and the wish for coital orgasm is plainly adaptive biologically. Manipulation of the external female genitalia does not bring about pregnancy and childbirth, the final affirmation of what Erikson (1964) called "woman's productive inner space."

Sherfey (1966) offered an explanation for the clinical observation that few women resort to digital stimulation of the lower vagina during masturbation and why this is not a preferred source of arousal in foreplay despite wishes for vaginal penetration. Considerable distension of the vaginal orifice is necessary to exert traction on the labia and carry the physiological mechanism of arousal past the initial point of vasocongestion of the pelvic area and transudation of fluid into the vagina. Repeated thrusting into the vaginal barrel brings two actions to bear on the clitoris: first, friction on the glans is maintained by movement of the prepuce of the glans; second, the shaft of the clitoris is relaxed, then retracted, in response to each thrust. Thus, the more thrusting, the greater swelling of the prepuce, the more pressure on the glans, the more flexion of the shaft, the greater arousal. Digital stimulation of the glans clitoris alone is not sufficient for the fullest arousal leading to the reflex mechanisms that bring about maximum contractions, expelling the blood collected in the venous plexuses and giving rise to the experience of orgasm. Obviously, fingers are not adequate substitutes for the erect penis in stimulating the female genitalia from the most external to the deepest zones.

Sexual desire in women with a well-established capacity for orgasm, reinforced by satisfying coital experience, is often described by them in terms of a longing to be entered vaginally. Pleasure in clitoral stimulation by touching or rhythmic massage may be incidentally exciting or may even climax in an orgasm characterized by short, sharp spasms experienced as localized "outside." Typically, this kind of orgasm is reported by women as "not deep enough," and the woman is left feeling unsatisfied, sometimes specifically feeling empty, or as if a part of the body within needed to be filled or rubbed.

Relatively nonneurotic women describe fantasies in coitus of being restored completely, filled, united with the beloved. The wishes are profoundly receptive and may coincide with the expansion of the vagina described by Masters and Johnson in the initial excitement and the plateau phases when the vaginal barrel increases in size and becomes engorged with venous blood. Deep vaginal penetration may be represented mentally by fantasies that at climax the penis reaches and kisses the cervix. One patient described the feeling that her vaginal barrel was very cozy, and she imagined that it was experienced by her lover as it if it were lined with velvet so that it cuddled his penis. I have heard the fantasy that the head of the penis nuzzles at the cervix like a baby nuzzling at the breast. This is not the kind of fantasy or the experience that the same women have in masturbation, although self-stimulation may lead to physical release.

If there has been appropriate genital stimulation in the course of development, the normal adult woman is potentially capable of responding sexually in coitus and of welcoming pregnancy and childbirth. Sensations from clitoris and vagina overlap and become fused in a total sexual experience. Mature female sexual orientation, however, is always dominated more by visceral inner sensation than by sensations from the external genitals. For the final achievement of sexual maturity and capacity for orgastic discharge, a woman is dependent on repeated coitus with a nonincestuous love object. Clinical observation does not confirm an absolute correlation between the capacity for stable object relations and the capacity for full satisfaction through genital orgasm (see Ross, 1970; Sarlin, 1970), but as Kestenberg (1968b) said, "In order to achieve an adult feminine orgastic discharge, woman is just as dependent on man's performance as teacher and organizer of her sexuality as she is dependent on his performance as effective provider and giver of semen" (p. 482). Study of masturbation in adult women demonstrates that the functionally adequate penis of a lover makes the difference between sexual experience in masturbation and that in coitus.

REFERENCES

Barnett, M. Vaginal awareness in the infancy and childhood of girls. *Journal of the American Psychoanalytical Association*, 1966, *14*, 129–141.

Benedek, T. *Psychosexual functions in women.* New York: Ronald Press, 1952.

Benedek, T. Sexual functions in women and their disturbance. In S. Arieti (Ed.), *American Handbook of psychiatry*, Vol. 1. New York: Basic Books, 1959, pp. 727–748.

Bornstein, B. Masturbation in the latency period. *The Psychoanalytic Study of the Child*, 1953, *8*, 65–78.

Deutsch, H. The psychology of women, in relation to the functions of reproduction (1925). In R. Fleiss (Ed.), *The Psychoanalytic Reader*. New York: International Universities Press, 1948, pp. 192–206.

Deutsch, H. *Psychology of women: A psychoanalytic interpretation*, Vol. 1. New York: Grune & Stratton, 1944.

Deutsch, H. *Psychology of women: A psychoanalytic interpretation*, Vol. 2. New York: Grune & Stratton, 1945.

Erikson, E. H. Reflections on womanhood, *Daedalus*, 1964, *2*, 582–606.

Fraiberg, S. Some considerations on the introduction of therapy in puberty. *The Psychoanalytic Study of the Child*, 1955, *10*, 264–286.

Fraiberg, S. Technical aspects of the analysis of a child with a severe behavior disorder. *Journal of the American Psychoanalytic Association*, 1962, *10*, 338–367.

Fraiberg, S. Genital sensation in latency girls. *Bulletin of the Philadelphia Association of Psychoanalysis*, 1971, *21*, 261–262.

Freud, S. Three essays on the theory of sexuality. *Standard Edition*, 1905, *7*, 125–245. London: Hogarth Press, 1953.

Gillespie, W. H. Concepts of vaginal orgasm. *International Journal of Psychoanalysis*, 1969, *50*, 495–497.

Glenn, J., and Kaplan, E. H. Types of orgasm in women: A critical review and redefinition, *Journal of the American Psychoanalytic Association*, 1968, *16*, 549–568.

Greenacre, P. Special problems of early female sexual development. *The Psychoanalytic Study of the Child*, 1950, 5, 112–138.

Harley, M. Masturbation conflicts. In S. Lorand and H. Schneer (Eds.), *Adolescents: Psychoanalytic approach to problems and therapy*. New York: Hoeber, 1961a, pp. 51–77.

Harley, M. Some observations on the relationship between genitality and structural development at adolescence. *Journal of the American Psychoanalytic Association*, 1961b, 9, 434–460.

Heiman, M. Sexual response in women: A correlation of physiological findings with psychoanalytic concepts. *Journal of the American Psychoanalytic Association*, 1963, 11, 360–387.

Horney, K. On the genesis of the castration complex in women. *International Journal of Psycho-Analysis*, 1924, 5, 50–65.

Horney, K. The denial of the vagina: A contribution to the problem of the genital anxieties specific to women. *International Journal of the Psycho-Analytic Association*, 1933, 14, 57–70.

Jacobson, E. On the development of the girl's wish for a child. *Psychoanalytic Quarterly*, 1968, 37, 523–538.

Jones, E. The early development of female sexuality. *Papers on Psychoanalysis* (1927). London: Ballière, Tindall & Cox, 1948, pp. 438–451.

Kestenberg, J. On the development of maternal feelings in early childhood. *The Psychoanalytic Study of the Child*, 1956a, 11, 257–291.

Kestenberg, J. Vicissitudes of female sexuality. *Journal of the American Psychoanalytic Association*, 1956b, 4, 453–476.

Kestenberg, J. Menarche. In S. Lorand and H. Schneer (Eds.), *Adolescents: Psychoanalytic approach to problems and therapy*. New York: Hoeber, 1961, pp. 19–50.

Kestenberg, J. Phases of adolescence: With suggestions for a correlation of psychic and hormonal organizations. *Journal of the American Academy of Child Psychiatry*, 1967–1968, 6, 426–463, 557–614; 7, 108–151.

Kestenberg, J. Discussion of Mary Jane Sherfey: The evolution and nature of female sexuality in relation to psychoanalytic process. *Journal of the American Psychoanalytic Association*, 1968a, 16, 417–423.

Kestenberg, J. Outside and inside, male and female. *Journal of the American Psychoanalytic Association*, 1968b, 16, 457–520.

Kinsey, A., Pomeroy, W. B., and Martin, C. I. *Sexual behavior in the human male*. Philadelphia: Saunders, 1948.

Kinsey, A., Pomeroy, W. B., and Martin, C. I. *Sexual behavior in the human female*. Philadelphia: Saunders, 1953.

Kleeman, J. A boy discovers his penis. *The Psychoanalytic Study of the Child*, 1965, 20, 239–265.

Kleeman, J. The establishment of core gender identity in normal girls. *Archives of Sexual Behavior*, 1971, 1, 103–129.

Lampl-de Groot, J. On adolescence. *The Psychoanalytic Study of the Child*, 1960a, 15, 95–103.

Lampl-de Groot, J. On masturbation and its influence on general development. *The Psychoanalytic Study of the Child*, 1960b, 15, 153–174.

Masters, W., and Johnson, V. *Human sexual response*. Boston: Little Brown, 1966.

Masters, W., and Johnson, V. *Human sexual inadequacy*. Boston: Little, Brown, 1970.

Nunberg, H., and Federn, E. Discussions on masturbation. In *Minutes of the Vienna Psychoanalytic Society*, Vol. 3. New York: International Universities Press, 1974.

Panel. Frigidity (B. Moore, reporter). *Journal of the American Psychoanalytic Association*, 1956, 9, 571–584.

Panel. Masturbation (I. M. Marcus, reporter). *Journal of the American Psychoanalytic Association,* 1962, *10,* 91–101.

Panel. Female sexuality (W. J. Barker, reporter). *Journal of the American Psychoanalytic Association,* 1968a, *16,* 123–145.

Panel. Masturbation (J. Francis, reporter). *Journal of the American Psychoanalytic Association,* 1968b, *16,* 95–112.

Pearson, G. A young girl and her horse. *Bulletin of the Philadelphia Association of Psychoanalysis,* 1965, *15,* 189–206.

Reich, A. The discussion of 1912 on masturbation and our present-day views (1951). In G. Gero (Ed.), *Psychoanalytic contributions.* New York: International Universities Press, 1973, pp. 155–178.

Ross, N. The primacy of genitality in the light of ego psychology. *Journal of the American Psychoanalytic Association,* 1970, *18,* 267–284.

Sarlin, C. The current status of the concept of genital primacy. *Journal of the American Psychoanalytic Association,* 1970, *18,* 285–299.

Sherfey, M. D. The evolution and nature of female sexuality in relation to psychoanalytic theory. *Journal of the American Psychoanalytic Association,* 1966, *14,* 28–128. Discussion, 1968, *16,* 405–456.

Another Point of View

JOSHUA GOLDEN

Masturbation is coming out of the closet. Under the moralistic on-slaught of the 19th-century physicians and clergymen who blamed masturbation for everything bad that happened in the world, mastur-bation went into hiding. It probably had a vigorous role in the experi-ence of most men and almost as many women, but only the very brave or the very foolhardy dared to discuss their experiences openly. Cur-rent attitudes toward human sexuality have evolved into a more com-fortable and more scientific position. It is now all right to talk about, write about, and practice sexual activity.

Dr. Clower's paper raises fond hopes for some enlightenment on a subject of great interest, "Masturbation in Women." There has been so little information available on female sexuality in general and fe-male masturbation in particular that any contribution can be expected to add measurably to our meager and sorely needed knowledge. Un-fortunately, my hopes were disappointed. To begin, it is clear that she is a psychoanalyst and she cites as the basis for her information only authors who are psychoanalysts or who write in psychoanalytic jour-nals. Kinsey and Masters and Johnson are the exceptions. Much of the paper seems to be an apology for the much-belabored Freudian hy-pothesis that distinguishes between vaginal orgasm and clitoral orgasm: vaginal orgasm is good, mature, and normal; clitoral orgasm is not so good, immature, and less normal. The data from which her conclusions are drawn are mostly the speculations of other psychoana-lysts. Dr. Clower ignores or is unaware of the anatomical and physio-logical bases of sexual behavior. She fails to mention that the inner portions of the vaginal mucosa have relatively few sensory nerve end-

JOSHUA GOLDEN, M.D. • Director, Sexual Dysfunction Clinic, Department of Psychiatry, University of California, Los Angeles, California.

ings as compared with the richly endowed tissues of the clitoris and the introitus. One might explain how women masturbate on the basis of the sensations they receive. Dr. Clower attempts to account for the observed behavior on the basis of less parsimonious, more tortured explanations that derive from classical psychoanalytic theory.

My 15 years of experience in treating men and women with sexual dysfunctions has demonstrated enormous variation within the range of "normal" activities engaged in by men and women whom I and other colleagues consider "normal." The women I have seen, clinically, achieve orgasm most reliably and most intensively and forcefully by stimulation of the clitoris. Some normal women, who are capable of responding to intravaginal thrusting of the penis, prefer that method of reaching orgasm, at times. At other times, like "normal" people, they prefer other sexual activities. Some "normal" women regularly achieve orgasm from digital stimulation of the clitoris, but they never achieve orgasm from a penis or any other object's thrusting deeply or otherwise into their vaginas. Some very abnormal women, with a variety of diagnosable psychiatric disorders, are highly sexually responsive and orgasmic; other women, ostensibly very psychiatrically normal, are never or rarely responsive to sexual stimulation to the point of orgasm. Some nonorgasmic women enjoy sex; some orgasmic women do not. It is misleading and a disservice to those varied women to label them as pathological, immature, or any other pejorative term because their life experience fails to conform to Freud's hypothesis about female personality development. Freud based his ideas on a few cases, treated in psychoanalysis, not directly observed, with no more substantiation from empirical data than the repeated agreement of a series of his followers. Despite paying lip service to the impressive data of Kinsey, Masters and Johnson, and others, Dr. Clower seems to disregard the data and returns to her defense of ideas that Freud, a rigorously scientific empiricist, would probably have discarded long ago in the absence of supporting data.

At this point in our gathering of knowledge, there is still much more that we do not know than there are useful data. We have very little information about the social forces that inhibit or permit or perhaps encourage masturbation in women from infancy onward. We do not know at what age women are first able to experience orgasm, or what relationship that ability has to neuroendocrinological or neurophysiological status. We know that the potential for sexual responsiveness seems to reside in all humans, but that learning has to take place in order for sexual behavior to develop and become overtly expressed. Women and men learn to be sexually responsive, just as some learn to be unresponsive to sexual stimulation. The psychic stimuli that are effective in evoking responses are very clearly learned phenomena and vary tremendously from culture to culture and less widely, but still noticeably, among different individuals within a given culture.

Women usually experience orgasm first by masturbation. As a method of helping inorgasmic women to achieve sexual pleasure, teaching them to masturbate to orgasm has been extremely useful in clinical practice. Many women gain in confidence and motivation from their ability to experience orgasm by masturbation, and they then go on to learn how to respond to a partner's caresses, and commonly, but not as often as one would wish, they may become orgasmic through coital thrusting. The basic character structure and personality of these women do not change over the days, weeks, or months that they are learning to modify their sexual responses. The treatment that we employ is brief; usually, visits are spaced at weekly intervals and a course of treatment may comprise as few as 1 or 2 visits or up to 20 or more. Obviously, any human activity, including masturbation, may be pathological. One cannot fairly judge an act (like masturbation) or a sexual fantasy (such as one of being raped) out of the context of the whole life experience of the actor. In fact, judgment may be exactly what we should avoid. Understanding, based on an unbiased examination of observed data, is what we should strive to achieve.

The subject of sexual fantasy deserves some systematic consideration, and its customary association with masturbation suggests its consideration here. The relative power of psychic sexual arousal in comparison with tactile, physical stimulation has not been measured. Clinical observation supports the belief that psychological factors are a powerful influence on sexual arousal and responsiveness. Usually, we are concerned with the negative effects of psychological factors in suppressing desire, arousal, or responsiveness. Obviously, the effects of mental activity can also enhance sexuality, and sexual fantasy is the clearest example.

The symbols that our culture provides as exciters of sexual feeling are selected and determined in ways that we do not understand. What is sexually exciting varies from culture to culture and from place to place, as well as varying within a given culture from time to time. What we respond to as erotic or sexually arousing is a consequence of learning. Most people fantasize. The sexual socialization of women is still more inhibiting than of men. The result is that more women than men feel guilty about sexual fantasies or repress them more completely. Still, the majority of women respond to sexual fantasies with arousal, and overtly or covertly, women use fantasies to enhance sexual pleasure, in masturbatory activities as well as with partners.

The characteristics of women's fantasies are quite varied, yet some themes appear consistently and are used by many women. At the present level of our ignorance, we can only speculate about explanations. Women often fantasize themselves in situations where they are helpless, overwhelmed, and forced, seduced, or otherwise coerced into sexual activities that they find highly erotic. It is important to distinguish clearly between what is exciting in fantasy and what might be abhorrent if it were to occur in reality. Fantasies of being raped are examples of this phenomenon. A possible explanation for the arousing power of such a fantasy is that it allows women to enjoy sex without having to take the responsibility for initiating either the activity or their pleasure seeking. Since the culture's message is that women are not supposed to be sexually aggressive, the fantasy allows for pleasure and conformity to the cultural ideal, both at the same time. However, the role of women is changing rapidly, and it is increasingly common that women are more sexually aggressive, initiate activities, and experience erotic feelings from fantasies of being the sexual aggressor, the seductress, or the wanton, uninhibited lover. There is a strong link between what is forbidden and what may be arousing. What we are free to do is less exciting than what we should not or must not do.

The clinical relevance of sexual fantasies is in their application to the solution of sexual problems, particularly as clues to what may be erotic for a given individual. They can and are used to enhance arousal and responsiveness. They can also provide a fascinating window through which one can begin to see the nature of our culture's influences on our social and sexual development. In time, we may come to learn and perhaps control the sources of sexual excitement in our efforts to help people live enjoyably.

Chapter 9

The Misnamed Female Sex Organ

MILDRED ASH

INTRODUCTION

In every medical book on human anatomy, the female external genitals are called the *vulva*. Yet, the term *vagina* is almost universally used when the speaker refers to the pubic region of the girl or woman. Laypersons are not alone in making this error. Sex educators fail to teach the correct term. Professionals in the mental health field, including physicians, use the term *vagina* inappropriately. Lexicographers make errors revealing emotional reactions leading to intellectual confusion. In some instances among laypeople, the error is due to miseducation. However, I feel the conclusion is inescapable that the word *vulva* causes psychological discomfort. It is repressed by a substantial portion of the population, most significantly, a substantial portion of the professional population. Substituted for it is the name of an internal organ, the vagina. An examination of the practice of using the word *vagina* instead of *vulva* should reveal psychological problems related to female sexual anatomy and the anatomical differences between the sexes.

PARENTS CALL IT THE VAGINA

Embarrassed parents, unaccustomed to the use of medical terms and unable to be frank about sex, tend to limit their communication with a child by naming the fewest possible sex organs necessary to answer questions. With regard to the female genitals, the most obvious

---

MILDRED ASH, M.D. ● Psychiatrist and Psychoanalyst in Private Practice, Palo Alto, California.

need is to name the organ through which the baby passes from the uterus during the birth process and the organ that contains the penis during sexual intercourse.

The child's first question about sexual matters often is "Where does a new baby come from?" After being told that new life grows in the mother, the child asks, "How does the baby get out of the mother's body?" The parent answers, "The baby gets out through the vagina." The more sophisticated child becomes interested in how the process got started and is told something about seeds and Daddy. Of course, the next question is, "How does Daddy plant the seed?" The answer is "Daddy puts his penis in Mommy's vagina." It is easy to bypass the vulva when the child asks, "The boy has a penis; what does the girl have?" The parent answers, "The girl has a vagina." There is a correct aspect to this answer. When the child discovers that the sexes are not exactly alike, an assumption is made that there is complementarity. Penis and vagina are complementary organs—a fact that contributes to the error being discussed.

Often lay adults remain ignorant of the word *vulva*. When the parent supervises the little girl at her bath, the girl may be instructed to wash her peepee, down there, that, number one, or creasy. The list of euphemisms has by no means been exhausted. A Jewish patient reported that her external genitals were called *poopick*; since the same name was used at table for the chicken gizzard, she assumed the name for gizzard was applied to her genitals because of the similar configuration. That left her wondering what the real name of her genitals was. *Tushy*, a Yiddish diminutive for the Hebrew word for "bottom" (not "buttocks"), and the English word *bottom* are used frequently by parents for the buttocks of either sex. The meaning of *bottom* is often extended to include the external genitals of little girls. Health educator Rosalind Singer of the Albany, California, school system discovered during PTA meetings designed to acquaint the parents with the anatomical terms that would be taught their children, kindergarten through eighth grade, that parents were uniformly amazed that the female external genitals are not called the *vagina*. Lerner (1976) reported, "Many of these parents think the word vagina means both the internal and external genitals." Kestenberg (1968) quoted four-year-old Gigi, who complained, "My vagina hurts," and commented, " 'Modern' mothers, in their zeal to be enlightened parents, introduce this word for the female genital before the child is aware of her inner organ." Fraiberg (1972) has observed, "Little girls will use 'vagina' in global terms, referring to the entire genital region and including the urethra."

SEX EDUCATORS CALL IT THE VAGINA

What do sex education books teach young people? There is a beautiful book (Gordon and Gordon, 1974) from which one reads to children in the early grades: "If the baby has a vagina, it's a girl." The accompanying drawing of a naked girl shows her vulva!

A preschool teacher (Waxman, 1976) found it necessary to write a sex education textbook for her very young pupils. The genital differences are illustrated both by photographs of nude children and adults and by drawings made by very young children. On one left-hand page, the question "And, what is a girl?" is followed by a child's drawing on the right-hand page. A nub labeled *vagina* is added by the child artist onto the large circle composing the trunk. On the next page, left side, the question that I quoted above, "And, what is a girl?" is answered: "A girl is someone with a vagina." On the facing page is the photograph of a sturdy toddler standing proudly on a beach, her fat legs parted like a miniature Colossus of Rhodes to show her vulva. Above the photograph is the caption, "Every girl has a vagina." Of course, the girl's vagina is not visible. A subsequent photograph of a nude woman is preceded by the statement, "Every woman has a vagina." Since only the woman's pubic hair is visible, the author implies that region is named the vagina.

It is obvious from the foregoing that many laypeople use the incorrect term for the female external genitals because they have been misinformed by authoritative sources. What is visible is given the name of a hidden organ. Information that is available to anyone who looks at a medical textbook is not obtained. Behind the scenes are colleagues who have tested the teaching materials, and editors and publishers who have let this error go unchallenged. It is the exceptional textbook on sex that names the vulva. In their book for older children, Hofstein and Richmond (1967) included in their list of female genital organs, "The folds of skin and flesh at the opening constitute the vulva," and the vulva is labeled on the diagram. In the American Medical Association pamphlet (Lerrigo and Southard, 1970), all of the sexual parts are named as well as written phonetically to ensure correct pronunciation. Curiously, on the clearly labeled diagrams, the vulva is not indicated.

Even college-level textbooks manage to avoid using the word *vulva*. Beck (1969) described human development from birth through adulthood. His book includes such impressive chapter headings as "The Pituitary Gland at Puberty" and "Chromosomes, Genes and Heredity." X and Y chromosomes are explained, and DNA and RNA are discussed. The word *vulva* does not appear in the text or the glossary. In *Essentials of Life and Health* (1977), *vulva* does not appear in the text or the glossary. The word is avoided while the organ is described:

> Covering the vaginal opening are two soft, sensitive, wrinkled flaps of skin called labia minora, or smaller lips. Covering the labia minora are two broad, less sensitive, hair-covered folds of skin called labia majora.

Judging from this college-level material, we can see that the errors of omission or commission of the parents, teachers, and juvenile sex education books remain uncorrected for many students reaching college. It is a cause for wonder that the college-student population has society's permission for sexual activity, the use of contraceptives, and access to abortion but has not been allowed to learn the correct name of the female external genitals. It is the exceptional college textbook that names the vulva. Katchadourian (1972) clearly differentiated between what is visible and what is invisible under ordinary circumstances:

> The external genitalia of the female are known as the vulva, which means "covering," or the pudendum, which means "a thing of shame"! They include the major and minor lips, the clitoris, and the vaginal introitus, which is normally concealed from view.

Masters and Johnson (1966) did not use the word *vulva* in their trailblazing book, *Human Sexual Response*. In the chapter entitled, "The Female External Genitalia," the component parts are listed. The labia and other parts are minutely described. The clitoris has a chapter of its own, reflecting the complexity of this organ and its importance in the female sexual response. Here Masters and Johnson verified Kinsey's (1953) insistence that every female orgasm achieved by whatever means is a vaginal orgasm. In the chapter on the vagina, Masters and Johnson described their important discoveries: (1) the means by which the vagina becomes lubricated in response to sexual stimulation and (2) the manner in which the orgasmic platform develops at the distal third of the vagina. Surely, Masters and Johnson have no psychological blocks against the use of any anatomical term. I feel that their avoidance of the word *vulva* reflects its lack of acceptance by other sex educators, amply demonstrated above, and the sensitivity of Masters and Johnson to its absence from the vocabulary of the general public.

Nancy Friday (1977) probed the mother–daughter relationship more deeply and more correctly than most psychoanalysts can and do. Surprisingly, she not only failed to use the word *vulva* but also repeatedly used the word *vagina* when she meant *vulva*. For example, she referred to the pubescent girl who "wants hair on her vagina." She vehemently protested against women's ignorance of their genitals, again using the wrong word: "If you cannot call a vagina a vagina, you are in trouble with your own body." How could this educated, sophisticated, and psychologically courageous woman avoid learning the word *vulva*? How could the other authors quoted have avoided looking at a medical textbook on anatomy?

PROFESSIONALS IN THE MENTAL HEALTH FIELD CALL IT VAGINA

There are people who use the word *vagina* for *vulva* despite their required study of anatomy. Among those of my patients who have had training in medical terminology, most use the term *vagina* erroneously. For example, a woman marriage counselor described stimulating herself in childhood by rubbing near her clitoris. Her nursemaid interrupted this activity and cautioned her against danger of damage to "my vagina." In another instance, a male physician recounted an episode from his childhood when his mother emerged from the bathroom nude: "I saw my mother's vagina and I was frightened of all that dark hair." When questioned, both patients replied that *vagina* was the term for the external female genitals taught them by their parents. Obviously, professional training did not enable them to correct this error. To put it another way, they were more comfortable using the word approved by their parents. In childhood, the physician had consulted a dictionary for more information whenever he heard a new sexual term. When he found the derivation of vagina was the Latin word for sheath, he realized that beyond the "hole" he had seen in mutual exhibition games with little girls was a "tube." The average collegiate dictionary describes the vagina as an internal organ connecting the uterus with the outside of the body. The vulva is not always named in the definition of the vagina in dictionaries of the sort one might find in a home, depriving the child of a cross-reference to it. *Vulva* does appear as a separate entry.

Compilers of dictionaries of slang and obscene language can be diffident about sexual terms. The discrepancies in Wentworth and Flexner (1960) due to a shift in the definitions of the female external genitals reveal their discomfort. They define *hair pie*, "The vulva, esp. as considered the object of cunnilingus"; *dark meat*, "The vagina of a Negress"; and *white meat*, "The pudendum of a white woman." *Pudendum* and *vulva* are correct terms, while the word *vagina* in this series is wrong. Eric Partridge (1970) confessed in the preface of his dictionary:

> My role, in the matter of unpleasant terms, has been to deal with them as briefly, as astringently, as aseptically as was consistent with clarity and

and adequacy; in a few instances I had to force myself to overcome an in-
stinctive repugnance.

Although psychoanalysts regard the sight of the vulva as being
crucial to the personality development of children of both sexes, the
term *vulva* is rarely used in the literature. Castration anxiety is one of
the basic concepts of psychoanalytic theory and arises in part from the
recognition of the anatomical differences between the sexes. Discussions of castration anxiety occur, for example, around symbols for the
vulva that may appear in dreams such as of the cat and the spider.
Many real and fantasized genital qualities are symbolized by these
two creatures. The cat typifies the soft, furry feel of pubic hair as well
as the appearance of it. The cat also represents the primitive fear of
males that the vulva or the vagina can make quick movements, like a
cat catching and eating a mouse, to seize and consume the penis. The
slang word *snatch* incorporates this fear. The spider, visually frightening because of its many hairy legs and its quick movements, symbol-
izes the child's awe of female pubic hair. (One of my patients had a
frightening dream of a spider covered with red down; her mother had
red hair and red pubic hair.) Spiders also represent the dangers of
being stung or eaten, fears associated with the woman's "hole" (a
mouth) and emphasized so often by male homosexuals, who can never
forget that the female spider eats the male who fertilizes her.

In the psychoanalytic literature, we can find that professionals
who should know better use the word *vagina* in error. A typical example occurs in a paper by Carlson (1977). The male patient reports
part of a dream: "I saw her breasts and vagina." There is no comment
on this error, demonstrating that the use of the term *vagina* for what
one sees is so natural that it is not noted.

I was astonished when I watched Paul Mazursky's movie *Bob &
Carol & Ted & Alice* (1969) because the psychiatrist in the movie con-
fidently substituted the word *vagina* for Alice's euphemism (*teetee*) for
her vulva. Greenfield (1970), in an article about Paul Mazursky, author
of the screenplay, revealed that the actor who played the psychiatrist
is a real psychiatrist. This is another example demonstrating that professional education does not overcome psychological blocks in some
instances.

DISCUSSION

I have reviewed the curious absence of the word *vulva* from our
vocabulary. It remains unknown and unheard, unspoken in polite society, while the word *vagina* passes with almost as much ease as the

word *penis* into common use. The word *vulva* is not being taught to children early in life, so it cannot become acceptable as the word *penis* is. When and if the word *vulva* is learned, it is unpleasant to use, for it evokes fears of the little girl's lack of a penis as well as fear of the woman's impressive thatch of pubic hair hiding a mysterious opening. These reactions are uncomfortable and encourage repression of the correct name for the organ and the substitution of an incorrect name.

Why do women tend to prefer the word *vagina*? Apart from the sensitive clitoris, which until recently was ignored by parents, the vulva of the little girl is considered a "nothing" organ (Lewin, 1948; Abrams and Shengold, 1974), distinguished only by its lack of a penis. Mothers are eager to teach their daughters that they are identified as girls by a "something" organ, the vagina, as was noted by Lerner, Kestenberg, and Fraiberg.

Why do men tend to prefer the word *vagina*? Shapiro (1965) described what he called hysterical cognition as it applies to children when they are startled by their recognition of the anatomical differences between the sexes. Thinking back to the case of the male physician who insisted on using the word *vagina* for *vulva*, we can follow Shapiro's theory as it applies to boys. Shapiro feels that instead of really seeing that there is no penis on the girl and repressing that information, the boy instead avoids making a careful scrutiny of the little girl's external genitals. He quickly imagines something positive to replace what he experiences as the emptiness. It is this need for something to be where there is seemingly nothing that accounts for the persistence of the substitution of the word *vagina* for *vulva* among men.

In a paper noting the avoidance of the word *clitoris* and the absence of slang names for it, Blau (1943) theorized, "The absence of a word . . . may be indicative of a widespread process of repression." His point was that since the clitoris is the seat of sexual sensations in childhood, "This imperfection in language must indicate a form of cultural evasion." Blau attempted to explain why the clitoris was so ignored at the time he wrote his paper that it did not have any slang names and that even the scientific name was hardly used. He felt that children of both sexes are disturbed by what appearr to be an inadequate penis, that they repress knowledge of the clitoris, and that they fail to give it a name even when they grow up. Thus, unrecognized, the clitoris seems not to exist.

Similarly, the vulva undergoes a "cultural evasion" by being given the name of an internal genital organ, the vagina. Many laypeople are unaware of the word *vulva*. Professionals all too frequently use the vernacular *vagina* to denote the vulva. This misnaming contributes to difficulties in the personality development of the little girl. She cannot see her own genitals, while the boy can see much of his. Hers cannot be held in her hand in the satisfying way a boy can hold his. Nor is the mother's personal involvement and touching required (which gives the boy pleasure and implied permission to touch) when the little girl urinates as it is when the little boy first urinates standing up. Yes, she sits while he stands, and she cannot direct a discrete urinary stream so accurately. She gets intense pleasure from her clitoris, yet she is often disheartened by the difference between what is to her an invisible organ and the little boy's very visible penis.

Granted that it takes years for children to develop concepts to back up the words they learn for the girl's sexual parts: the vulva (with its labia), the clitoris, the vagina, the uterus, the Fallopian tubes, the ovaries, and the potential breasts. Respect for the girl's future development is communicated. Translation of the concepts into correct mental images for both boys and girls can begin with the proper naming of the parts. Obviously, this statement applies to the proper naming of all of the boy's sexual organs as well. We cannot prevent all of the psychological vicissitudes of childhood, but the frightening mystery about sex that handicaps the emotional and intellectual development of so many children (and adults) of both sexes can be to some extent prevented by the correct naming of the genitals.

REFERENCES

Abrams, S., and Shengold, L. The meaning of "nothing." *The Psychoanalytic Quarterly*, 1974, *43*, 115–120.

Beck, L. F. *Human growth*. New York: Harcourt, Brace & World, 1969.

Blau, A. A philological note on a defect in sex organ nomenclature. *The Psychoanalytic Quarterly*, 1943, *12*, 481–485.

Carlson, D. Dream mirrors. *The Psychoanalytic Quarterly*, 1977, *46*, 38–70.

Essentials of life and health (2nd ed.) New York: Random House, 1977.

Fraiberg, S. Genital arousal in latency girls. In R. S. Eissler, A. Freud, M. Kris, and A. J. Solnit (Eds.), *The psychoanalytic study of the child*, Vol. 27. New York: Quadrangle Books, 1972.

Friday, N. *My mother/my self*. New York: Delacorte Press, 1977.

Gordon, S., and Gordon, J. *Did the sun shine before you were born?* New York: Joseph Okpaku Publishing Co., 1974.

Greenfield, J. Paul Mazursky in wonderland. *Life Magazine*, September 4, 1970. Chicago: Time, Inc.

Hofstein, S., and Richmond, J. B. *The human story: Facts on birth and growth and reproduction*. New York: Scott, Foresman, 1967.

Katchadourian, H. *Human sexuality: Sense and nonsense*. Stanford, Calif.: Stanford Alumni Association, 1972.

Kestenberg, J. Outside, inside, male and female. *Journal of the American Psychoanalytic Association*, 1968, *16*, 457–520.

Kinsey, A. C., Pomeroy, W. B., Martin, C. E., and Gebhard, P. H. *Sexual behavior in the human female*. Philadelphia: W. B. Saunders, 1953.

Lerner, H. E. Parental mislabeling of female genitals as a determinant of penis envy and learning inhibitions in women. *Journal of the American Psychoanalytic Association*, 1976, *24*, 269–183.

Lerrigo, M. O., and Southard, H. *Parents' responsibility*. Chicago: American Medical Association, 1970.

Lewin, B. D. The nature of reality, the meaning of nothing, with an addendum on concentration. *The Psychoanalytic Quarterly*, 1948, *17*, 524–526.

Masters, H., and Johnson, V. *Human sexual response*. Boston: Little, Brown, 1966.

Mazursky, P. *Bob & Carol & Ted & Alice*. Burbank, Calif.: Columbia Pictures, 1969.

Partridge, E. *A dictionary of slang and unconventional English*. New York: Macmillan, 1970.

Shapiro, D. *Neurotic styles*. New York: Basic Books, 1965.

Waxman, S. *What is a girl? What is a boy?* Culver City, Calif.: Peace Press, 1976.

Wentworth, H., and Flexner, S. *Dictionary of American slang*. New York: Thomas Y. Crowell, 1960.

Chapter 10

Finding Self in the Lesbian Community

Barbara Ponse

Common sense usually assumes a direct relationship between sexual activity and identity. With reference to gay identity, some writers such as Simon and Gagnon (1966, 1967) and Barry Dank (1971) noted the influence of the gay community in providing strength and support for a transition from heterosexual identity to gay identity—thus acknowledging a period of incongruity between sexual activity on the one hand and sexual identity on the other. However, these writers assumed, as do other analysts of homosexuality, that there is a correspondence between identity and activity—albeit that there may be a delay in the acceptance of gay identity. My own study of identity in the Lesbian world is based on three years of fieldwork in both secretive Lesbian and political-activist Lesbian communities, conversations with hundreds of women in those communities, and 75 in-depth interviews. This study demonstrates that, indeed, there is no automatic or necessary correspondence between sexual activity and sexual identity, that the identity resolutions of women who relate sexually and emotionally to other women are diverse and problematic. (I am using the terms *identification* and *identity* to indicate *conscious* designations of the self as like another or as a member of a particular category.)

The women who participated in this study were identified generically as "women-related women," indicating women who currently have, have had, or anticipate having sexual–emotional relationships with other women, *regardless* of whether they define themselves as Lesbian, bisexual, gay, straight, or heterosexual, "sexual," or celibate. The term *women-related women* encompasses the above identifications

Barbara Ponse, Ph.D. • Psychotherapist in Private Practice, Los Angeles, California.

and yet allows new distinctions to be made among them, distinctions that derive from the experiences of the women they typically are used to name.

My purpose in this paper is to analyze the interrelationship of behavior, experience, and identity in the context of the ways in which women-related women make contact with lesbianism. Before an individual defines herself in any way related to lesbianism, she must first come into contact with—either abstractly or through direct association—persons who so define themselves (or who are so identified by others). Thus, she must make contact with the idea of lesbianism and share a set of meanings about her behavior and feelings with others. Second, she must see herself as fitting the description of lesbianism that she encounters. She must see a fit between her own biographical experiences and the biographical norms of the gay community. This article will explore the ways in which contacts between individual women and lesbianism typically take place and the identity resolutions that may eventuate from such contacts.

HIATUS IN IDENTITY

Women who experience themselves as not fitting the mold of heterosexuality may begin to define themselves in opposition to, or in contrast to, the heterosexual patterning around them. They may feel or believe that they are *not* like these heterosexual others and yet be without a clear notion of what it is they *are* like, thus creating a hiatus in identity. They may begin a search—conducted with greater or lesser intensity—for explanations or rationales that can terminate the identity hiatus.

THE SEARCH FOR IDENTITY

Women who say they had identified themselves as Lesbian prior to any contact with other Lesbians or Lesbian subcultures typically state that they had always experienced themselves as different from heterosexuals. This difference was experienced in several ways and with varying degrees of specificity. Some young women experienced themselves simply in oppositional terms, as *not* being interested in boys as they saw other young girls were. Others experienced a positive interest in girls accompanied by the perception that other young girls were interested in boys. In the absence of any information about a Lesbian interpretation of these feelings, these girls experienced a hiatus in self-identification that led them to search for a framework within which to interpret their feelings.

In his study of "coming out" in the male homosexual world, Dank (1971) supported the idea that the acknowledgment of gay identity often signifies the end of the search. This search may take the form of looking in the library for information—in novels or in psychiatric and psychological literature—or other such "disembodied" sources of contact with lesbianism. A woman in search of identity might look closely to her surrounding world for cues and explanations of herself.

Styles of Contacts with Lesbians and Lesbianism

There are three basic ways in which women may come into contact with Lesbians or lesbianism. These are, first, "disembodied" contact with the social category or idea of lesbianism; second, through contact with a particular partner in a couple relationship; and third, through contact with the Lesbian community.

Once she has information about lesbianism, an individual typically makes one of three types of conscious identity resolutions. First, she may identify herself as Lesbian positively and not accept the negative imagery as descriptive of herself. She would typically formulate new meanings of lesbianism. Second, she may identify negatively because of stereotypical meanings prevalent in our society. And third, she may feel that the category *Lesbian* does not pertain to her at all. The first type of resolution was most prevalent among the women I interviewed: these women identified with the category *Lesbian* but changed or modified the meaning of the category. Each of these three ways of handling a stigmatized identity will be considered in the discussion that follows.

Disembodied Contact. Contact with lesbianism in the absence of direct contact with a Lesbian group or community means that there must be access to sources of information about lesbianism. Disembodied access includes contact through literature or media presentations. Some women first "recognize" their own lesbianism through such disembodied contact. Such persons may call themselves Lesbians without being so designated by others and in the absence of contact with actual Lesbians or without sexual contact with other women. Women who come to identify themselves as Lesbian or homosexual before actually meeting any Lesbians, and prior to Lesbian relationships, usually do so in response to subjectively perceived feelings or attributes that they interpret as having Lesbian significance from what they have read and seen. Symbolic self-labeling as Lesbian through disembodied contact typically takes place in childhood or adolescence but may occur in adulthood as well. Among the women I interviewed, about 20% began to identify themselves as Lesbians at a very early age, during prepuberty or puberty, through such disembodied contact. Disembodied contact and identification in adulthood is more likely among women who are geographically isolated from the gay subculture.

Some women labeled themselves Lesbians when they came into contact with positive information about Lesbians, such as Sappho's poetry or European novels that portray Lesbians favorably. Such women may have developed a sense of connection with a noble Lesbian tradition as evidenced in the following recollection by a 78-year-old poet:

> You see, as I told you, I didn't have any educational advantages, and everything I've learned has been through reading—through associating with my kind of people. I think I was about seventeen when I first heard of Sappho, so naturally I read anything I could find about her. Lesbianism has an honorable tradition. It meant—someone who lived on Lesbos, the women who lived on Lesbos—a great many of whom were Sapphic. . . . *Lesbian* to me is a perfectly honorable and beautiful word and I like it. I've no objection to Lesbos being my spiritual home in a sense. (Tape-recorded interview)

The Well of Loneliness, a novel that has a Lesbian as its center character, has been frequently cited as a source of information through which some women came to identify themselves as Lesbians. Identification as Lesbian through reading this book was sometimes experienced as traumatic, as the following account illustrates:

> I read *The Well of Loneliness* and I knew I was Lesbian. I tried to kill myself. I thought, "Shit! Who wants this life?" (Tape-recorded interview)

For other women, however, reading the same book led to their identifying themselves as Lesbian with positive feelings about it. Such women changed the connotation of lesbianism for themselves.

Other women discovered the concept of lesbianism later in life. One woman came across *The Well of Loneliness* and the idea of lesbianism quite by accident. She had been married for many years and had never even heard about lesbianism. Reading this book started her on a search for other related material. She kept her Lesbian interests secret from her husband and her three children. After her husband died, she moved to another city, where she approached a gay organization, met a woman, and finally had her first Lesbian experience, 20 years after she made her initial identification:

> I picked up a book off the bookshelf, and I read *The Well of Loneliness.* That was the very first time—this is an orange book sitting here, and I picked it up, and I read it, and I said, "Well, what in the world do women want—to do together," 'cause I never had any concept. I knew of men, you know, so I didn't know what women did together. But the book was so fascinating,

and as I went along, I read it, and I began to feel some kind of desire, you know. . . . And I had three children, and I simply did not understand that, and I had a husband. As the years went along, we just drifted sort of apart, you know. We were getting older, I was getting older, and so was he. . . . Well, what I did was I started groping around in the bookstores and looking for literature. As the years passed, it was coming up, 'cause I never came upon anything like that. . . . So then I just really wanted to—it just got to be an obsession with me. I wanted to see what I could—find somebody that I could have that sort of relationship with. (Tape-recorded interview)

For yet other women, merely learning about the concept of lesbianism was definitive of their identities:

I first became aware of being different, loving, being attracted to other women when I was eight or nine years old, and it just wasn't some impulsive idea that went through my mind. It made such an impression on me that it became part of my identity. Somehow I knew, when I heard the word *homosexual* that that was me. At that young age, I didn't know anything about it. . . . For a while it didn't figure as important. I remember though, I was very intense, and some of my little girlfriends said, "You act like a boy." I was a tomboy, but they meant something else. (Tape-recorded interview)

Symbolic self-labeling as Lesbian through disembodied contact may involve ascribing masculinity to the self. Because of their sexual object choice and popular notions of Lesbians as masculine women, these women identify themselves not only as Lesbians but as "masculine" as well:

I guess I assumed that I would take the butch [masculine] role and proceeded to act in that fashion. I assumed I was masculine . . . an overgrown tomboy. My attitude toward it at that point had to be very stereotyped. It had to do with duck haircuts and leather jackets and all that stuff. . . . I was more masculine than feminine. . . . I considered myself as masculine. (Tape-recorded interview)

Later, following more extensive contact with the gay community, women like the one quoted above may conclude that lesbianism and masculinity are not necessarily linked.

Other women, who later come to identify themselves as Lesbians, initially handle the stigma associated with the category by rejecting the category as not fitting the self. As one woman expressed it, "They said homosexuality was sick; I knew I wasn't sick, so therefore I couldn't be a Lesbian." Such women reported that lesbianism might apply to them, but because of the images of sin and sickness, they would not accept it. Some of these women continued to experience themselves in a hiatus of identity. They felt that they did not fit in the heterosexual patterning of male–female relations but were unwilling to accept the alternative self-definition of Lesbian because of its negative implications. Others felt that their sexual and emotional experiences did not have identity implications and continued to assert that they were heterosexual. Yet others identified themselves as bisexual.

COUPLE RELATIONSHIPS. For many women, the critical event in beginning to identify as Lesbian was an emotional and sexual relationship with another woman. Some established such a relationship with prior knowledge about lesbianism; others had no prior knowledge about lesbianism.

Couple relationships, defined as emotional–sexual relationships between two women, can be considered under two principal types: isolated relationships that take place outside the Lesbian community, and those that take place in the context of community or in contact with specific groups in the Lesbian community. Couple relationships may be interpreted by participants as having or as not having implications for identity. In the latter case, such relationships are usually perceived as situational and temporary arrangements, or the gender of the partner is considered "coincidental" and unimportant. For others, sexual behavior *does* carry identity connotations.

ISOLATED COUPLES. Three general types of isolated-couples relationships can be identified as characteristic: (1) isolated young experimental couples; (2) isolated commitment to a unique relationship; and (3) Lesbian or homosexual contacts in the context of a heterosexual relationship. All three types generally carry the presumption of ignorance about Lesbians and lesbianism.

Type 1: Young Experimental Couples. Tripp (1975) stated that among young women or adolescents, where lack of information about homosexuality is most likely to occur, sexual contacts are often experienced by participants as a type of conformity. This observation is corroborated by the reported experiences of women in this study. Heterosexual socialization typically does not address the issue of lesbianism. In contrast, it emphasizes the taboo against premarital heterosexual activity, which may allow young girls to enter into relationships with one another not knowing of the homosexual significance of such relationships. The meaning given to these early same-sex experiences is contingent on the satisfactions that may or may not accrue to such relationships and their subsequent repetition in concert with learning the social meanings of sexual contacts with one's own sex. Such isolated relationships may lead to further experimentation with the same sex or they may not.

A woman currently engaged in an ongoing relationship with another women described how she interpreted her early experience with women and men:

> I think . . . I was 16 when I first got sexually involved for about four years on and off. . . . Then she came to college, we were in different sororities. . . . It really tapered off because she got interested in a guy who she married. . . . I never thought of homosexual as relating to women, only thought of it as related to men, and I really had no idea of what two women did together. Our sexual relationship we kept to ourselves, and I was more excited about it than anything else. I just thought it was a delicious secret. And at the same time, I had a mad crush on a guy. I didn't think of it as being anything weird. I just thought of it as being neat, really something terrific—I didn't feel sneaky. I just felt appropriate . . . I thought it was a unique thing we were doing. (Tape-recorded interview)

This woman did not view her early relationship as "Lesbian." She subsequently married, had children, and was reintroduced to relationships with women in a *menage à trois* with her husband about 15 years after her initial experience. She describes herself as basically heterosexual during that period of her life. Now, in an ongoing primary relationship with a woman, she views herself as bisexual.

In the absence of further couple relationships or contacts with the Lesbian subculture, isolated experimental relationships may be experienced as a "phase," a part of the heterosexual developmental process. For other women, such relationships may lead to a continuing interest in relationships with women. A third possibility, more characteristic of the women I interviewed, is that these earlier relationships come to be reinterpreted in the light of later experience as precursors to Lesbian identity, which may have been unrecognized at the time.

Type 2: Commitment to a Unique Relationship. Isolated commitments to a unique relationship differ in intensity and duration from young experimental relationships. However, like young experimental relationships, a long-term commitment to a same-sex relationship may or may not have implications for identity in the absence of contact with the Lesbian community. The definitive factor in determining identity implications is whether the relationship is perceived by the participants as a unique and situational relationship in which the gender of the participants is perceived as incidental (that is, the person, rather than the gender, is stressed) or whether the relationship is seen as an expression of a thoroughgoing preference.

Generally speaking, women in ongoing, unique relationships that originate outside the Lesbian community will, slowly and over time, begin to label themselves Lesbian symbolically through making contact with other Lesbians. Precisely because of their isolation and lack of social validation in the heterosexual community, couples may eventually begin to seek out others like themselves:

> I still think that if X had been a man, I would still love her. . . . I never felt sexually different from other women. X and I are pretty much loners, and except for a few people we keep looking for, that we can have really good friendships with, we're destined to stay that way. We were together for seven years before we met any gay people. . . . It came to the point where we wanted to acknowledge ourselves as a couple, and that was part of the reason we became involved in gay groups. (Tape-recorded interview)

Lesbian identity, then, may follow Lesbian behavior by many years. Indeed, Lesbian identity and Lesbian associations may be adopted not because of a perceived connection between identity and sexual behavior but because of the need for an accepting milieu.

Type 3: In the Context of Heterosexual Relationships. Individual contacts with lesbianism, isolated from the Lesbian community, may occur within heterosexual relationships.

> My husband and I got involved with another couple, and actually my husband got involved with this woman . . . and the two couples spent a lot of time together and so the four of us, actually the four of us got sexually involved with each other . . . so we would have foursomes. That way I could be with her [the wife] sort of. And she didn't relate to me exclusively. She related mostly to my husband. I used my husband as a vehicle to get to her, and, at the same time, I think I used her to get to him. (Tape-recorded interview)

If, in such relationships, emphasis remains on the heterosexual relationship and the Lesbian relationship is seen as secondary, the likelihood is that the women involved will continue to think of themselves as heterosexual. If, however, the relationships become equally important, the women participants may come to define themselves bisexual. The third possibility is that a relationship may bring about a reevaluation of the self and facilitate identification as Lesbian.

LESBIAN SEXUAL ACTIVITIES AS AN AVENUE OF IDENTIFICATION

Sexual activities between women are implicit in the discussion of dyadic relationships. However, there is no necessary correspondence between particular sexual activities and affiliation with the category *Lesbian*. Sexual activities between women should be understood in relation to the *meanings* these experiences have for the women involved. If women experience fulfillment and satisfaction in relationship to each other, such relationships may be the fulcrum of identity; however, it should not be assumed that sexual activity has specific or unidirectional implications for identity.

The study showed that women-related women did not talk graphically about their actual sexual activities. Rather, emphasis was on the *quality* of relationships between women. They described mutuality and closeness, particularly emotional closeness. This emphasis in describing intimate relationships is not substantially different from the way that heterosexual women talk about their intimate relationships: they do not routinely talk in explicit sexual details about their experiences but also tend to talk about the quality of relationships. Klaich (1974) similarly found that most of the women-related women she interviewed did not refer directly to their sexual activities.

The respondents in this study reported various individual preferences regarding sexual activities. They said that mutual satisfaction was more important than any specific technique. Some expressed a preference for manual penetration and manipulation; others preferred oral–genital sex; more preferred to combine these techniques. Yet others preferred tribadism, or simultaneous genital stimulation. Regardless of the particular sexual practices engaged in, none of these appeared to be a *sine qua non* of a Lesbian identification. In sum, the respondents engaged in a wide variety of sexual behavior with other women and identified themselves in a variety of ways—as Lesbian, as bisexual, or as heterosexual.

For the women I studied, engaging in sexual activity with another woman was only infrequently reported as the basis for identification as Lesbian. In fact, isolated-couple relationships among women were often not conceived of as Lesbian relationships at all. Thus, it would appear that homosexual activity does not unequivocally lead to Lesbian identity.

Community Contacts and Identity

Prior to having come to a Lesbian resolution of their own identities, women in the Lesbian community are likely to experience both covert and overt subcultural pressures toward adopting a Lesbian identity.

Individual or couple contact with the Lesbian community presupposes some knowledge of the community and is usually accomplished in one of four ways: (1) friends within heterosexual networks who reveal themselves as being Lesbian or gay; (2) a mutual interest in feminist issues; (3) gay bars or gay meeting places; and (4) gay activism or politics. Overt Lesbian groups are more accessible to the novice than are secretive groups and may be sought out by women who are tentatively exploring the idea of lesbianism, as well as by individuals who have already symbolically labeled themselves as Lesbian.

GAY FRIENDS IN HETEROSEXUAL GROUPS. For some women who eventually become part of the Lesbian community, contact with gay people takes place within the context of heterosexual groups. Gay persons may be openly gay in these groups, but more typically they pass for straight. The disclosure of gay identity to the "potentially" gay person may occur for social reasons or within the context of an intimate relationship.

Contacts with gay people in the heterosexual world may be the occasion for entry into the gay life for the potentially gay woman and may result in more extensive contacts with the gay community. These contacts and relationships may continue over time within the context of the heterosexual community, or initial contacts with other gay people in straight settings may lead to affiliation with the Lesbian community.

CONTACTS WITH LESBIANISM THROUGH FEMINISM. The feminist movement spans both the heterosexual and the Lesbian worlds and sometimes provides an avenue of contact with lesbianism and Lesbians for the potentially gay woman. Contacts with the feminist Lesbian community may be the occasion for solidifying a commitment to a Lesbian identity for women who were previously identified as bisexual or heterosexual as well as for those who had previously made an identification as being Lesbian.

For some women, the women's movement served to change the meaning of the category from negative to positive and to promote identification with that category:

> I was thirteen years old when I had my first experience [with a woman]. I had no category for it at that time. I was involved in religion, and what I was doing had to be the A Number One Sin! And in addition to that, the very person who brought me out wouldn't even dare say the word *gay* or *Lesbian* or whatever. We were just different and meant to be together. It was very, very oppressive. It was so difficult for me . . . to get over the feeling that I was what everybody said I was: scum of the earth, perverted, sick—myself—that's what really drove me over the edge—the terrific conflict of knowing that I really was okay, and I was right, and I had a perfect right to be however I was, and it was a tremendously important aspect of my life to me, and yet I wanted other people to like me. I really wanted acceptance. We would avoid any people we thought were gay; we would never know, of course, because we'd never say anything, and they would never ask anything. The most important thing for me in accepting myself was getting involved with the movement—seeing people who had their heads up—it was so important to me—it gave me pride. In the closet, I was very, very fragmented. Now I feel like I have sisters instead of just having acquaintances. (Tape-recorded interview)

Thus, the women's movement may facilitate access to the Lesbian world and may be the framework for initial experimentation with Lesbian relationships. Contact with the Lesbian community through feminism may serve to support a tentative self-definition as Lesbian and be the source of positive meanings of Lesbian identity.

SEEKING THE LESBIAN COMMUNITY. It should be emphasized that finding the community can be very difficult indeed, particularly for the isolated gay woman. Gaining entry into a Lesbian friendship network is sometimes dependent on meeting people in straight settings and establishing trusting relationships with them.

Some women actively seek out the community after having become aware of the social category of Lesbian and after having labeled themselves Lesbian. Other women make a tentative identification with the social category or simply want to investigate gay life and themselves in relation to it. I would concur with Simon and Gagnon (1969) that emotional–romantic relationships usually precede the overt sexual aspects of relationships among women. However, some women do set about seeking the community in order to make sexual contact:

> I was ready, I went to my first gay bar all by myself to meet other women. I was a minister's wife. I didn't even drink. I was scared shitless. I was so scared. My rationalization before going into the bar was that if there were any men in there, they wouldn't want to have anything to do with me, and if there were any women who wanted to do anything to me, I'm sure it can't be anything that I haven't done in my head. Because I had been suffering for two years because I was trying to conform to something I just couldn't get into. So my initial feeling was one of great excitement, because I knew I wasn't going to be alone and I thought if I'm going to go to hell I might as well have a good time doing it. I was actively seeking a relationship with a woman. . . . I'd gone into the bar thinking I would sleep with someone that night because I felt Lesbians were really into sex. But it wasn't that easy; I had to go again to meet someone who wanted to be with me, and it didn't matter who she was or what she was, she was a woman, right? I wasn't falling in love, I was really into meeting a woman. It turned out she was a butch—we spent some time together before we finally got to bed. And I was into my aggression. I really wanted a woman. It was two years of pent-up emotion. (Tape-recorded interview)

Gay bars are a relatively accessible avenue of contact with the Lesbian community and frequently provide normalizing experiences for newly identified Lesbians. Bar contacts also may provide contacts with friendship networks in the community. In addition to gay bars, access to parts of the Lesbian community has been provided in recent years by gay organizations and feminist groups.

Gay organizations derive from a variety of concerns with gay life. These include educating the public and providing social services to gay clientele. Whatever their stated purpose is, these organizations serve as an avenue to the gay subculture. For some women, gay organizations provide the initial introduction to the life of the Lesbian community. As the following example illustrates, the gay organization may serve as a clearinghouse for information about various special gay groups in the community. The following account refers to the Daughters of Bilitis (DOB). Founded by Del Martin and Phyllis Lyon in 1956, it is the oldest Lesbian organization in the country. Some of its many purposes are education, providing an alternative meeting place to the gay bar, and altering the public image of the Lesbian. The following account is from the woman quoted earlier who had come upon the idea of lesbianism through reading *The Well of Loneliness*. She subsequently sought to find the Lesbian community through contacting the DOB:

> R: Somewhere along the line I read about the DOB, and on a late-night interview I saw this woman from the organization. And she spoke about the DOB. Well, that never left my mind. . . . But I had seen it in a newspaper that it would be on TV and I stayed up and watched it. So we had come here to visit, and one of the first things I did was I looked in the telephone book and found the DOB, and my husband was with me when they [Lesbian activists] were having a march down by the city hall there, and they were all gathered up there, and there were all the signs . . . and I said, "Oh boy, what's going on here? Let's stop and go see!" (*Laughter*) Somebody in the car said, "Oh, that's those women," you know. And I said, "Well, I'm interested. I'd like to know what they—what it's all about." But anyway they wouldn't stop and it just stayed in my mind from then on—that one day I'd go back to San Francisco where I could really be free and find out. And so that's what I did. The first thing I did—it took me about six months. I'd go every other week or so, and sometimes I'd just pass it five times in one night. (*Laughter*.) And I'd go down the street a little farther, and then I'd come back and I'd stand at the door, and I'd say, "Well, just go in." And then I'd say no. I can't go in there. And then I'd get on the bus and I'd come home. And I'd do it again and again. And finally I said, "Well, I'm going in here tonight," and I did. . . . Once I went in there, all I could see was just young kids. They were nice and friendly and accepting, but they were young. I asked if there was any older group . . . and she said yes and gave me a telephone number. Anyway, after I did that that night, well, it took me another month to call, and I did call. And in the conversation, she told me there was a group of women who called themselves SOL—Slightly Older Lesbians—and she gave me a telephone number . . . and then in the conversation I asked her—this is going to sound awful—anyway I asked her where or was there somebody that she could recommend to me for counseling, you know, because I had begun to feel that maybe I'm nuts, you know.
>
> I: What made you think you were nuts?
>
> R: Well, here I am. I was way past fifty, and I'd never done anything like it before, and I knew none of my family to be oriented this way. (*Laughter*.)

Contact with the social category *Lesbian*, with gay people, or with the gay subculture may take place in different ways, but it may ultimately raise the issue of personal sexual identification. Identity—the response to the question "Who am I?"—looks to the data of personal history and experience for an answer. The most personal level of experience, the experience of the self over time, shifts and changes according to present demands. Reconstructed biography is used to support and sustain a current identity status. It may demonstrate that one's identity is grounded in the past and that it makes sense in terms of the past. On the other hand, biography may be used to demonstrate that one is not the person whom others think her to be. Before going into these specific uses of biography in the personal historical level of affiliation with lesbianism, I shall define *biography* as I am using the term here.

BIOGRAPHY. Though the term *biography* is usually used to indicate the sum or sequence of events over the lifetime of an individual, my use of this term is more specialized and has three main features: reconstruction, reinterpretation, and continuity.

All biographies, especially autobiographies, are *reconstructions* of the past on the basis of present demands, interests, problems and questions. Biographical reconstruction involves culling out events and experiences from one's life and shaping these into an ordered sequence organized with respect to present purposes.

Reconstruction is to be distinguished from *reinterpretation*. With biographical reinterpretation, current meanings given to previous life experiences are different from the meaning of those life experiences at the time they happened. Current meanings are superimposed on past events in such a way that these events are now seen as always having pointed to the present state of affairs. Thus, reinterpretation of biography implies a reformulated and superimposed *consistency* and *congruence* of personal history, creating a consistency between past and present as the basis of the current identity, and demonstrating congruence between past and present identities and actions. What is to be included in a biography as well as the meanings imposed on biographical events depends on the present frame of reference. Individuals assess, reassess, and reformulate their biographies in such a way that their present seems continuous with the emergence from the past. They attribute importance to events in personal histories in such a way that they become congruent with present truths.

Within the Lesbian world, three modes of biographical reconstruction result in three different resolutions of identity. The first is the *primary Lesbian*, who presents in her biographical reconstruction an actual continuity of experience. She has had a consistency of identity throughout her life, which is manifested in such statements as "I was always that way." The second mode of biographical reconstruction characterizes what I designate the *elective Lesbian*. She reinterprets discontinuous life experiences so that they demonstrate a true, underlying Lesbian identity. The third mode characterizes women-related women who have *idiosyncratic identities* and some who have Lesbian identities. They are not concerned with biographical continuity and consequently have no strain toward biographical reinterpretation. Their reconstructed biographies lack the reinterpreted continuity found in accounts of elective lesbians.

Primary Lesbians. The following, typical of the biographical statements of primary lesbians, illustrates the congruence between biographical reconstruction and gay biographical norms as well as continuity between past and present identities:

> I first fell in love with a woman when I was about fifteen or sixteen. I fell in love with a woman who was about a year older. I don't know whether I used the term Lesbian then; I knew that I loved a woman, and that was where I was and where I wanted to be. I didn't fall in love with men. I don't dislike or hate men, whether homosexual or otherwise. I've had many more men friends in my early life, and I have all my life, than Lesbian friends. It just happened that way in my work, I guess. It was not difficult—it was far from being difficult for me to accept myself as a Lesbian. It was a joyous thing. I like the way women look. I like women as people, and I wanted to have women as lovers and I love women. (Tape-recorded interview)

This woman was unique in having a bohemian, artistic group of friends and a family who admired her for her artistic achievements as well as for her personal qualities. They were reportedly unconcerned about her sexuality. She was therefore not subjected to the pressures about her lesbianism that many Lesbians report.

Elective Lesbians. The elective Lesbian generally comes to identify herself as a Lesbian at a later time in her life than does the primary Lesbian. She may do this during her 20s, 30s, 40s, or even 50s. She has had heterosexual experiences, often extensive ones. And she usually has had a heterosexual identity prior to her identification as a Lesbian. She may also have had a bisexual identity.

The distinguishing features of the biographical reconstructions of the elective Lesbian are, first, a discontinuous or "mixed" history of sexual–emotional relationships (often heterosexual experiences followed by homosexual experiences) and, second, an imposition of continuity of meaning through retrospective reinterpretation. The elective Lesbian reviews her heterosexual past and finds it fraudulent, obscuring her true Lesbian nature.

For example, a 52-year-old woman who had been heterosexually married and so identified for 22 years has identified herself as Lesbian for the past three years. In talking about how she came to relate to women, she reflected on her past and found evidence of lesbianism in her early childhood:

> I began at this point to become involved with women's consciousness-raising groups, and I began to hear . . . of the idea of women being turned on to each other. It was the first time I heard about it in terms of people that I knew. . . . I met a woman who said in a workshop: "Well, there are older women who are finding other options for themselves." . . . I was receptive, but there was no previous, immediate history. . . . To think of it in terms of an older woman saying it was very exciting to me. . . . And then, of course, when that happened I got in touch with my own background and remembered that I had had these kinds of thoughts as a high school kid, that I had had two small sexual experiences with women, and both were cases where I had touched their breasts. And there was a period in my all-girls' high school where I had worn men's shirts, and my mother was so scared by it that she took me to my social worker aunt to get me straightened around. (Tape-recorded interview)

Biographical accounts of elective Lesbians reflect a basic discontinuity in their identities and the content of their life events that is resolved by reinterpreting events that are perceived as incongruous with Lesbian identity and by selectively recounting events compatible with Lesbian identity.

Idiosyncratic Identities. The biographies of a number of women-related women in the Lesbian community do not fit with gay biographical norms. These women do not strive to approximate a continuous Lesbian past. Some identify themselves as Lesbians though they identified themselves as heterosexual in the past. These women do not see lesbianism as an essential identity, and they experience their identification as Lesbian in terms of a "conversion" or a change: "I used to be heterosexual, now I'm a Lesbian." Or they call themselves Lesbian only while they engage in Lesbian lifestyles and relationships. They see Lesbian identity as situated and temporary. Still other women, despite the fact that they are engaged in what they describe as meaningful Lesbian relationships and are affiliated with the Lesbian subculture, remain obdurate in identifying themselves as heterosexual, bisexual, or just plain "sexual."

Though fewer in number than either primary or elective Lesbians, and in the face of many pressures to assume Lesbian identity, these women do not identify as Lesbian. Their biographical reconstructions exhibit a discontinuity in their sexual–emotional lives as well as an apparent lack of strain toward continuity. These women do not draw the identity conclusion that would ordinarily be drawn by both heterosexual and Lesbian worlds.

The woman quoted below is currently involved in a long-term relationship with a woman. Although she uses the term *gay* to de-

scribe some of her relationships, she has also had several emotional–
sexual relationships with men.

> It feels to me that bisexual is essentially what I am. I must be bisexual—
> that's how I've lived my life. I don't just relate to women; I have not just
> related to women. Although I'm with a woman now, for a long period of
> my lifetime I was relating just to men. And sexually that's been most of my
> life. . . . Right now I'm not having any relationship with a man, but I cer-
> tainly have the proclivity for it. I don't think of myself or my friends as
> Lesbians. They just seem to me like people who just love one another. And
> that almost seems accidental. And for me also. That is my most comfortable
> view of the whole thing, that it is really accidental . . . and it's just where
> you happen to find yourself and who you happen to be turned on to.
> (Tape-recorded interview)

Women-related women with idiosyncratic identities, then, continue to stress the circumstantial, accidental, and situated features of
their Lesbian relationships.

Women who make these three types of identity resolutions conceive of lesbianism differently. Whether it is seen as determined or as
a choice relates in part to rhetorics available in the Lesbian world. The
idea of lesbianism as a choice is relatively recent.

The primary type typically sees lesbianism as an orientation or
condition that informs the whole character of herself. While elective
Lesbians may come to view lesbianism as a condition or an orientation, they are more likely to use the term *preference* with respect to
their sexual–emotional behavior. Though elective Lesbians attribute
an essentiality to lesbianism (as does the primary Lesbian), unlike
primary Lesbians they see lesbianism as a voluntary choice.

Women-related women who have idiosyncratic identities, on the
other hand, may hold that lesbianism is the essential, pivotal feature
of the identities of other women. However, lesbianism describes only
an *aspect* of themselves or refers to situated and circumstantial behavior that does not have identity implications.

ETIOLOGICAL ACCOUNTS. Primary and elective Lesbians propose
different etiological, or causal, accounts for lesbianism. The primary
lesbian is most likely to offer a genetic or hormonal theory. Such an
explanation ignores the heterosexuality (and the children) of other
Lesbians. However, primary Lesbians typically formulate lesbianism
in such a way as to exclude the possibility of heterosexuality.

The elective Lesbian holds similar beliefs about the etiology of
lesbianism, regarding its naturalness, its inborn quality, and its place
in the world. However, she must explain a heterosexual past while
maintaining the essentiality of lesbianism. This requirement involves

positing different levels of reality, the most apparent of which is not the most real. Consequently, the elective Lesbian is likely to maintain that her heterosexual past was not "really" pertinent. Reality is attributed to fantasy life or to the previously unrealized character of the self. The elective Lesbian may state that she was not acting in accord with her real feelings when she led a heterosexual lifestyle.

The etiological accounts of lesbianism from the perspective of women-related women who have idiosyncratic identities have greater applications to others than they do to the women themselves. That is, these women may hold the belief that lesbianism is an essential quality of the self for those whom they term "real Lesbians" and may posit a genetic, hormonal, or social learning theory with reference to others. However, the woman with an idiosyncratic identity would focus on the personal and idiosyncratic qualities of relationships, regardless of the gender of her partner:

> I guess you might say I'm person-oriented, as opposed to being heterosexual or homosexual. I personally can't relate to the idea of being only with women or only with men. It depends on the person. One of the most important love relationships of my life was with a man, and I can only say that I would be with [my lover] whether she was a man or a woman. It is her as a person that I love. It doesn't matter to me what sex a person is, but what kind of person they are. (Tape-recorded interview)

The idiosyncratically identified woman tends to discount considerations of etiology with respect to her own behavior and identity. Her own involvement in Lesbian relationships is accounted for more in terms of attraction to a particular personality, though she may well express deep commitment to her relationship with women. It should be noted that the idiosyncratically identified woman, like the primary and the elective Lesbian, is influenced by the negative and pejorative connotations attached to Lesbian behavior and may have gone through a period of questioning whether or not the label *Lesbian* or *homosexual* applied to her.

Most of the women in this study presented reconstructions of their lives that were in conformity with the biographical norms of the community. A number of women, however, conformed neither to the identity rules nor to the biographical norms of the community. Identity resolutions are possible only through learning the social meanings attributed to behaviors and persons. But, as illustrated, this fact by no means necessitates a perfectly isomorphic relation between personal identity and available definitions. The individual is not only acted upon but acts and, in so doing, may accept, reject, refine, synthesize, or even fundamentally change the meanings of self and world.

REFERENCES

Becker, H. S. *Outsiders, Studies in the sociology of deviance.* New York: Free Press, 1963.

Berger, P. L., and Luckmann, T. *The social construction of reality.* Garden City, N.Y.: Doubleday/Anchor, 1967.

Blumer, H. *Symbolic interactionism: Perspective and method.* Englewood Cliffs, N.J.: Prentice-Hall, 1969.

Blumstein, P. W., and Schwartz, P. *Lesbianism and bisexuality,* unpublished manuscript, University of Washington, 1974.

Brecher, E. History of human sexual research and study. In A. M. Freedman, H. I. Kaplan, and B. J. Sadach (Eds.), *Comprehensive textbook of psychiatry,* Vol. 2, Baltimore: Williams & Wilkins, 1975, pp. 1352–1357.

Caprio, F. S. *Female homosexuality, A psychodynamic study of lesbianism.* New York: Citadel Press, 1954.

Chesler, P. Patient and patriarch: Women in the psychotherapeutic relationship. In V. Gornick and B. K. Moran (Eds.), *Women in a sexist society.* New York: Basic Books, 1971, pp. 362–392.

Dank, B. Coming out in the gay world. *Psychiatry,* May 1971, *34,* 180–197.

Douglas, J. D. *American social order.* New York: Free Press, 1971.

Emerson, J. Nothing unusual is happening. In T. Shibutani (Ed.), *Human Nature and Collective Behavior.* Englewood Cliffs, N.J.: Prentice-Hall, 1970, pp. 208–222.

Freud, S. *Collected papers,* Vol. 2. New York: Basic Books, 1959.

Freud, S. The psychology of women. *New introductory lectures of psychoanalysis.* New York: Norton, 1933, pp. 153–185.

Freud, S. *Three essays on the theory of sexuality,* J. Strachey (trans.). New York: Basic Books, 1962.

Gagnon, J. H., and Simon, W. *Sexual deviance.* New York: Harper & Row, 1967.

Glaser, B., and Strauss, A. Awareness context and social interaction. *American Sociological Review,* 1964, *29,* 669–678.

Goffman, E. *Stigma. Notes on the management of spoiled identity.* Englewood Cliffs, N.J.: Prentice-Hall, 1963.

Goffman, E. *The presentation of self in everyday life.* Garden City, N.Y.: Doubleday, 1959.

Gordon, C. Self conceptions: Configurations of content. In C. Gordon and K. J. Gergen (Eds.), *The self in social interaction classic and contemporary perspectives,* Vol. 1. New York: John Wiley & Sons, 1968, pp. 115–137.

Hall, Radclyffe. *The Well of Loneliness,* New York: Covici, Friede. 1928.

Hooker, E. The adjustment of the male overt homosexual. In M. Ruitenbeek (Ed.), *The problem of homosexuality of modern America.* New York: E. P. Dutton, 1963, pp. 141–161.

Hopkins, J. H. The Lesbian personality. *British Journal of Psychiatry,* 1969, *115,* 1433–1436.

Hunphreys, L. *Out of the closets. The sociology of homosexual liberation.* Englewood Cliffs, N.J.: Prentice-Hall, 1972.

Humphreys, L. *Tearoom trade, impersonal sex in public places.* Chicago: Aldine, 1970.

Johnson, J. *Lesbian nation. The feminist solution.* New York: Simon & Schuster, 1973.

Katz, J. Deviance, charisma, and role-defined behavior. *Social Problems,* 1972, *20,* 187–202.

Katz, J. Essence as moral identities: Verifiability and responsibility, in imputations of deviance and charisma. *American Journal of Sociology,* 1975, *80,* 1369–1390.

Klaich, D. *Woman + woman. Attitudes toward lesbianism.* New York: William Morrow, 1974.

Larkin, J. Coming out: "My story is not about all Lesbians." *Ms.*, 1976, *9*, 72, 84, 86.

Leif, H. I. Introduction to sexuality. In A. M. Freedman, H. I. Kaplan, and B. J. Sadock, (Eds.), *Comprehensive textbook of psychiatry*, Vol. 2. Baltimore: Williams & Wilkins, 1975, pp. 1349–1352.

Lemert, E. *Human deviance, social problems, and ·social control.* Englewood Cliffs, N.J.: Prentice-Hall, 1976.

Lofland, J. *Analyzing social setting.* Belmont, Calif.: Wadsworth, 1971.

Lofland, J. *Deviance and identity.* Englewood Cliffs, N.J.: Prentice-Hall, 1969.

Lyman, S. M., and Scott, M. B. *A sociology of the absurd.* New York: Appleton-Century-Crofts, 1970.

McCall, G., and Simons, J. L. *Identities and interactions.* New York: Free Press, 1966.

McIntosh, M. The homosexual role. *Social Problems*, 1968, *16*, 182–192.

Marmor, J. *Sexual inversion: The multiple roots of homosexuality.* New York: Basic Books, 1965.

Martin, D., and Lyon, P. *Lesbian/woman.* New York: Bantam Books, 1972.

Mills, C. W. Situated actions and vocabularies of motives. In J. G. Morris and B. N. Meltzer (Eds.), *Symbolic interaction, A reader in social psychology,* (2nd ed.). Boston: Allyn & Bacon, 1972, pp. 393–404.

Money, J., and Ehrhardt, A. A. *Man & woman, boy & girl: The differentiation and dimorphism of gender identity from conception to maturity.* Baltimore: The Johns Hopkins University Press, 1972.

Ponse, B. *Identities in the Lesbian world: The social construction of self.* Westport, Conn.: Greerwood Press, 1978.

Ponse, B. Secrecy in the lesbian world. *Urban Life,* October 1976, *5* (3).

Raphael, *Coming out, The emergence of the movement Lesbian,* Ph.D. dissertation, Department of Sociology, Case Western Reserve University, Cleveland, Ohio, 1974.

Rosen, D. M. *Lesbianism, A study of female homosexuals.* Springfield, Ill.: Charles C Thomas, 1974.

Rule, J. *Lesbian images.* Garden City, N.Y.: Doubleday, 1975.

Schutz, A. *Collected papers. Studies in social theory,* Vol. 2, Arnid Broderson (Ed.). The Hague: Martinus Nijhoff, 1971.

Shelley, M. Gay is good. In K. Jay and A. Young (Eds.), *Out of closets. Voices of gay liberation.* New York: A Douglas Book, 1972, p. 34.

Simmel, G. *The sociology of Georg Simmel,* K. H. Wolff (trans. and ed.). New York: The Free Press, 1950.

Simon, W., and Gagnon, J. H. Femininity in the Lesbian community. *Social Problems,* 1966, *14*, 212–221.

Simon, W., and Gagnon, J. The Lesbians: A preliminary overview. In J. Gagnon and W. Simon (Eds.), *Sexual deviance.* New York: Harper & Row, 1967.

Simon, W., and J. Gagnon, J. H. On psychosexual development. In D. A. Goslin (Ed.), *Handbook of socialization theory and research.* Chicago: Rand McNally, 1969.

Strauss, A. *Mirrors and masks.* New York: Free Press, 1959.

Szasz, T. S. *The myth of mental illness.* New York: Harper & Row, 1961.

Tripp, C. A. *The homosexual matrix.* New York: McGraw-Hill, 1975.

Warren, C., and Johnson, J. A criticism of labeling theory from the phenomenological perspective. In R. A. Scott and J. D. Douglas (Eds.), *Theoretical perspectives in deviance.* New York: Basic Books, 1972.

Warren, C. *Identity and community in the gay world.* New York: Wiley Interscience, 1974.

Warren, C. *Labeling theory: The individual, the category, and the group,* unpublished manuscript, University of Southern California, 1976.

Warren, C. Observing the gay community. In J. D. Douglas (Ed.), *Research on deviance.*
New York: Random House, 1972, pp. 139–163.

Warren, C. The use of stigmatizing social labels in conventionalizing deviant behavior.
Sociology and Social Research, 1974, *58,* 303–311.

Warren, C. Women among men: Females in the male homosexual community. *Archives
of Sexual Behavior,* 1976, *5,* 156–175.

Discussion of Chapter 10

Random Comments

B. F. RIESS

{EDITOR'S NOTE

Homosexual behavior belongs in a volume on women's sexual life, since there are women who are not defined by themselves or by others as Lesbian but nevertheless have had homosexual experience. Many, perhaps most, defined Lesbians, on the other hand, have had considerable heterosexual experience, including marriage, and a substantial number have had children. These data are important in emphasizing the variability and changeability of object choice in women as compared with gender identity, which appears to be much less subject to discordance in women than in men. In their sexual identity and behavior, women are neither mirror images nor copies of men; they are simply different, and they follow a unique female model of development.

Dr. Riess points out the difficulty in comparing his data with Dr. Ponse's. There is also a problem in comparing his data with Dr. Bieber's. Self-reports on questionnaires, no matter how carefully prepared and honestly answered, do not provide information about psychological events or mechanisms of which the reporter is unaware. One can tabulate how people answer, but not what the answers mean. Sociological data are the exception, and consequently, some social factors can be identified. The psychological mechanisms underlying gender identity for object choice, heterosexual or homosexual, remain only partially understood, since they operate so early in life (around 18 months to 2½ years) and simply do not reveal themselves by these methods. I believe Dr. Ponse's and Dr. Riess's articles are important

---

B. F. RIESS, Ph.D. • Adjunct Professor of Clinical Psychology, New School for Social Research, New York, New York.

because they help to wipe away the mystery, prejudice, and ignorance surrounding homosexual behavior and encourage a more rational approach to the study of all female sexual development.}

Dr. Ponse's chapter is an interesting attempt to develop a taxonomy of lesbianism and Lesbians. Her descriptive system is based on her fieldwork with "hundreds of women in those [secretive lesbian and political-activist Lesbian] communities and 75 in-depth interviews." Unfortunately, this methodology is reminiscent of the anecdotage of a field of inquiry. The reader is left either to believe in the generality of the quoted interview material or to ask how many of the "hundreds" fell into the identified groups. Dr. Ponse asserts that identification of self as part of a woman–woman relationship comes either from an ideational, conceptual source ("disembodied"), from an experiential contact with another woman experienced more as a person that as a sexual partner ("contact"), or from immersion in one or more of the homosexual political-activist or social communities.

As one who has for over a decade been involved in trying to get a foothold on female gender identification, either homosexual or heterosexual, I find it difficult to accept Dr. Ponse's attributions, since I have no information about the people who were in the hundreds studied in the field. One wonders how many of Dr. Ponse's respondents were white, middle-class, young, married, single, etc. How does Dr. Ponse define *lesbianism?* There is no clear description of her definition. It seems to include youthful experimental couplings, brief samplings of adultlike sexual experiences, and relationships with women begun at a later life stage. The stability, duration, and emotional involvement in and of like-sexed relationships are not either quantitatively or qualitatively mentioned. These criticisms are made not to challenge the accuracy of the findings but to suggest that the chapter would be more seriously appreciated if there were more factual material included in it. Even in clinical psychology, we have moved away from case description to more specific analyses.

If I now present the findings of our own investigations (Gundlach and Riess, 1968, 1973), I trust that our data will not be read as contradictory of Dr. Ponse's work. We have no way of comparing or contrasting the subjects of our two approaches since Dr. Ponse gives us no leads on which to base a comparison. It is the purpose of what follows to show a difficult and more quantitative probe into the difficult terrain of self-identification and choice of love partners.

Our story begins with the involvement of my closest collaborator, Ralph Gundlach, in the work of Bieber and his co-authors (Bieber, Dain, Dingle, Dreilich, Grand, Gundlach, Rifkin, Wilbur, and Bieber,

1962). Their work culminated in the volume called *Homosexuality: A Psychoanalytic Study of Male Homosexuals*. Because this volume devoted itself exclusively to males and to that selected sample of males who were in psychoanalytic treatment, we decided to embark on a study of homo- and heterosexual women, some of whom were in psychotherapy and some of whom were not. We also framed our research instruments so as to provide data that made possible a comparison with Bieber *et al.*'s men.

The first step was to define, for our study, what we would call a homosexual relationship. Our definition was explicitly limited to an adult (21 or older) experience of more than six months' duration with another mature woman. Thus, to start with, we eliminated the transitional, experimental, and exploratory sexual behaviors of adolescents and young people.

Our second step was to develop a cohort of Lesbian subjects. This was made possible by the magnificent cooperation of the Daughters of Bilitis, a woman's homophile national organization. We thus had a source of homosexual women drawn from all the major areas of the United States.

The comparison group of heterosexual women was obtained from colleagues, friends, and various social and professional gatherings. For each self-identified Lesbian, we were able to get data from a heterosexual woman matched with the homosexual woman for age, educational level, and geographical distribution over the United States. The population thus selected numbered 226 homosexual and 234 nonhomosexual women. The anonymity of the respondents was guaranteed by a method that additionally made possible continuing contact for subsequent tests and data collection. Within the samples, there were 90 Lesbians and 98 non-Lesbians in therapy.

From the respondents, we obtained retrospective information on early family attitudes and experiences and relationships with father, mother, friends, school, and teachers. In addition, there were items on sex, first crushes, tomboyism, and hetero- and homosexual behavior and material on current love relationships. Both groups of subjects answered the same questionnaire of 450 items.

In addition, human-figure drawings were returned by over 100 people in each group. These were scored for field dependence and independence. A semantic-differential denotation of the meaning of the concepts *mother, father, woman, man, friend,* and *lover* was also obtained. The questionnaire data on the 188 persons in therapy were checked for reliability by the therapists in question. This check gave some indication of the reliability and validity of the retrospective questionnaire.

In the space allocated to me, it is difficult, if not impossible, even to summarize our findings. These have been described in a number of publications (Gundlach, 1972; Gundlach and Riess, 1968, 1973; Riess and Safer, 1979). We certainly did not find any conclusion that described the etiology of homosexuality in women. We also found that the Bieber *et al.* description of the family origin of male homosexuality did not appear even in mirror image among the women. The semantic-differential test provided some fascinating hypotheses. All of the 460 responses were thrown into one pot, and a factorial study was made of the data. Only one factor identified a group of homosexuals, with only one heterosexual included in the subsample. This group had good mother and good father responses but was very negative about the concept *man*. In addition, in an article on birth order and sex of siblings (Gundlach, 1972), Lesbians predominated in the "only-child" category and were overrepresented as the eldest in small families (2–3 children). Conversely, in large families (4–12 children), the homosexual women were found at the tail end of the sibling order. All of these findings point to a social etiology for Lesbians and certainly point away from a genetic or even an ideational, idealized causation.

In finishing this presentation, I wish to return to the definition of homosexuality. In a recent review (Riess, 1977), I stated that

> Homosexuality fails as a diagnosis because it does not describe a uniform set of signs and symptoms, because the dynamics of the preference vary among individuals rather than having a common core, and finally because the causes of the sex preference are so varied. In fact there would be no diagnosis of homosexuality—only the myriad forms of homosexual behavior would be recognized—if the bigotry of the righteous did not force the belief (shared even by the homosexuals) that a distinct essence—homosexuality—exists.

It then becomes a minimally important question to ask how women identify as homosexuals.

Since we are therefore not dealing with a condition called homosexuality but with a variety of choices of like- and unlike-sexed love partners, what is there to say about the many comparisons possible from our data? We have responses from female homosexual nonpatients, female heterosexual nonpatients, female homosexual patients, female heterosexual patients, and a special group of male homosexual and heterosexual patients. With all this richness of possibilities, one conclusion stands out, namely, that, as usual, there are greater differences on most items within each group than between groups.

In comparing the nonpatient homosexual with heterosexual nonpatients, it seems that Lesbians have had more attachments to a like-sexed teacher, a later development of genital sex, greater frequency of adolescent heterosexual play and exploration, less guilt about sex, and greater self-identification as homosexual in partners by choice. Tomboyishness was about equal in both groups of women. "Platonic" relationships were slightly greater among homosexuals. The duration of a relationship was about the same in the married heterosexuals and in the coupled homosexuals. Perhaps the most significant finding is that the overt signs of pathology among the nonpatients were at the same low level in both groups. The same finding of equivalence of symptomatology holds for the patient groups. Thus, there is some substantiation for the position of the American Psychiatric Association that homosexuality is not necessarily pathological or sick.

In our study, among other findings, there were some indications that family patterns and parental expectations were different for homosexual and heterosexual women. The child who became Lesbian was more frequently neglected and ignored by her mother, who treated the daughter impersonally and in many instances without love. At the same time, the father selected the Lesbian child as the least favored. Fewer fathers of Lesbians were warm and affectionate, and more were indifferent and acted like strangers.

The lack of clear-cut patterns distinguishing the total Lesbian and non-Lesbian groups suggests that there are many more ways to homosexual behavior among women than among men. The unique events in the history of each female that led to homosexual activity were far more scattered than with Bieber's males. Girls in our society are caught in the confusion of changing patterns of sexual relations. For them, there is a conflict between the older definition of feminine roles centered on marriage and family and masculine roles of being strong and of being successful in achievements and in decision making. This conflict contrasts with publicity about equality, new ideas of sexual freedom, and equal opportunities for vocational choice-making. Few of our Lesbians identified themselves as "masculine." Sexually, the Lesbians more often said that they attained orgasm easily but that sexual intercourse was not as frequent as among the heterosexuals. What was more valued by the Lesbians was warmth, tenderness, and close physical contact. Loss of the love partner was more frequently described as "losing part of me," a "tearing experience," by the Lesbians than by the heterosexuals.

It is then possible to conclude that emotional health is no worse among homosexuals than among heterosexuals, that good interpersonal relationships are very important to Lesbians, that sex is no real problem, that guilt is less, and that rape is more frequently the cause of antimale feelings. How women identify as homosexual or heterosexual is not clear except that for the homosexual, the causation is

more frequently mentioned as derived from bad family and male–
female experiences. Genetic factors, specific sexual aversions, and constitutional structure play almost no role among the Lesbian women,
contrary to the mythology of the field.

REFERENCES

Bieber, I., Dain, H., Dingle, P., Dreilich, M., Grand, H., Gundlach, R. H., Rifkin, A.,
    Wilbur, C., and Bieber, T. *Homosexuality: A psychoanalytic study of male homosex-
    uals.* New York: Basic Books, 1962.
Gundlach, R. H. Data on the relation of birth order and sex of siblings of Lesbians.
    Annals of the New York Academy of Sciences, 1972, *197,* 179–181.
Gundlach, R. H., and Riess, B. F. Self and sexual identify in the female: A study of
    female homosexuals. In B. F. Riess (Ed.), *New directions in mental health,* Vol. 1.
    New York: Grune & Stratton, 1968.
Gundlach, R. H., and Riess, B. F. The range of problems in the treatment of Lesbians. In
    G. Goldman and D. Milman (Eds.), *The neuroses of our time: Acting out.* Springfield,
    Ill.: Charles C Thomas, 1973.
Riess, B. F. (Book review) Stoller on perversion. *Journal of Homosexuality,* 1977, 2(3),
    290–291.
Riess, B. F., and Safer, J. Homosexuality in males and females. In E. Gomberg and V.
    Franks (Eds.), *Gender and disordered behavior.* New York: Brunner/Mazel, 1979.
Safer, J., and Riess, B. F. Two approaches to the study of female homosexuality. *Interna-
    tional Mental Health Research Newsletter,* 1975, *17*(1), 11–14.
Safer, J., Riess, B. F., and Yotive, W. Psychological test data on female homosexuality.
    Journal of Homosexuality, 1974, *1,* 71–85.

Chapter 11

Daughters and Lovers

Reflections on the Life Cycle of
Daughter–Father Relationships

Rudolf Ekstein

{Editor's Note

Although the current psychodynamic understanding of personality development was founded on the child's perception of the father, his protection and his power, the father himself was presented in static terms. He was there, and the child responded, projected, misperceived, incorporated, and wove a sequence of age-appropriate fantasies around its reactions. The mother, however, as her primary role was discovered, was conceptualized in much more dynamic terms: not only was she there and subject to the infant's psychical uses, but she was "schizophrenogenic," "binding," "seductive," "inadequate," "overprotective," "abandoning," "cold," or, at best, "good enough." The dynamic interaction with fathers has yet to be codified. This chapter and the next are presentations by two fathers, a child psychoanalyst and a child psychiatrist, who describe and reflect their personal and professional experiences with the fathering of daughters.}

Some 67 years ago, D. H. Lawrence wrote his classic *Sons and Lovers,* and Alfred Kazin (1962), who wrote the introduction to a later edition, suggested that it was an autobiographical novel, "written in order to demonstrate freedom from the all-too-beloved mother." He described

Rudolf Ekstein, Ph.D. • Clinical Professor of Medical Psychology, University of California Medical School, Los Angeles, California; and Training and Supervisory Analyst, Los Angeles Psychoanalytic Institute and Southern California Psychoanalytic Institute, Los Angeles, California.

the sons of that time as growing up "in bondage to their mothers." He
suggested that the novel could be considered a symptom of that hectic
time before World War I that initiated many young men's struggle for
their emancipation from the mother.

One might well say that these cries for emancipation have never
stopped and that the dominant problem today consists of the increased struggle of women for their own emancipation, including
emancipation from their fathers. One might wonder whether another
novel, perhaps entitled *Daughters and Lovers*, might be written by a
feminist in the women's movement, another triumph of art that might
give her and us lasting satisfaction. Alfred Kazin suggested that:

> Art could not fulfill Lawrence's search, and only death could end it. But the
> ecstasy of a single human relationship that he tried to reproduce never
> congealed into a single image or idol or belief. Imaginatively, Lawrence
> was free; which was why his work could literally rise like a phoenix out of
> the man who consumed himself in his conflict with himself.

Kazin recalled that Freud (1917/1955) wrote once that he who was the
favorite of his mother becomes a "conqueror." Freud wrote at that
time about Goethe's experience with his mother, which gave him ultimate confidence. Obviously, he referred indirectly to his own relationship with his mother. He was indeed her favorite.

Usually, we try to highlight a problem such as the relationship between fathers and daughters by trying to turn to incidences of severe
psychopathology or to outstanding examples of such relationships,
which, like a beacon in the night, are to bring us light and insight. But
that beacon in the night can hardly substitute for the light of day and
does not help us to get beyond the specific and arrive at the generic.

Maybe we are overawed by Pallas Athena (Slater, 1968), who
jumped out of the head of Zeus, fully armed, full of wisdom, obviously fully identified with him, carrying out his mission and inspiring Pericles' leadership of free Athens.

Ordinarily, when we use the clinical method, we concentrate on
the inner life of a patient. We try to understand the inner situation by
tracing back to earlier events the symptoms, the maladaptations, the
strengths, and the weaknesses and by eliciting the meanings that the
patient gives to old relationships. Usually we find traumatic situations
that seem to explain the patient's problems. We frequently find that
the patient's early traumata, the infantile neurosis, and the relationships to significant adults in the past, are reflected in the transference neurosis, and thus we frequently get a magnified picture of early
constellations, a view that is, of course, also influenced by the kind of
magnifying glass, the theoretical position, that the psychotherapist

uses in order to help the patient. It is important to remember that Freud's first insights into the mental development of the child and the adolescent came from material gained in listening to adults who suffered from neurotic conflicts. These early insights into child life were supplemented later by direct observation and the study of educational processes and thus allow us to revise the first preliminary views that the study of psychopathology afforded.

Just as Freud (1905/1953) developed the stages of psychosexual development, the phases of the development of aggression, others turned to study other aspects of the stages of life, for example, Charlotte Bühler in *Der menschliche Lebenslauf* (1959), about the human life cycle, and Erikson in *Childhood and Society* (1950), about the eight stages of life.

These authors always looked at one person, the *Homo psychologicus,* the *monad,* at the inner life of a person, while I look at *dyads* in order to reexamine some of these issues in terms of changing relationships within changing social realities.

I recently suggested (1977) that we should look at the life cycle of a marriage, the specific tasks and crises that a couple face as they move from courtship and engagement and through the different phases of the marriage, such as parenting, postparenting, and old age. Not always does the life cycle of the marriage become consummated. Rarely can we speak of the last stage of the marriage as if it were the fulfillment of the Greek myth of Philemon and Baucis, who were turned into trees by the grateful gods, and who whispered throughout eternity to each other without having to lose each other through the death of one of the partners.

That gentle view of marriage does not quite fit into contemporary society, which seems to know little about the continuity of relationships and today is facing other forms of living: disruptions, separations, divorces, and discontinuities full of anxiety and pain that some people refer to as differing lifestyles.

Nevertheless, if we speak about normal development—an impossible concept, perhaps—we usually try to work out a scheme, an *epigenetic scheme,* as Erikson suggested.

His epigenetic scheme of 1950 gave us the stimulus to fill out the empty blanks of his eight stages, the postcursors and the precursors of each of the stages he developed, following indirectly Freud's phases of psychosexual development.

I suggested such a scheme, which would allow us to have better insight into the vicissitudes of the life cycle of the marriage; and I propose to outline a scheme now concerning *the life cycle of the father–daughter relationship.*

One might well say that this father–daughter unity starts before the daughter's birth. It is as yet an undifferentiated unity. It is all in the mind of the father-to-be. In the musical version of Ferenc Molnar's stage play *Liliom,* the touching and sensitive song of Richard Rogers and Oscar Hammerstein tells us what goes on in the mind of Billy Bigelow, that handsome and proud barker, inviting customers to ride the carousel. Julie Jordan, his wife, is pregnant, and Billy Bigelow daydreams about the child-to-be in his soliloquy of anticipation. This father–daughter unity, and perhaps it will be a father–son unity, has to accomplish the task of constructing basic trust between father and child. At present, however, the task of course, is one-sided. It is the struggle in the mind of the father-to-be. Does he want the child? Does he trust himself? Will he be able to maintain the marriage and provide for the child, or does he feel like running away from the task to be undertaken? He is anxious and hopeful. He wonders whether he and his wife are ready to move toward parenthood. If he were ready to have a child, would he want this child to be a boy or a girl? Does he need the child in order to have someone to be like him, to carry his name, to imitate him and identify with him? Or is he afraid that he will set a bad example or that the son will disappoint him? But perhaps he does not want a son. He might reject a boy, and he really wants a girl. What does he think about the task of fathering now? Can he provide for her, protect her, truly love her? What does it mean to love the girl, and what does it mean to love the boy? Is the girl the replica of his own mother? Does he see in her the miniature of his wife?

Much of what he thinks now about the role of the daughter in his very inner life depends, of course, on previous experience, on the quality of the marriage, on the existing conflicts, and on the capacity of both mother and father to let the marriage of two grow into the triangle of a family of three, the child being a girl. Do his narcissistic needs require a boy, an heir and successor in the old-fashioned way, someone to be like him? Will the disappointment then create an obstacle in the development of the relationship between a baby girl and the father?

In any case, at present, the relationship exists only in the mind of the father. The child is as yet unborn. It is a fantasy relationship, a fantasy that implies a psychic task, the capacity to develop trust in his capacity for the kind of parenting that is required in a father–daughter relationship. Usually, we say that the question of basic trust is two-sided. He has basic trust who can trust the other person and who at the same time can trust himself. It cannot be blind trust, and since the child is not yet born, the trust of the father-to-be is a kind of blind trust. Predictions of his capacity to develop toward mature fatherhood can be made, perhaps, on the basis of his trust relationships in the past, the one with his wife, the one with the first family in his life, his own parents, the siblings, etc.

The trust in himself, of course, one-sided as it is, is filled with uncertainty, with anxiety, with questions, since he does not know as yet what the child will be and what tasks it will put before the parents, and the question of trust, the question about the capacity to love, can be resolved only in the moment that extrauterine life for the girl child starts. The process of physical separation from her mother and her slow psychic separation and individuation will lead her more and more to the discovery of the father. She will respond to him and set new tasks for herself as well as for him.

We need not stress that in different cultures, this meeting of the minds—the mind of the adult, the father, and the mind of the growing girl—is a slow and sometimes awkward, certainly always different process. How will the fantasies that the father has about the little girl influence his ways of dealing with her? What will he do to make these fantasies into self-fulfilling prophesies? In older days, we stressed primarily the Oedipal situation between father and daughter. The earlier struggle concerning the acquisition of autonomy and basic trust was frequently described in terms of the existing—and at the same time, changing—relationship of the very small child and the mother. But this, indeed, was an oversimplification, even in those cases where the father hardly entered the nursery. In today's culture, the father frequently participates much more actively in the early stages of development. Certainly, he is not left out in questions of nurture and control, the struggle that leads to a balance between trust and distrust and between autonomy and control. We do not want to overlook the fact that this sharing of providing for the child and of educating her will lead to complex imitations and identifications on the part of the little girl. To what degree will she identify with father and with mother, and to what degree will she slowly take in the events that go on between mother and father and form an internal representation of marital tasks and conflicts that later becomes, perhaps, the prototype of her own capacity to deal with others?

But during the Oedipal phase, a more distinct separation of the father and the mother images begins.

A little illustration, funny on the surface, makes a serious point concerning certain psychological tasks that are hidden below the surface of the Oedipal fantasies of daughter and father. In a previous paper (1950), I described a little girl, Jean:

> About the age of five, Jeannie was sitting with her parents in the living room. With a side glance at her mother, she said to her father, "Daddy,

I want to marry you." Her father told her that he was already married to her mother and that he could not marry her. Jeannie thought perhaps he could marry *both girls*. Her father told her that this was not possible. Jeannie looked thoughtfully out the window, then decided with determined resignation, "Well, then I am going to marry Nolan." Her father wondered what she wanted to marry her kindergarten playmate for. Jeannie said, "Because I want to have a baby." The father's curiosity about the sex knowledge of the child was increasing at this moment and he asked her, "If you want to have a baby, what do you need Nolan for?" Jeannie was not puzzled for long and answered, "I want to marry Nolan so he can take care of the baby while I go out and play."

Whether the father's premature curiosity forced the child to answer defensively, to hide her secret knowledge of how babies are made, or whether she identified with a certain division of labor between her father and her mother, having observed that he actually took care of her while her mother went out, is difficult to say. But it is clear that the relationship between daughter and father, never free from the influence of the ever-present mother (in fact or just in the mind of father and daughter), goes partly beyond the core idea concerning the little girl's sexual wish for the father and her potential resentment against the mother. She is willing to share with the mother, and she even indicates that she would be satisfied if the father would marry—that is, accept—both girls. At that moment, the father was perhaps more curious than he should have been, and that curiosity also says something about the complexities of the relationship, which is a love relationship that expresses acceptance on the part of the father but at the same time sets limits. To be sure, this is only the conscious part of the relationship, and much may go on in the minds of both that does not come to the surface verbally. Both father and daughter must contend with their own private sexual fantasies about each other and must face the task of mastering these fantasies.

There is an indication, though, that the child is starting to move away from her primary love objects, is making new attachments with peers, and is acquiring knowledge about the use of people, at times a selfish use and at times a sharing use. As she wishes to *go out and play*, she moves toward more autonomy, toward an initiative not yet undermined by guilt. She is curious about the world, and she will experiment. We can predict that she will be a good student in elementary school, that she is about to pass into the phase of latency (the school age), and that her relationship with the father will now be one in which she wants to prove that she can function well and that she learns, and her overt and covert conditions for acquiring love from him will change and mature.

As the little girl starts to go to school, the very early *learning through play* will change into *school learning*. While all play can be considered a kind of psychic work of inner accomplishment, we may also see that work has in it elements of play. Much of learning in school and earlier is actually based on identification with the adult world. Very early, Jeannie developed new dimensions in her relationship with her father, and he did the same, of course, in his relationship with her. He was a professional person and she wanted to be a doctor, too. That wish filled him with pleasure, playful pleasure, and he watched her imitating his teaching functions as well as the way in which her own teachers in elementary school worked with children. She wanted to be like them. She gathered some younger children around her and played school. She was very effective with the children but really also very bossy, a caricature of the grown-up world. One can see that the child's problem in relation to the father had also to do with her inability at that time to read him completely right. She saw him and the teachers, so to speak, via projection and childish distortion. She distorted her view of the adult world. If she saw her mother as someone who would *go out and play,* she, of course, invested her mother with her own play activities and did not see what her mother really did. When she made teaching into a cruel persecution of children, she invested the adult world with versions of teachers created in her own not-fully-developed mind, displaying certain ways of dealing that were age appropriate but that showed that her identification with the adult world was undermined by the projection of her own basic drives and untamed wishes.

But there is the wish to identify with the father, the male. Helene Deutsch (1969) has described the wish for identification with the father, the male element, in adolescent girls. One can see the precursor of this identification much earlier, as the previous illustration suggests.

The same Jean who, at the age of five, wished to be a doctor like her father answered at the age of 15, when he asked her whether she still wanted to be a doctor, "Oh Daddy, one doctor in the family is enough." She was then struggling with individuation, with the wish to be herself, and her father—though he must have dreamed at times as all fathers do, that she might take on features of his as part of her own life—recalled how, while she was in kindergarten, she had taken great delight in a little song that she had learned and often repeated:

> Everybody says I look just like my mother,
> Everybody says I am the image of Aunt Beth,
> Everybody says my nose is like my father's,
> But I want to look like me.

Of course, in later years, she wanted not only to look like herself but to be a person on her own, with goals of her own and an occupation of her own, and thus she changed the conditions for a positive relationship with her father.

The girl's early primitive wish to marry her father, to be close to him, and to be fully (including sexually) loved by him—an impossible condition of love, to be sure—changes slowly, provided the father's response to the Oedipal demands of the little girl is not a neurotic reaction but is the response of a father who is capable of parenting.

Even in the girl's early years, we hear about child abuse and about incestuous bondage between a father and a daughter that might be acted out in one form or the other. Some primitive cultures allow intimacies between fathers and child daughters that we, today, would consider child abuse but that are naively practiced and become part of group and family life.

If, however, the father–daughter relationship takes its normal course in the life cycle within the average environment of today, we see that the conditions for love change. During the school years, the conditions change slowly from overt and covert demands for direct sensual gratification toward demands for achievement, such as the accomplishment of tasks at home and in school. And even though these demands are derived from earlier, more primitive wishes and strivings, they are now centered on tasks that a growing and maturing ego can fulfill. The mutual love expresses itself now in mutual interests on a higher level, whether they be interest in school tasks, in recreational tasks, or in achievement in sports. More and more, the father becomes a teacher, in part an ego ideal and in part the living conscience. The wish for sensual gratification from father is slowly replaced by and supplemented with a wish for his inspiration and guidance.

It must be stressed, and cannot be stressed often enough, that not only are we dealing with interpersonal relationships and interpersonal conditions for love and acceptance, but both father and daughter must acquire psychological functions that make the new turn of events possible. For both of them, the father–daughter relationship is not only an external event, an external happening, but is to be understood in terms of internal achievements, internal permanent representations of that relationship, so that each of them lives up to these demands, internalized as they are now and represented as they are by stable internal representations of the love object and its demands and rewards. One might well say that each has the other in his or her head, along with a psychic replica of the actual relationship.

It must be understood that these internal achievements are not merely based on maturation but are developmental achievements, based on internal and external struggle and the solution of each task as well as the resolution of each conflict. Both give up the early intima-

cies and develop new forms of intimacy, age appropriate and subli-
mated.

An adult patient was once asked during a consultation why she
thought she needed intensive analytical work. She started to cry and
recalled an event that took place when she was 10 or 11 years old. She
recalled being in the bathtub. Her father was present. He wanted to
leave and she tried to keep him back, but he left and she suddenly experienced a panic attack. She was sure after he left the bathroom that
he had died. She would never see him again. And ever since, she had
been full of fear that her parents might die. As she lay in the bathtub,
unable to free herself from the panic and from the dreadful fantasy,
she suddenly thought that all the warm water was flowing out of the
tub and that she would turn colder and colder, that the tub would turn
into a coffin, and that she would lie there dead.

This event, a dramatic and powerful fantasy, condenses within a
few powerful images the inner tasks of the latency-age girl. The warm
water and the warm relationship with the early father of more sensuous days and sexual fantasies, a father who often used to give the
child a bath, moved suddenly toward the panicky ending. One might
well think that this fantasy, remembered as it is together with the terror and the fear, condenses a variety of situations that happened over
and over again in some similar fashion. The fantasy can be considered
a kind of simile for the growing-up process, the developmental task
that has to be accomplished by both father and daughter. He realizes
that she is growing up and that he has given in much too long to her
and perhaps to his own desire for the pleasurable bathroom play. She
should wash and dry herself now. She is not to need the father any
longer. He is tempted to stay and is angry with himself for being
tempted, and he finally breaks up the love game. He does not want to
stay any longer and he leaves against her will. The disappointed and
angry girl has the sudden thought that her father has died, that she
has lost him forever, that he does not love her any longer, and her rage
against him turns into the thought that he is dead. Now, she is full of
guilt, and she gives up the warm-water play and the wish for gratification and punishes herself. She should finally get out of the tub. But
the fantasy life, dreamlike as it is, turns the emptying of the tub, the
loss of the warmth, the loss of the father, into a cold coffin and the
thought of her own death.

In Grimm's fairy tale "Snow White," the struggle is between the
hated stepmother and the little girl, who, while the dwarfs (the little
men) are absent, is poisoned by the jealous stepmother's apple. She is
now frozen. She is beyond childhood life, cannot move, and is seemingly dead. But she is beautiful, a girl to soon be awakened and sex-

ually aroused, not by the father but by the prince. She rests as if dead for a while in the coffin, waiting to change once more her inner relationship to the father and to move toward awakening adolescent life and later toward a fulfilling, adult life.

In the story of our patient, though, the dominant conflict was not between mother and daughter but between father and daughter. The awkward and painful time must come when the father cannot treat his daughter any longer as a little girl. She cannot sit on his lap and he cannot carry her around. He cannot give her a bath, and he must cease to yield to her more childlike demands. Over and over again, he might say, "You are too big for that." This is now a new and disastrous disappointment. The relationship is now dominated more and more by ambivalence. The rage against him and the tender yearning for him are in violent conflict. Jean's playful thought that she could give up the marriage with her daddy and marry Nolan characterizes the father–daughter relationship in a different way than does the story of the patient who thought that the father who left her was dead, who was terrorized and saw herself dying in the bathtub while the warm water flowed out. Both incidents have a similar structure but served different tasks. Jean moved into latency, while the patient continued to have a very stormy latency, a kind of prelatency, and found herself, suddenly, at the beginning of puberty in a painful conflict leading to severe symptom formation.

Jean's relationship with her schoolmate Nolan was very different from the relationship to the prince, the fantasies about the man who is to give adult autonomy and an adult relationship.

The place of the father in both instances was different.

Also, it should not be forgotten that, somewhere, there is always the mother in the background. Jeannie will not marry Daddy. She knows that both her father and her mother love her. She lives within the context of a triad.

The girl in the bathtub thought she had lost the love of the father and saw nowhere the maternal figure, except that she assumed that her father left her for her mother.

Snow White faces an angry stepmother and a seemingly absent father.

Jean's parents permitted her to find little Nolan and play with him, and they guided her toward latency, toward a relationship in which the condition for love had now become different. The love referred now to the solution of tasks and the offering of identity models. Jean moved from the gratifying parental love object to the parental role model.

The adolescent girl faces intensive struggle as she tries to find her own identity and to bring about another step in the separation from the father. He is seen as ideal, as someone who guides but who also prevents. Is he jealous? Can he let her go? Will he be prohibitive, or will he be understanding? In any case, she moves now toward intensive experiences that remind her of the early intensive strivings, of sexual fantasies and desires that are fed by a society that is very different from earlier days. What was in earlier days a drama on the stage, such as Ibsen's *A Doll's House*, expressing the ideas of the women's rights movement, has become more and more an accepted and open opportunity as well as a hidden danger. Job opportunities and sexual freedom, previously availably only to males, have led to the adolescent girl's equality with boys. Free love and marriage arrangements and new birth control means have driven adolescents into opportunities much too overwhelming, into risks that they cannot master. And many of these risks are characterized in the crisis relationships that exist now between the girl and her father.

Will the father, by sanctioning the new sexual freedom, act as an *agent provocateur*, or will he know that the growing girl can maintain her psychic equilibrium only if she experiences the father as a supportive figure who allows her to identify with the adult world rather than to act out a premature pseudoadulthood.

Helene Deutsch (1969) spoke about the conflict that the girl meets as she becomes a young woman, struggling between motherhood and professional achievement. She can identify with the pre-Oedipal father, may wish to have a profession like him and to have the same rights as he has, and may be a free woman but unable to acquire maternal ideals. The triangle—daughter, father, and mother—may become lopsided, and then a new equilibrium has to be established.

Helene Deutsch asked whether the new social situation will allow the girl to identify not only with the father, with the males, but also with the mother, and to develop a socially appropriate feminine ego ideal. The achievement of equality, based on individual difference, is the task of the adolescent girl.

The father, one would assume, can help her with the task only if he has a way to maintain the daughter–father–mother triangle and to help her develop her new adult self out of double identifications with both father and mother.

How difficult that would be in split families, if the girl, instead of being backed up by both parents, becomes the center of parental disharmony, of divorce and discontinuity of family life.

The daughter's relationship with the father is maintained if she succeeds in maturing to the point where she can give up her infantile bondage and create a new bond of love between herself and her father that allows for separation and further individuation. He must let her go and must "give her away" (as expressed in the marriage ceremony). But this letting go and this giving away is not really a giving up. It is merely a change in the relationship, a maturation in the relationship. The father remains in the head of the daughter, and the daughter remains in the head of the father. Their emotional relationship and their bond continue even though its quality has changed. It is now an adult relationship.

Often, the father finds it difficult to let go of the daughter, particularly if other aspects of his life are unsatisfying. But if things go right, their relationship becomes even deeper. Freud once said to Reik (1940), who could not quite let go of him as they said good-bye to each other, "People who belong together do not need to be glued together." That, to be sure, would be the new character of the father–daughter relationship. They may enjoy each other now on a different, higher level. If she marries and has children, he will become a grandfather and enjoy her offspring. Whatever that may mean to him consciously and unconsciously, it will again deepen the love to an entirely new level. Again, in some ways, she will make demands of him as she hopes and expects that he will be a good granddaddy. But she will not want him to take over the parental function. And he will have to learn that grandparenting is an entirely new role that he has not yet acquired. The struggle and the growth, the task solving and the conflict resolving never stop for either.

And always, somewhere in the picture, there is the mother, the wife. She only *seems* to be invisible. She is, of course, a powerful and important aspect of the father–daughter unity.

The daughter grows older and the father grows old. Some aspects change now. As his life moves on and as he sees his daughter settled in her own life career, perhaps in her own family and her own task of mothering, he recedes into the background. In tender ways, they remember their past history. They remember together her childhood and his parenting. And many a story is exhanged and remembered. That, too, is a psychic task and a psychic opportunity for both. It gives both of them renewed love and value. They still, in some ways, live for each other. And as he grows older, the father–daughter life cycle moves toward the other end. In the beginning, the father–daughter relationship exists merely in the mind of the father. He fantasizes about the future. A little later, the ever-changing father–daughter unity, with the mother in the background, begins in a fuller sense. That unity moves through the different phases of the life of both, forming a characteristic life cycle that usually ends with the passing of the father. As he becomes older, he needs the daughter in a different way. Sometimes, she almost becomes a mothering figure in the life of the aging man. He needs her help, her advice. Sometimes her anxiety mounts, since now she feels that she may lose the father, but, this time, she experiences not the loss of his love but the loss of the object.

At the end of the musical *Carousel*, Billy Bigelow is pictured in heaven. His daughter is an adolescent girl, deeply in trouble, feeling herself rejected. She has lost the father and thinks no one will ever love her. But here he comes, for but one day, back from heaven, and appears as a strong memory from the past in the mind of the daughter. She experiences his renewed love as he gives her a star. And faith is restored in her.

The touching end of this musical version of *Liliom* refers to the psychological fact that the relationship between daughter and father, after all, is also an internal achievement, an acquisition in her. There are moments of doubt and she feels rejected. And then she brings back a memory of a loving and trusting father. This golden star—as if she were a little girl in nursery school who acquires gold stars—is the equivalent of a loving superego inherited from the father, his way of bringing her up. She feels that he is with her. She thinks of the dead father and knows that he is internalized, that he is in her mind, and that therefore he will protect her. The life cycle of the father–daughter relationship seems to have come to an end. But not quite so. Even though he is physically dead, he is psychologically alive in her for the remainder of her own life cycle.

In the beginning, she existed in his fantasy and was psychologically alive in him even though she was not yet born. Of course, even in his fantasy, the mother was in the background of that relationship. Now that he is no more, having himself returned to Mother Earth, he is nevertheless alive. In the beginning of the life cycle of that relationship, he was thinking of the future. And she, now at the end of the physical aspect of that life cycle, thinks about the past. In the beginning, there was anticipation, and toward the end, there is memory. Both are functions of a healthy ego, of a growing and maturing self in both the daughter and the father. And as she thinks of him lovingly, she is capable of fulfilling the functions of an adult woman, perhaps the functions of mothering, when the mother is again in the background. The basic triangle never leaves us.

Ordinarily, in the daily pursuit of our life work, we clinicians see disturbances in the life cycle, traumatic events, premature losses, the catastrophic events that disrupt the life cycle of relationships. We see so many trees that we do not notice the forest. As I try to give a blueprint of that life cycle, the father–daughter relationship with the mother in the background, I develop a happy fairy tale, a positive myth, where all good behavior, all good identifications, and all good love are finally rewarded. This is a kind of mythological belief in normality.

I have created an ideal measure, a yardstick, a blueprint by means of which a father-and-daughter relationship can be better understood.

I think of the picture that I have given of that life cycle as a kind of model. I do not consider this a model of perfection, like a fashion model, but rather a kind of basic yardstick, by means of which we may evaluate the real relationships that may exist between fathers and daughters. My epigenetic scheme is meant to be as "real" as Erikson's eight phases, leading from basic trust to wisdom. We do not expect to find these phases in pure culture, but we use these schemata in order to bring our data together, to fill the empty spaces, and to explain the vicissitudes, normal or abnormal, in the ever-changing relationship between daughter and father within the triad of father, mother, and child. Such epigenetic schemes permit us not only to compare pathology with the normal but to set tasks for both as they move through their own life cycles. In our society of uncertainties and discontinuities, we speak frequently about the *generation gap*. Such concepts seem to suggest that there can be continuity only between people of the same generation. Actually, continuity and growth require the generation gap. The daughter, without the father and without the mother in the background, cannot move through childhood, adolescence, and adulthood. She needs the father in front of her. And he cannot move from young adulthood toward parenting and grandparenting and all the skills that are thus acquired unless there is that generation gap. It is not only that children need parents but also that adults need children. They need them for inner completion. They do not need children merely or necessarily in the biological sense, but they need to exist in the mind of the grown-up as a task set for completion. Life would otherwise be half empty.

While this communication stresses the role of the father and the role of the daughter vis-à-vis each other and tries to give a picture of the relationship's life cycle, I do not want the reader to get lost and think of me as believing that there are only Zeus and his daughter Pallas Athena. In the background, to be sure, in spite of all the magic powers she conceded to Zeus, there was Hera. Behind the dyad is the triad. We have made the mother less visible only in order to put the spotlight on the life cycle of the father–daughter dyad. The mother is not meant to be forgotten as we wonder about the development of the girl child. I merely meant to highlight the father in order to understand his role better and to restore his place, which he so often seems to have given up. Between the father's soliloquy of anticipation and the daughter's soliloquy of remembrance is the dialogue of the living, ever-developing, and ever-changing life cycle of the daughter–father relationship.

References

Bühler, C. *Der menschliche Lebenslauf als psychologisches Problem.* (The human course of life as a psychological problem). 2 Auflage. Göttingen: Verlag für Psycholigie, 1959.

Deutsch, H. The contemporary adolescent girl. *Seminar in Psychiatry,* 1969, *1*(1), 99–112.

Ekstein, R. Sexuality and aggression. In H. Herma and G. Kurth (Eds.), *Elements of psychoanalysis.* Cleveland & New York: World Publishing, 1950, pp. 105–20.

Ekstein, R. Normality and pathology in marriage. *Modern Psychoanalysis,* 1977, *2*(1), pp. 35–42.

Erikson, E. *Childhood and society* (1950). New York: W. W. Norton, 1964.

Freud, S. Three essays on the theory of sexuality (1905). *Standard edition of the complete psychological works of Sigmund Freud,* Vol. 7. London: Hogarth Press, 1953.

Freud, S. A childhood recollection from *Dichtung und Wahrheit* (1917). *The standard edition of the complete psychological works of Sigmund Freud,* Vol. 17. London: Hogarth Press, 1955, pp. 147–156.

Kazin, A. Introduction to D. H. Lawrence, *Sons and lovers.* New York: Modern Library, 1962.

Reik, T. *30 years with Freud.* New York: Farrar & Rinehard, 1940.

Slater, P. *The glory of Hera–Greek mythology and the Greek family.* Boston: Beacon Press, 1968.

Chapter 12

Role of the Father

Christine Adams-Tucker and Paul L. Adams

{Editor's Note

Freud, who gave scientific validation to the woman's sexual needs, saw the father, through his protective role, as the primary figure of a child's life. This view was repeated in his writings up to 1921. He identified the role of the penis as an organizer of infantile emotion and personality. Despite Otto Rank and others who stressed the role of the mother, it required the work of a woman—Melanie Klein, who worked with very young children—to establish for psychoanalysis the primary role of the mother, who, through her nutrient breast, acts as the earliest organizer of infantile emotional life and personality.}

Sexism is a term that we shall use often to denote gender-based discriminations, in both attitude and overt behavior, whether made by women or by men, by boys or by girls. *Gender* is simply maleness or femaleness or some intervening state, such as "intersex" or hermaphroditism. Sexism, thus, is inequality (believed and practiced in institutional forms) based on gender. Both ideologically and institutionally supported, sexism pervades the lives of all individuals in U.S. society. Although not as strong as the oppression of children, sexism joins with racism and economic injustice as a widespread oppression. Sexism cuts across class lines, ethnic lines, IQ lines, age lines, and religious lines to produce an impressive, weighty homogeneity of beliefs and practices. Sexism is a form of oppression learned in the family of orientation and buttressed by subsequent experiences outside the person's family of origin. Even when gender differences are quan-

CHRISTINE ADAMS-TUCKER, M.D. • Fellow in Child Psychiatry, Department of Psychiatry and Behavioral Sciences, University of Louisville, Louisville, Kentucky. PAUL L. ADAMS, M.D. • Professor and Vice Chairperson, Department of Psychiatry and Behavioral Sciences, University of Louisville and Louisville Veterans Administration Medical Center, Louisville, Kentucky.

titatively or objectively meager, sexism underlines the dissimilarities and vaunts those differences. Having defined our terms, we shall look at fathers relating to their daughters and shall try to see what roles fathers play in the "sexual development" of their female offspring.

Sexual development may mean many things: *gender* formation, *gender identity* progression, *sex-role* induction and elaboration, the stirrings of *lust or sex drive, sex-partner preferences, sexual orientation* (as coming to choose predominantly autoerotic, homosexual, or heterosexual involvements), and *sex-act preferences.* The father's role in many of these facets of sexual development is, in truth, little known and understood but is often made the subject of pontifical assertions by traditionalists and innovators alike. Psychiatrists show a professional weakness to overgeneralize from the individual case, and, alas, even one case is seldom thoroughly studied. One Lesbian is often set up as typical of all homosexual females, and, furthermore, implicit comparisons are made with the given writer's mental images of what a "typical" heterosexual female surely must be. Everyone is an expert, everyone a discoverer, everyone original, when there is talk of women's gender, gender identity, sex role, lust, sexual orientations, and sex-act preferences. The trend toward overassertion is one that we hope partly to counter in this chapter in order to give a total impression of the diversity that we know and celebrate in an air of humility and questioning. We share the ignorance of many other writers on this topic of fathering the female. Who can really say dogmatically what a female is, what a father is, and what a father can do in the project of developing full personhood in his daughter?

Our discussion will give our working view of the biological chemistry relevant to female gender. At the biochemical level, the father seems to rise to a role that is equal to the mother's for a very limited, brief period; we feel that genetics and chemistry should introduce the topic of the father's role with father equal to mother, since as a biological parent (Latin, *parens,* "source"), he is a potent figure. Following a consideration of biochemistry, we move to the societal pervasiveness of gender dimorphism, of stereotyping as it pertains to both father and daughter; next, to the father's part in the girl's developing gender identity; then to the father's influences on her sexual preferences for both sex partners and acts; and prior to concluding, we consider the more-highly-prevalent-than-anyone-guessed incest between father and daughter.

CHEMISTRY OF CONCEPTION AND EARLY GESTATION

Carrying X chromosomal material from both the mother and the father (XX), the egg, once it is fertilized, that will go on to elaborate a female fetus is programmed as much by the father's genetic contribution as by the mother's. That particular episode in sexual programming, in the view of Money and Ehrhardt (1972), although critical, is short-lived: the two X chromosomes, coming one from each parent, influence the undifferentiated genital tubercle to develop as female. Thereafter, the XX chromosomes "retire" and relay the lion's share of the next task to the now-differentiated female gonad. This happens in about the sixth week of fetal life.

The fetal ovary then proceeds to elaborate hormones that promote the regression of the Wolffian ducts and the progressive development of the Müllerian ducts as well as the subsequent formation of external genitalia over a range of normally female anatomy. If the ovary does not take up its task of making the fetus female via its hormones, Nature seems to adopt a "never-mind" attitude, for the development of female genital apparatus will occur *either without ovarian hormones or with them*. All that seems uniquely able to alter this embryonal imperative toward femaleness is the presence of testosterone, since *the absence of testosterone* is all that it takes to get a female morphological pattern.

Likewise, the brain pathways dealing with female lust and gender develop apace *if* there are no testicular hormones to break up the advance to femaleness. What is true of the brain, notably the hypothalamus, is also true of the peripheral nerves supplying the genital structures of the female embryo. Without testosterone, the embryo's femaleness is assured. Therefore, the father's early genetic contribution of X instead of Y has some far-reaching consequences for the embryonal female: to induce the genital tubercle to become female. Having become female, the genital tubercule elaborates female hormones in the embryo, thereby induces Müllerian progression, and finally, orients the brain and the nervous system toward female lust and behavior. In Turner's syndrome, where one X chromosome only is present, the girl is only phenotypically female and does not have female gonads. That she never achieves menarche shows the importance of X chromosomes from both parents.

To say that brain pathways mediate the embryo's "feminization" is tantamount to saying that forever more the brain, the body's principal organ of learning, will take over the regulation and control of femaleness. The organ of learning achieves such control before birth occurs. Forever afterward, the sex of the female is subject to the influences of others—is subject to learning. All too often, we keep biologizing, playing down the importance of social learning. Her brain has been feminized *in utero* (unless an excess of exogenous androgens brought on a masculinization of the central nervous system at that time). It seems sensible to use the terms *feminization* or *masculinization* in this context because, increasingly, data are amassed to prove that intrauterine determinants of gender identity do limit the work carried on by the postnatal program (including the father's input).

POSTNATAL MILESTONES

The postnatal program (in which the father can be absent or present, active or inactive) uses the materials present at birth to forge the core gender identity of the female (or the male), and that identity is formed between the ages of 18 and 30 months. The little girl is socialized or reinforced—partly by her father—in playing the culturally prescribed female role from the time of birth onward; her girlish or feminine activities unfold under this tutelage for the first time when she is around five years of age. Her sexual orientation—that is, her choice of preferred sex partners (*sex objects* is a gruesome term to us) and what she likes to do with them—may gel only in her late 20s. Sometimes, her special preferences are to be indelibly stamped by the more-or-less accidental contingencies surrounding an infantile orgasm, or an orgasm in preschool, elementary school, preadolescence, or adolescence. Or perhaps her specific tastes will crystallize only with the serious commitments of adulthood or even in the casual one-night stands of old age, if the authors are to believe the reports of our female patients of diverse ages and social backgrounds.

GENDER DIMORPHISM PERVASIVE

Throughout the several childhood portions of the postnatal life cycle, a girl is given gender-specific upbringing: she is spoken to, rewarded, punished, flirted with, dressed up, taught to sit down to urinate, taught to wipe her behind from front to back and not back to front, and instructed in modesty and keeping her panties on during playtime. As a result of all of this induction, conditioning, and socialization, she is channeled, ineluctably, into one society's view of femaleness. By age four, she even can say with a very high degree of accuracy (or self-fulfilling prophecy) whether she will be a mommy by age 30 years! The die is truly cast . . . but only between 18 and 30 months of age. Until then, fathers (as well as mothers) behold in their daughters a "nature, half created, half perceived."

Her father will be coy and courtly with his little girl, imagining a full dish of femininity and an eyeful of beauty, long before other observers (except the mother) will give confirmation to these paternal fantasies. Fathers play more gently with their daughters and do more roughhousing with sons, according to Lynn (1974). Other observers, however, begin to see what her parents see by the time a little girl is three, four, and five years old. Beverly Birns (1976) summed up the emergence of sex differences in preschool children in this statement:

> . . . preschool boys engage in more aggressive play, manipulate toys more, and are more exploratory. Girls are more sedentary, imitative, persistent, and attentive. Cognitive differences in coding and in memory are not observed, but differences in field independence, characteristic of males in adolescence and adulthood, favor females in the preschool years. The hypothesis that sex differences begin to emerge only in the preschool years appears supported.

That means that boy–girl differences, even if known, are not actualized in the girl's behavior until she is a preschooler. And that is surprising when we recall that the father's genitalia (being externally placed) are not unknown to her and that the mother's breast and pudendum are usually part of the consciousness of a two-year-old girl. It seems odd that she delays confirmed girlishness (as a contrast with boyishness) until nursery-school or kindergarten age.

POLARIZING, A FRAME OF MIND

The girl, for her part, in her early years learns to categorize and polarize with a vengeance. The polarities of her loving mentors are adopted in toto—and many of them without her knowing what is being shaped in her own awareness. She learns certain crude categories and schemata initially, and, if fortunate, later on she will learn to derepress, to modify and refine crude distinctions, to question, and to unlearn the easy stereotypes from childhood. Ultimately, she will forsake even her mother and father.

In the little girl's (as in the little boy's) cognitive grasp of her world, she effects polarization between a number of *either-this-or-that* concepts: male–female, adult–child, good–bad, ingroup–outgroup, beautiful–ugly, yummy–"yucky," macho–sissy. This dichotomization (Aristotelian logic) provides a crude sorting out that helps a girl to get some sense of mastery over the chaos of percepts that she holds of things around her and enables her to "place" herself amid all the constructs she is learning. The father's precepts and examples are influential even if far from decisive at this stage.

Only the part of her schematizing and polarizing that jibes with adult categories and values—in some part due to the child's own dogged tenacity of personal judgment—has a chance of surviving. Dichotomizing may serve some useful purposes during her early childhood; it may be related to the splitting between good me–bad me that Kleinian analysts have written about so much. However, we must recall that dichotomies always entail dissociation, oversimplification, "false consciousness" and outright cognitive distortion. Partly because they are so distorting, we (fathers included) outgrow our infantile bent to think in dichotomies.

We, including little girls, abandon many of our early dichotomies but not all of them. Our sex-role dichotomies retain partial immutability, under the strengthening and reinforcement of cultural values. It is for this reason that sensible adults who have forsworn dichotomies and stereotypes concerning race, religion, ethics, aesthetics, and economic class frequently cling to sex-role behavior that is stereotyped for gender.

Cognizant that sex-role stereotypes, even if irrational, may be used to support certain fragile personalities, Harriet E. Lerner (1978) and others have summoned arguments that sex-role stereotyping may be a "needed fiction" of some persons, especially those whose basic gender identity is poorly formed. The argument runs thus: those who are weak in gender identity must stereotype, and those who are strong can move toward androgyny.

Although the matter has been subjected to little research, it seems plausible to contend that the father plays a heavy role in this shaping of his daughter according to sex-role stereotypes. In fact, when the shaping is not fraught with problems, the father may play a key role in his daughter's developing identity within her sex role. The reader will please note that we do not contend that all of her identity is wrapped up in her sex role, but since some is, it merits consideration.

FEMALE IDENTITY AND FATHER'S ROLE

The newborn baby girl is announced as a girl and assigned to being female, as little or as much as that must mean from the standpoint of either nature or nurture. Ultimately, she develops a picture of herself as female.

At first, she is generically a baby, but also a girl baby. Although much of the parental reaction refers to her from a childist perspective (i.e., a perspective that is demeaning to children), somehow she is more than just baby because she is a girl. The parents' equilibrated relationship may require considerable retuning and readjustment—simply because of her new presence *as offspring* and sometimes more so because of her presence *as girl.* She is more human baby than otherwise at the outset, but if the father is pervasively sexist (as he is childist), the father will not rest easy with what he may see as an imperfect, incomplete baby—simply because she is not male. Lynn (1974) reported a preference for a male child among expectant fathers.

The father has been proclaimed by the Freudians as harboring deep-seated misogynist complexes; he has also been encouraged in this view by one of the mightiest churches: a woman cannot be a priest, Catholics say, because she does not have the same genitalia as Jesus Christ. We get visions of Irish priests racing to get circumcised and cosmetic surgery to look like Jesus, the little Jew.

Or another example: the father who has little religion of his own but decides to adopt, when in mourning for a dead parent, the rituals of his parents' religion. He goes to synagogue each morning and utters repetitively those male-chauvinist words that demean his own wife and daughters, as he prays orthodox thanksgiving to Jehovah that he was not born an inferior female!

If the father has been thoroughly indoctrinated in misogyny, buttressed by the status quo in religion, economics, politics, family life, and all the rest, that father will not rest content with a daughter as his heir. He wants a son, much as a Turkish male psychiatrist says he has no children, meaning that he has only daughters. A father may want a son because he believes that only his Y chromosomes will give the immortality he longs for—a son, an heir to one's name, one's lineage, one's seed. Postpartum depressions in fathers may have this fact of gender disappointment as an ingredient of their evolution, although Wainwright (1966) reported more psychopathology in fathers following the birth of a son.

Most fathers seem to make an accommodation to the sex (gender) of the girl baby within the first several weeks of the baby's postnatal life. The baby's growing attachment to the parents, her obvious dependence on adult caregivers, and the increasing signs of her fitting in with the family group all help the father to move toward love for the baby girl, even if he started with a moderate number of sexist reservations. There are other things that help him to develop a loving bond to his baby girl: not only does she serve as a reminder to the father of the infantile part of the generically human life cycle, but she also specifically helps him to replay his own dependent condition and his own "femininity."

A father may actually hold the female in considerable respect, if not awe, for her being complementary to his maleness and, above all, for her being able to carry a baby inside her belly. The woman's special reproductive capabilities—gestation and delivery—spur some womb envy in most of the males we have known. Similarly, most mature males have transcended their hang-ups sufficiently to be comfortable with their own feminine identifications and tendencies. Lots of men get "broody" unabashedly when they see or cuddle a little baby.

Maybe it would be better to ask a question: Who on earth could refrain from identifying with a little girl baby who needs one's love and care? What father could deny his fascination with a delightful little girl? As we see it, this is a question not of gushing sentimentality but of a father's willingness to let go in his empathic identification with his little daughter. A father is just a father, but that could be a lot.

HOTHOUSE FAMILIES

Some families, often middle-class in reality or in outlook, constitute a high-temperature incubator of eroticized interactions between parents, between or among siblings, and between parents and siblings. Loving and fondling, virtues during the little girl's first year or two of life, are continued despite her own wishes to be let go in developing her own autonomous behavior. These parents are not empathetic but intrusive, meddling, overpowering, and "overprotective" in a special way. The father may become so enamored of his little daughter's flirtation that he finds himself, a grown man, feeling pridefully puffed up by his daughter's attentiveness to him, to his genitals, to his body. He may imagine more than is actually there and see her every kiss or proposal of marriage as a seductive move. In short, he is narcissistic; he is also exhibitionistic, calling it natural nudity; he is seductive, calling it freedom; he is using projective identification—attributing "evil" adult motives to a three- or four-year-old girl. With all these rationalizations and distortions, he may take the step to outright molestation of his daughter, which we consider in the later section on incest.

A love cult provides the glue that holds a contemporary superheated family together: not the love of "brotherliness" (or sisterliness), *agape*, but of *eros* and its ins and outs, its distortions. Children of these parents work for love and are punished by love's withdrawal, the parents may sexualize their punishment of the children, and the ideal breeding ground for Oedipus and Electra complexes is prepared. Paul Chodoff (1966) endorsed the view of Frieda Fromm-Reichmann that these emotional hothouse families were class-bound, ethnic-bound Viennese families very conducive to Oedipal formations, as the Freudians attested, but certainly not to be found universally, or even widely, and certainly not behind every neurosis or every type of human discomfort. A father can help his daughter's sexual development when she is a preschooler if he lets her have her own sexual longings, fantasies, and feelings and does not try to colonize her mind, being neither too seductive nor too guilt-inspiring.

When she does go to school, the father can help both girl and mother to release her to the care of her teacher and the company of her peers. He can trust his daughter to make friends, especially in later elementary-school years, irrespective of parental prejudices, knowing that what his daughter does to get loving validation from her chums and crushes is more important now than that she please her family's members. The father can have a good function, from the schoolgirl's standpoint, if he serves as a mere alternative to the mother—sometimes, as a less abrasive tutor who helps with school assignments; again, when the girl at seven years old, for example, uses her father as a friend, for she feels her mother hates her; sometimes, as one who approves of the racially or economically different chum whom the mother caustically discredits. School-age girls (and boys) who are not very disturbed emotionally seem to have a freer, less sticky interaction with their fathers than do children of the same age who are more seriously disturbed; also, the fathers of these children seem more empathetic to the children. That is only a correlation, however, not necessarily a cause–effect connection (Adams, 1965).

In Erikson's (1959) terms, the father can aid his young daughter, if he wishes and knows how to achieve it, in her learning during earliest infancy the lessons of trust, of confidence that sustenance and pleasure come from others—in itself an important lesson for later sexuality—and during the second year of life (the so-called anal stage), how much good feeling comes from doing something for oneself even if despite others. During the so-called phallic stage the father potentially aids his daughter's guiltless genitality and high initiative in all areas of her functioning, again without exploiting her or persecuting her. During the school years, he helps her consolidate her industriousness and to develop in mastery and competence; this help, too, will be useful to her adult sexual being in those later years—when the imperiousness of sexual lust is muted ony because it is felt in a context of middle-aged "latency," the subduing of the sex drive through integration into a life of work and serious commitments to adult projects, a world of human values. In preadolescence, he can affirm her love for the chum, thereby giving a boost to her emancipation from her family (that will be top item on her agenda in just a few more years); he can also approve and validate her impending womanhood, observe her menarche with congratulatory comments, and make encouraging reference to her breast development. And he can do all this as a healthy father who loves her, not trying to seduce or exploit her.

By the time she is reaching puberty and adolescence, the older girl characterizes her gender behavior as a woman-to-be. In large part, she can learn this behavior from her father by identifying with him and thereby internalizing his view of appropriate gender behavior for a young woman. After all, fathers treat girls femininely, as girls and not as boys. Such feminine treatment by fathers of their daughters can contrast well with the father's own more masculine behavior. This counterbalancing provides an older girl or a young woman with a firm concept of appropriate femininity, alongside the more traditionally masculine attributes of assertiveness and goal orientation. By modeling, the father can impart both feminine and masculine traits to his daughter while providing an appropriate guide for her gender behavior as a woman. Perhaps women's libbers should take another look at fathers in particular and not overly scorn fathers' contributions to the making of young women—even those who struggle for women's liberation.

During her adolescence, in addition to condoning her progressive movements outside the nest, the father may welcome his daughter's choice of the vocation that will use her talents best. He will not coerce her into a coarcted life-calling that is "a woman's work," her lot in life, somehow inferior, but something she opts for because she does not want to "have people think you are trying to be a man."

During the daughter's adolescence, a father might not only offer understanding and protection against her sexual exploitation by her age-mates but also uphold the viewpoint that adolescence is a time for sexual experimentation, lest she wither into a compulsive virginity that will not serve her well for the rest of her life. Occasionally, the selfsame father who has behaved well toward his daughter prior to her adolescence becomes possessive, untrusting, and pernicious during her adolescence. There come to mind several fathers we have seen who call their teenage daughters whores when they come home half an hour late from a date, who inspect their daughter's panties for tell-tale signs of sexual secretions or ejaculate, and who envision adolescence as an unending orgy of promiscuity. Another type of father, at least in his overt actions, is the one who becomes cold and distant, moving away because of his own incestuous attraction to his now-grown daughter, a woman.

There are abundant assertions in writings of the 1970s that the less-constricted, less-stereotyped sex-role functioning a young woman has, the better she will fare in terms of assuming the responsibilities of career, marriage, child rearing, or all three (Lynn, 1974; Money and Ehrhardt, 1972; Lerner, 1978; Badaracco, 1974). Increasingly, we learn that the father has a vital role to play: he has the dual role of imparting feminine images as well as masculine ones to his daughter. The more she can incorporate into her repertoire of gender behavior all those qualities (of others and herself) that she enjoys and that fulfill her, the happier, the more capable, and the less emotionally ill she will be.

Only the father who has not held down his daughter can know the delight to be derived from seeng her achieve capable womanhood, not as a separate species of humanity but as a variant of humanity in all its fullness.

Sexual Preferences: Paternal Influences

There are several fathers whom we have encountered who decry all sexual activity for their daughters, subscribe vociferously to the cult of virginity, and bend over backward to keep their daughters from trying any sexual expression at all. Such hard-won virginity hardly seems virtuous, and our experience is that these daughters sustain a defensively low level of sex drive most of the time, sometimes punctuated by panicky periods when they feel they must be homosexual "deep down." Patently, such chastity is not virtue at a peak level. On the other hand, as hard as it is for psychiatrists to reckon with, there are women, noble women indeed, who have elected to be celibate. They feel (and we would not dispute them on the basis of what we have seen up to now) that celibacy is a happy ("blessed") way to deploy their total energies for human welfare (Goergen, 1974). Such chastity soon loses (if it ever had) its character of defensive renunciation and seldom relies on a misogyny that hates sexually active women in order to exalt the Virgin Mary, for example.

A feminist could be anti-Lesbian only with great feats of casuistry and self-deceptive legerdemain. Why should not a woman love a woman? Similarly, we feel, a father who truly respects and appreciates women would be hard put to repudiate a daughter who developed in her sexuality along Lesbian lines—or heterosexual or any other lines (including the bisexual or androgynous). Any preference, if it does not diminish her own worth or infringe on the rights of other persons, should be accepted as appropriately fulfilling until proven otherwise.

From a psychiatric standpoint, there are many more hideous things than lesbianism or celibacy for a young woman. There are worse traps than heterosexuality, too, or bisexuality. As sexually preoccupied as we psychiatrists may be, we do not believe that a person's sexual preferences are determinative of her character structure. The situation is quite the reverse, and it is her character structure we must focus on as psychiatrists. From character, sexuality flows.

A heterosexual woman can be very unhappy; one does not have to be celibate, bisexual, or Lesbian in order to be miserable! Compulsive "gay" behavior (not a woman's invention, assuredly) is just as questionable from a psychiatrist's perspective as compulsively "jock" or macho carryings-on. The same is true of the determined butch and her opposite. Perhaps the strongest case can be made, as the Freudians have claimed (as well as the Jungians and many Oriental and Western religiophilosophical traditions), for being noncompulsive and accepting of our bisexual feelings as natural and for being as unmarred by convention as possible so that we may have a sexuality worthy of us all as human beings. The case for androgyny is appealing.

At all events, a father who does not feel alien to any form of uncompulsive sexuality is a father who can best sustain a relationship as coequal and friend with a grown daughter who is being her own person in the sexual sphere. That is a rather weak generalization, but it is a considered statement. The fact is that the *general* role of the father in his daughter's sexual preferences is uncertain, for it is only in the single case that we can make sensible and plausible attempts to reconstruct credible scenarios of father–daughter interactions.

FATHER–DAUGHTER INCEST

Up to now we have considered some of the optimal possibilities for a father-and-daughter interaction. Now, we turn to a more sordid, destructive topic.

Incest between father and daughter does occur almost from birth onward, not in a majority of families but more frequently than was formerly thought. Father–daughter incest is, in many communities, the principal form of sexual abuse of children, the *last* frontier of child abuse (Sgroi, 1975).

Incestuous relationships are hardly new in human history. They are as old as other forms of child exploitation: murder, sodomy, neglect, abuse, abandonment, and physical torture (corporal punishment). Sophocles, Racine, and Freud were only the chroniclers of incest. They did not invent it. The Oedipus complex of boys and the Electra complex of girls are now joined extensively by the Phaedra complex of stepchildren, lusting for their stepparents. The very way we describe these complexes tells a lot, since we put the onus on the children instead of on the adults in our definition of each complex. Psychiatrists tend to do this again, for example, when they describe girls who are molested by their fathers as "incestuous daughters."

Although living in an era when a certain chic brand of victimology assigns blame to the victim instead of the oppressor, we do not view incest as a harmless form of father–daughter interaction. We see it as a sickness—a father who is already sick and a daughter who is fated (barring long-term help) to be sick in a sociomoral context that is also sick. Incest is destructive of the family's integrity, and we do not agree with the opinions of those workers from Philadelphia and San Jose who declare that The Family is of foremost importance. We believe that a family in which a father molests his daughter is no longer a salvageable and viable family. To too many therapists, *family* really means "parents." A family of father–daughter incest is an odoriferous fragment of a true family, if the latter is to be considered an instrument for the nurturance and protection of children. Of course, if the family is for patriarchal jollies at any cost then incest is best, as the joke proclaims.

Our experience in Louisville, Kentucky, and elsewhere suggests that incest has extremely dire consequences for the little girl. The pathological sequels are compounded when the mother does nothing to help her daughter should the girl tell her mother of the incestuous attack. Many a young woman looks back with a killing hatred of her mother, who stood by, proclaiming a superior interest in her own meal ticket, when her little girl reported the father's rape. In our estimation, incest with a minor is always rape. Even the statutes portray it as statutory rape, a heinous crime. It entails a bad relationship with the father as well as with the mother under those conditions. Among the personal problems that may ensue in the adult life of the incestuously assaulted girl are homosexuality, frigidity, promiscuity, prostitution, and problems in marriage and sexual functioning too diverse for easy listing, as is shown in the writings of James (1977), Peters (1976), and Poznanski and Blos (1975).

Fathers who commit incest with their daughters are very cunning individuals. They usually show a pattern of maneuvers and strategies, including, first, denial and verbal or physical abuse of the daughter who "told"; second, trying to threaten the mother into complicity against the child so that both parents will be united in trying to divert the "authorities" from any action against the child-molesting father; third, making a counteraccusation that the child invited it, brought it on; fourth, stating he did not know what he was doing because of his distress with a frigid wife or because of temporary insanity or because of being under the influence of alcohol or other drugs. If the case is ever prosecuted, there usually lie ahead only the barbarities of a long prison term for someone who merits consideration and therapy even while society, and his daughter especially, is being protected from his attacks. Incestuous fathers are slippery, mendacious, and resistive to psychiatric treatment, however, and, unfortunately, the entirety of the portrait of father–daughter incest is an ugly one. The picture is given with crystal clarity in papers by Bender and Grugett (1952), Chaneles (1967), Finch (1973), Ford (1977), Hayman and Lanza (1971), Laury

(1978), Lewis and Sarrel (1969), Lukianowicz (1972), Rosenfeld, Nadelson, Krieger, and Backman (1977), and in Sexual Survey #12 in *Medical Aspects of Human Sexuality* (1978).

Concluding Discussion

A father can be a strong force for good or ill in the sexual development of his daughter. Our intention has been to be realistic, by citing at first some of the facts of biological paternity; considering the father's ways of participation in the making of a healthy baby girl, a wholesome toddler, preschooler, schoolgirl, preadolescent, and adolescent; also considering some of the nonwholesome and counterproductive things a father can do with regard to his daughter's sexuality; and finally, citing briefly some of the most awful consequences of incest, the epitome of sickness in a father–daughter relationship.

We could be wrong in our assertion that realism inheres in or accrues from the approach taken, namely, to present capsules of fact, of idealized possibilities and of sordid pathology. We trust that by our panorama we have enlarged on the usual painting of father–daughter relations: often a self-consistent vignette that shows either a bland or utopian or degenerate scene. We think a more useful approximation of truth lies in the depiction of all three scenes.

References

Adams, P. L. Empathic parenting of the elementary school child. *Southern Medical Journal,* 1965, *58*(5), 642–647.

Badaracco, M. R. Recent trends towards unisex: A panel. *American Journal of Psychoanalysis,* 1974, *34,* 17–23.

Bender, L., and Grugett, A. E. Follow-up report on children who had atypical sexual experience. *American Journal of Orthopsychiatry,* 1952, *22,* 825–837.

Birns, B. The emergence and socialization of sex differences in the earliest years. *Merrill-Palmer Quarterly of Behavior and Development,* 1976, *22*(3), 229–254.

Chaneles, S. Child victims of sexual offenses. *Federal Probation,* 1967, *31*(2), 52–56.

Chodoff, P. A critique of Freud's theory of infantile sexuality. *American Journal of Psychiatry,* 1966, *123*(5), 508–517.

Erikson, E. H. Growth and crises of the healthy personality. *Psychological Issues,* 1959, *1,* 50–100.

Finch, S. M. Adult seduction of the child: Effects on the child. *Medical Aspects of Human Sexuality,* March 1973, pp. 170–187.

Ford, S. Incest. *Courier-Journal,* October 23, 1977.

Goergen, D. *The sexual celibate.* New York: The Seabury Press, 1974.

Hayman, C. R., and Lanza, C. Sexual assault on women and girls. *American Journal of Obstetrics and Gynecology,* 1971, *109,* 480–486.

James, K. L. Incest: The teenager's perspective. *Psychotherapy: Theory, Research, and Practice,* Summer 1977, *14*(2), 146–155.

Laury, G. V. Quiz. *Medical Aspects of Human Sexuality*, November 1978, pp. 99–102.

Lerner, H. E. Adaptive and pathogenic aspects of sex-role stereotypes: Implications for parenting and psychotherapy. *American Journal of Psychiatry*, 1978, *135*(1), 48–52.

Lewis, M., and Sarrel, P. M. Some psychological aspects of seduction, incest, and rape in childhood. *Journal of the American Academy of Child Psychiatry*, 1969, *8*, 606–619.

Lukianowicz, N. Incest I: Paternal incest. *International Journal of Psychiatry*, 1972, *120*, 301–313.

Lynn, D. B. *The father: His role in child development*. Monterey, Calif.: Brooks/Cole Publishing, 1974.

Money, J., and Ehrhardt, A. A. *Man & woman, boy & girl: The differentiation and dimorphis of gender identity from conception to maturity*. Baltimore and London: Johns Hopkins University Press, 1972.

Peters, J. J. Children who are victims of sexual assault and the psychology of offenders. *American Journal of Psychotherapy*, 1976, *30*, 398–421.

Poznanski, E., and Blos, P. Incest. *Medical Aspects of Human Sexuality*, October 1975, pp. 46–76.

Rosenfeld, A. A., Nadelson, C. C., Krieger, M., and Backman, J. H. Incest and sexual abuse of children. *Journal of The American Academy of Child Psychiatry*, 1977, *17*(2), 327–339.

Sexual Survey #12: Current thinking on sexual abuse of children. *Medical Aspects of Human Sexuality*, July 1978, pp. 44–47.

Sgroi, S. M. Sexual molestation of children—The last frontier in child abuse. *Children Today*, May–June 1975, pp. 18–44.

Wainwright, W. H. Fatherhood as a precipitant of mental illness. *American Journal of Psychiatry*, 1966, *123*(1), 40–44.

Chapter 13

Sex Education versus Sexual Learning

Elizabeth J. Roberts

{Editor's Note

In this article, Ms. Roberts describes the need for a reconceptualization of "sexuality" and issues related to sexual development and sexual learning. She calls for a fuller examination of the breadth of human experience relevant to understanding sexuality and goes on to suggest that learning about sexuality is a lifelong process. Sexual learning occurs in many environments, and much of the learning that influences how we experience and express our sexuality is informal, indirect, and unintentional. In brief, Ms. Roberts believes that "sexuality is more than sex" and that learning about sexuality is more than sex education.}

We Americans evidence enormous interest in "sex." Our movies, television programs, and magazines attest to this. The wide distribution of pornography, do-it-yourself sex books, and the how-to-improve-your-life literature proclaim it. Given this national preoccupation with the topic, one might expect the American population to be well on its way to achieving sexual fulfillment, understanding, and happiness.

Not so.

The reports of three national commissions—the Commission on Population Growth and the American Future, the National Leadership Conference on Venereal Disease, and the President's Commission on Obscenity and Pornography—stress the importance of sexuality in our lives, yet document the fear and uncertainty that permeate our attitudes and influence our behavior. The studies prepared for these com-

ELIZABETH J. ROBERTS, M.A. • President, Population Education, Inc.; and Executive Director, Project on Human Sexual Development, Cambridge, Massachusetts.

missions revealed that ignorance and myth about sexuality are widespread in our society and suggested that both contribute to negative self-image, faulty communication between men and women, and uninformed or irresponsible sexual decision-making.

These reports concluded that millions of individuals of all ages in our society need and want help in understanding sexuality. But such an understanding will not come easily. The term itself is imprecise. The issues are emotionally charged. Clichés and oversimplifications often cloud discussion. And public attention is focused primarily on sexuality as a source of social problems rather than as an essential and important part of our identity. As a result, despite our presumed "sexual openness," we have not been able to hold full, rational, honest dialogue about the meaning of sexuality or the complex process of sexual learning.

Most distressing of all, the situation is self-perpetuating. A population that deals uneasily with sexual issues is not likely to guide the sexual learning of young children meaningfully and effectively. In response to this dilemma, many national and community policy planners point to school-based sex-education programs as a primary source of sexual learning. However, this form of education, when it is available, is little more than "reproductive education." It usually presents facts about the function of the Fallopian tubes, the development of secondary sex characteristics, and the means for preventing conception. Rarely does it involve a discussion of the many attitudes and experiences that shape our sexuality or give meaning to our sexual expression.

Indeed, the results of a study of over 1400 parents in Cleveland, Ohio, on their attitudes toward and perception of childhood learning about sexuality (Roberts, Kline, and Gagnon, 1978) reveal that the mothers and fathers surveyed exhibited little faith that formal "sex education" courses were an effective source of their child's sexual learning. Parents were asked, "Other than from you, where do you think your child has learned the *most* about sexuality?" and were given several possible answers from which to choose. Even though they could select more than one source of learning for their child, school programs did not appear in the list of the top five most frequently mentioned sources. (Note, however, that when mentioned, schools were cited among the most accurate sources of information.) Almost half of all parents felt that their children learned the most about sexuality from television. The next three highest-ranked sources in this survey were other young people: siblings, peers, and older children.

The majority of young people themselves usually report learning most about sexuality from their peers (Gagnon, 1965). Neither parents nor young people, then, seem to find the traditional authority figures (such as teachers, doctors, or clergymen) major sources of sexual learning. These responses should not surprise us because most formal "sex education" programs in this country are narrowly defined, limited in content, and late in coming. At their worst, they are simply irrelevant. How can we expect a formal, compartmentalized educational or social program to capture the essence of what is effectively a life-long developmental process?

Our society, formally and informally, treats sexuality as if it were an activity apart from most others. To most people, the word *sexuality* typically means sexual intercourse and brings to mind a brief and limited encounter that begins and ends at a certain time, occurs with a certain person in a certain place, involves specific parts of the body, and frequently results in conception.

Sexuality, however, involves considerably more than sexual intercourse, reproduction, or physiological development. In a professional publication, the American Medical Association (1972) stated:

> Human sexuality is involved in what we do, but it is also what we are. It is an identification, an activity, a drive, a biological and emotional process, an outlook and an expression of the self. . . . It is an important factor in every personal relationship and every human endeavor, from business to politics.

This statement, along with similar statements by the World Health Organization (WHO), Sex Information and Education Council of the United States (SIECUS), The Project on Human Sexual Development, and professionals from various fields, indicates that our sexuality is part of our basic identity. It encompasses our total sense of self as male or female. It involves our attitudes, values, feelings and beliefs about masculinity and femininity; how we feel about our physical selves—the limits, the joys, and the embarrassments of our bodies. It is the integration of our needs for affiliation and intimacy, and our expressions of love and affection, as well as our fears, fantasies, and decisions regarding our erotic conduct. Human sexuality is expressed in our full range of interactions with others. It influences and is influenced by our interpersonal relationships, our family roles, and our social life-styles. Thus, sexuality is integral to the establishment of self-image, self-understanding, and personal identity and to the formation of human relationships.

If we accept the broad-based meaning of sexuality in our lives, then education in sexuality includes considerably more than a sixth grade course in the "facts of life," the once-only parent–child conversation, the sex-education book left in a visible place, or a guest lecture on contraception and family planning. Sexual learning is social learning. It begins at birth and occurs through life, in a variety of complex and subtle ways, in many different environments. Truly effective education about sexuality must be broad enough and profound enough to help people understand the physical, psychological, social, and moral implications of their sexuality as part of their total personality and its development.

Seen in this light, it is obvious that very little of the information relevant to understanding sexuality is learned by children or adults in a formal manner or through formalized sex-education channels. Learning about sexuality is an ongoing process. What is learned, how it is learned, and who the teachers are might be different at different times in the life cycle. However, sexual learning occurs all the time, everywhere. Beginning the day we are born, a complex set of roles, behaviors, attitudes, and values about sexuality are being conveyed and defined by our family, our society, and our culture.

SEXUAL LEARNING IN CHILDHOOD: THE CONTENT MESSAGES

The importance of the first years in a child's life for the development of physical, mental, and emotional capacities is well known. An integral component of this early growth is the child's sexual development. During these early years, children develop an awareness of the body and its functions; they begin to learn how to express feelings and develop a growing sense of psychological self; and equally important, they are learning socially sanctioned gender roles and an understanding of appropriate behavior in close relationships.

Very early in their lives, young children explore their own bodies and become interested in exploring the bodies of others. When parents or friends react to this behavior, they influence the sexual learning of that child. The message they convey may be warm approval, neutral acceptance, or anger and disapproval. Whatever the verbal or nonverbal message, the child learns what can be touched, who can be touched, and under what circumstances it is acceptable to see, show, or ask questions about the body. Many studies indicate that most children take specific notice of their genitals early in their lives. They may touch them, fondle them, or systematically stroke them. They may want to explore the genitals of others. In the study on family life and sexual learning cited earlier (Roberts *et al.*, 1978) approximately 85% of all parents reported that they believed that most young children explore their genitals or masturbate. Again, the reaction of parents, teachers, and friends to such activities is important. The child perceives the acceptance or lack thereof and links the reaction to these behaviors. While such genital play or masturbation in childhood may not carry the same meaning it does for the adolescent or the adult in our society, responses to it set the stage for a child's feelings of pleasure or guilt about his/her body and its function.

In addition to self-exploration, children learn important body messages from the ways in which they are handled and touched by their parents. While this learning may not be understood as "sexual" by any of the people involved, it carries messages about feeling good and about warmth and closeness. Some children receive the message that hugging and kissing and free-and-easy access to their parents, grandparents, and relatives are, if not wrong, unrewarded or frowned upon. Such children grow up with a different sense of their bodies from that of children who have been rewarded and praised for their open displays of physical affection. Liking one's body is part of liking oneself. Feelings of comfort with the body and its image become part of the way people see themselves as desirable or undesirable. All are important elements in the sexual learning of children—elements that may affect their actions and reactions in countless interpersonal negotiations during the rest of their lives.

In addition to learning about their bodies, young people also learn which ways of demonstrating feelings and emotion are approved by members of their family and society. Substantial research indicates that we accept, even reward, assertive and aggressive behavior in boys and tend to discourage it in girls. With girls, we are more likely to encourage nurturing and caretaking behavior. Thus, child development literature indicates that girls are more likely than boys to express affection through hugging and touching. Indeed, boys are often systematically discouraged from kissing, hugging, being gentle, or asking for comfort and help. For example, the Cleveland parents (Roberts *et al;* 1978) revealed that while 60% of parents reported that their daughters occasionally or often hugged their girlfriends, 60% of parents reported that their sons never hugged their friends of the same sex. It isn't surprising to discover from the same data that approximately 7 out of 10 fathers reported that they themselves rarely or never hugged their friends of the same sex, while 6 out of 10 women reported they often hugged their female friends. Again, this learning takes place informally, almost incidentally—as children observe who their parents touch and talk with, who is allowed to cry, and who can ask for support in the family.

Consider this finding from *Family Life and Sexual Learning* (Robert *et al.*, 1978). Although 90% of fathers participating in the survey reported that they wanted to communicate to their children that it was "good for men to cry," when offered a set of situations (death of a friend, movie, television/books, intense day, when frustrated, when depressed, weddings, making love, when angry) and asked in which of those situations they had cried, in every instance except one (when angry), fewer men than women reported crying. If children see men given respect for controlling their emotions or women rewarded for being expressive, they are learning behaviors that will have implications for their sexuality and the various ways of expressing it.

One of the most important aspects of sexual learning is the set of messages given to boys and girls about appropriate masculine and feminine roles. While still young, children begin to learn what traits and styles are considered acceptable for one gender and not the other. This gender-role learning is of paramount importance because the basic division of adult social roles in our society is based on these masculine and feminine personality qualities.

Perhaps the most significant element in this process of gender-role learning is the way in which we segregate boys and girls. Physically, boys and girls are often divided on the playground or in elective school curricula ("shop" and "home economics"), for example. More importantly, however, we also segregate them psychologically by reinforcing the notion that how one gender behaves, the other should not. Even the term *opposite sex* implies this segregation. Thus, if girls can cry, boys do not. If men are competitive, women are not. This gender training can have dramatic influence on the future sexual decision-making of our youth.

Let's take, for example, a hypothetical 16-year-old boy and girl considering intercourse and some of the messages they may have received in this area that could affect their decision. Let's say he was raised to learn as part of his gender role that for a man, growing up means to grow away from others, to be independent, and to make decisions. Perhaps he has had little training in being sensual or affectionate and was raised to see his body as something he must perform with and use to prove himself and his masculinity; perhaps he has been encouraged by his peers to be goal-oriented and to succeed at all costs, even in the bedroom. We should not be surprised, then, having taught him to identify masculinity with "being cool" and "scoring," having taught him that wanting to be touched or held or comforted might be week or unmanly, that our hypothetical 16-year-old boy decides that the only way he can express his masculinity or receive affection is by pressing for intercourse.

Now for our young girl. Perhaps she was raised to see as part of her gender role the importance of meeting the needs of others. Perhaps billboards, TV programs, parents, and friends have conveyed to her that the most important aspect of her body is its attractiveness to males. She has been raised to think that sex is something that happens to her, something she should not or cannot make decisions about. Perhaps she is ambivalent or frightened about her own erotic feelings, and the only information she has about male physiology is the inaccurate notion that boys are possessed by an uncontrollable sex drive. So we should not be surprised when, despite all the contraceptive information in the world, our 16-year-old girl has difficulty acknowledging to herself or to her boyfriend that sex is something she understands, has planned for, and accepts.

How can we expect the conditions of this learning to let both our girl and our boy have increased options? She doesn't have to pretend it all just sort of happened, "I was swept off my feet"; she doesn't have to worry, "Will my parents think I'm a bad girl if I use a contraceptive device?" He doesn't have to fear being viewed as less of a man if what he really wants is to be held; and they don't have to worry, "How in the world do we talk about all this?" This hypothetical example is not about intercourse. Rather, it is about the many messages—the sexual learning—that influence what we do and how we feel about what we do. It's about body image, about feelings of love and intimacy, about what we think is "sexy," and how we make decisions.

Gender-role development sets the framework for the process of sexual learning; learning about expressive behavior tells how to share our feelings and with whom; and body learning sets the parameters for feeling guilt or pleasure about our bodies and their use. There are certainly many other "messages" that shape a child's understanding of sexuality. However, I believe the three discussed above are important reference points for understanding the process of sexual learning.

Sexual Learning in Childhood: The Learning Environment

If we accept the premise that sexual learning starts at birth and that attitudes about one's sexuality are partially formed in childhood, then it follows that we must increase our understanding of these environments within which children grow and learn. Clearly, this means achieving a better understanding of family relationships and communication styles—because the family is one of the most important environments in which children learn.

Children learn not only from their parents but also from relatives, neighbors, and friends. They learn from the toys, books, and games that surround them, and they learn from the major institutions in this society: religious teachings, mass media, work requirements, health policies, and social welfare programs. All of these contribute to the child's understanding, acceptance, and expression of her or his sexuality (Roberts, 1980).

Some of these influences are subtle, yet remarkably effective because they are all-pervasive and are reinforced over extended periods of one's life. For example, the way in which the resources of time, money, space, and energy are allocated conveys powerful messages that influence sexual values and behaviors. In our culture "time is money"; it is to be spent wisely, not frivolously. So it is no wonder we have not learned to savor the delights of a leisurely dinner. And no wonder, also, that we cannot forget the passage of time long enough to enjoy the unhurried expression of affection . . . with our children, our friends, and our lovers. Rather, we have taught our young girls and boys in subtle and covert ways to believe in love at first sight and instant, simultaneous orgasms.

For many individuals, messages about the body, affective expression, gender roles, and specific sexual behavior are substantially affected by the many social and moral sanctions surrounding sexuality in our society. These sanctions frequently take the form of actual codified laws and statutes. Indeed, from one point of view, the criminal laws related to sexual behavior could be considered the governing sexual code in the United States. Primarily through exclusions and a series of "do not's," this legal code sets the boundaries for what is approved and acceptable sexual conduct. Although most formal sexual laws are neither widely known nor universally enforced (according to most survey data on adult sexual behavior, the majority of individuals in the United States are guilty of having broken one or more of the many laws governing sexual conduct), their presence on the books subtly communicates what is socially acceptable.

Perhaps more important to childhood sexual learning than formal laws are the numerous social and moral norms that circumscribe sexuality. Based on them are numerous value judgments about how we should feel, think, and behave sexually. In Western societies, the Judeo-Christian tradition has been most influential in shaping such sexual codes. Whether we subscribe to this tradition and its teachings or not, we cannot deny that these social and moral norms and codes exert a continuous influence on how and what children learn about sexuality.

Supplementing interpersonal communication, the allocation of resources, and social and moral codes, there is that endlessly intrusive, extremely influential learning tool that flickers and whimpers, sparkles and bellows in the corner: the television set. We do not yet fully understand the exact nature of this learning instrument in the development of sexual attitudes and values, yet we do know it has its impact. Research indicates that television has become one of the chief story-tellers of our society, supplementing and in many instances supplant-ing the teachings of the home, the church, and the school. Through its entertainment and dramatic programming, television makes our cul-ture audible and visible to its members. It encourages people to per-ceive as normal and acceptable what fits the established fantasies of our society. A growing body of literature suggests that individuals young and old use what they learn on television as the cultural stan-dard by which to judge the larger society. The role of television as the common socializer and storyteller has become particularly important in the conveyance of sexual messages. Consider these few examples of research findings drawn from over the past several years:

- Content analysis of television programs has revealed that when personality traits of male and female characters are compared, television males tend to be ambitious, competitive, realistic, vi-olent, independent, logical, dominant, unemotional, tall, and smart. On the other hand, television females tend to be affec-tionate, sensitive, romantic, incompetent, submissive, emo-tional, illogical, independent, warm, and young (Busby, 1974; Tedesco, 1975).
- Male interests tend to dominate the television set in many ways: approximately 75% of all major characters on television are male (Tedesco, 1974); 65% of all characters in situation comedies are male (Women's Division, 1976); and 85% of all characters on action–adventure programs are male (Women on Words & Images, 1975). Approximately equal percentages of men and women are in the age category "under 25," but men outnumber women four to one in the "over-50" age category (National Organization for Women, n.d.). Women on television are generally well groomed, under 40, and attractive (Long and Simon, 1974).
- As for marriage and close relationships, almost half of all close relationships on prime-time television are between men. Only the smallest minority of close relationships on prime-time tele-vision are between women (Gerbner, 1972). The majority of close relationships are between partners who work together; of these, 62% are between men, 7% between women (Gerbner, 1972). Less than 2% of television female characters solve prob-lems by themselves; 48% of television females have their prob-lems resolved entirely by others (McNeil, 1975).
- In televisionland, marriage and family life are primarily the

concern of the female: 70% of all women are shown in and
around the home (Long and Simon, 1974; McNeil, 1975); 64% of
female activities focus on the home and family relationships
(Long and Simon, 1974; McNeil, 1975). This finding contrasts
sharply with the fact that only 20% of male interaction focuses
on marital and family relationships (Long and Simon, 1974;
McNeil, 1975); and while single men on television are portrayed
as strong, adventuresome, and independent, most married men
on television are portrayed as stupid or bungling (Long and
Simon, 1974; McNeil, 1975). And finally, about 90% of all television characters have no children (Lemon, 1975).

These statistics by no means present a definitive picture of television programming, nor do they presume to demonstrate a direct link
between specific television content and "effects" on audience viewers.
They simply highlight some of the images of men and women, close
relationships, and marriage and family life presented on television. It
is obvious that many other images and messages that are difficult to
count and evaluate through standard research methods have an
equally strong yet subtle impact on the television viewer.

Messages about sexuality, then, are conveyed in many ways and
in many environments. Sexual learning takes place in numerous formal and informal situations. It is a living and life-long process, and
the messages we receive are often ambiguous or conflicting. For example, we say that it is adult (even desirable) to be sexy—but not too
sexy because that can get one into trouble. We say that bodies are
good; we should jog, exercise, and take care of them; however, touching or finding pleasure in them may be bad. We say to be a woman is
to be emotional and passive and to say "no" even if you mean yes; we
say to be a man is to be aggressive, in control, and sure of oneself
under all circumstances. And we say the conjugal bed will overcome
the ignorance and repair the damage caused by years of psychological
segregation.

The process of sexual learning is not organized like a textbook or a
lesson plan, where first we learn this and then we learn that. Rather, it
is often a chaotic and disorderly collection of learning that never quite
becomes completely integrated. There are volumes of sexual literature
and mountains of data available to us, but no one to discuss them
with, no one to help us appraise and evaluate them. Most people are
forced to make sense of their sexuality, and the frequently conflicting
sexual messages they receive, alone. Children, adolescents, and adults
are required to find their way to responsible sexual satisfaction with-

out ever talking about responsibility or sexuality or satisfaction. If these are the conditions of learning about sexuality, then the evidence that many persons find their own sexuality a source of difficulty should come to us as no surprise.

Nor is it a surprise that difficulties that individuals have in other aspects of their lives may be traced back to the influence of inaccurate and unintegrated sexual learning. The influence of sexual unhappiness on work, on communication between spouses, on the rearing of children, and on the relations between friends is an interactive process—becoming a self-perpetuating system. Those forces (from the smallest interaction to the largest institution) that shape us and our sexuality, in turn, become shaped by us and the experiences and expressions of our sexuality. We are at once student and teacher—always learning and educating others about sexuality. The implications of this perspective on sexual learning are many:

- We must acknowledge that people don't magically become sexual all at once—at birth, at puberty, or in marriage.
- Learning about sexuality must be seen as an ongoing, lifelong process.
- We must recognize the importance of early learning and provide parents, teachers, pediatricians, and counselors with both information and opportunities for the discussion of childhood sexual learning.
- We must carefully examine the nonschool environments that have an impact on our sexual learning and our sense of self; and we must evaluate the roles that major institutions play in this process.

Because we do not now look at the processes through which people become sexual and the role that sexuality plays in our lives, we remain fearful that if we do anything, something will go wrong. The net result is an increase in those problems we seek most to resolve. Discussion about sexuality and sexual learning must be brought to the attention of the public in a way that will dispel the fear, anxiety, and misinformation that permeate most attitudes. Sexuality needs to be legitimized; the full range of topics must be explored in a form and in forums that can facilitate thoughtful consideration.

That is no small task: putting a new idea on a national agenda. And it amounts to nothing less than having us think differently— about ourselves and the world in which we live.

Yet, that awareness is the first step toward an increased understanding of sexuality and improved sexual learning.

REFERENCES

American Medical Association Committee on Human Sexuality. *Human Sexuality*, 1972, 3.

Busby, L. J. *Sex roles as presented in commercial network television programs directed toward children: Rationale and analysis*, Ph.D. dissertation, University of Michigan, 1974.

Commission on Population Growth and the American Future. *Population Growth and the American Future.* New York: New American Library, 1972.

Gagnon, J. H. Sexuality and sexual learning in the child. *Psychiatry*, 1965, *3*, 212–228.

Gerbner, G. Violence in television drama: Trends and symbolic functions. In G. A. Comstock and E. A. Rubinstein (Eds.), *Television and social behavior*, Vol. 1. Washington, D.C.: U.S. Government Printing Office, 1972.

Lemon, J. L. *A content analysis of male and female dominance patterns on prime time television*, qualifying paper, Graduate School of Education, Harvard University, 1975.

Long, M. L., and Simon, R. J. The roles and statuses of women on children and family TV programs. *Journalism Quarterly*, 1974, *1*, 107–110.

McNeil, J. C. Feminism, femininity, and the television series: A content analysis. *Journal of Broadcasting*, 1975, *3*.

National Leadership Conference on Venereal Disease, 1974.

National Organization for Women, National Capital Area Chapter, *Women in the wasteland fight back: A report on the image of women portrayed in TV programming.* Washington, D.C., undated.

President's Commission on Obscenity and Pornography, 1970.

Roberts, E. J. (Ed.), *Childhood sexual learning: The unwritten curriculum.* Cambridge, Mass.: Ballinger Publishing, 1980.

Roberts, E. J., Kline, D. and Gagnon, J. *Family life and sexual learning.* Cambridge, Mass.: Population Education, Inc., 1978.

Tedesco, N. S. Patterns in prime time. *Journal of Communication*, 1974, *2*.

Tedesco, N. S. *Men and women in television drama: The use of two multivariate techniques for isolating dimensions of characterization*, A dissertation in communications, University of Pennsylvania, 1975.

Women on Words & Images, *Channeling children.* Princeton, N.J., 1975.

Women's Division, Board of Global Ministries, The United Methodist Church. *Sex role stereotyping in prime time television.* March 1976, *9*.

Chapter 14

A Sex-Information Switchboard

Margo Rila and Judith Steinhart

⦃Editor's Note

The hot line is an innovative attempt to provide information and support in a relevant and reassuring setting. There is personal contact, unlike the impersonality of the television set; specific questions can be asked and answered; and anonymity protects the caller from embarrassment or fear of punishment. Some communities are making use of this device to provide sex education and a nonjudgmental referral source.

Although the San Francisco group whose brief report follows had limited funds amd minimal publicity, in the first year and a half of 3-to-9 pm operation, over 10,000 calls were received.⦄

San Francisco Sex Information is a five-year-old nonprofit volunteer organization that gives free, nonjudgmental sex information and referrals to its anonymous callers. The original founders of SFSI, Toni Ayres, Carolyn Smith, and Maggi Rubenstein, recognized the importance of accurate information concerning sexuality, specifically women's sexuality. They also perceived the need for an anonymous sex-education service that would reach people who might not ordinarily attend a course or a workshop. From their work as sex educators, counselors, and therapists, they identified the relationship between information about sexuality and people's attitudes.

Before volunteers answer any calls, they are required to partici-

Margo Rila, D.A. • Faculty, The Institute for Advanced Study of Human Sexuality, San Francisco, California.   Judith Steinhart, D.A. • Clinical Assistant Professor, Department of Health Sciences, State University of New York, Stony Brook, New York; and Department of Health Science, Brooklyn College, City University of New York, Brooklyn, New York.

pate in an intensive 40-hour training program. The program is based in part on the Sexual Attitude Restructuring process developed by the National Sex Forum, which has been training professionals as well as the general public in sex education, counseling, and therapy for the past 10 years. The National Sex Forum states that appropriate topics for a program in sex education consist of "what people do and how they feel about it."

The three components of SFSI training include:

Didactic and personal presentations
Use of explicit sex-educational material produced primarily by the
    National Sex Forum
Communication and small-group sharing

Disclosure of personal experiences and lifestyles contributes to the educational process of both trainees and staff. They learn not only to view themselves and one another as valuable resources, but also to appreciate each other's unique experiences and choices.

Women have played the primary role in the development of SFSI. Training has always been planned and conducted primarily by women, and over half the trainees are women. Consequently, a feminist and egalitarian perspective affirms a woman's right to be sexual, affects the ways that male volunteers and callers relate to women, and encourages both men and women to be themselves, with their own individual wants and needs. In addition, the training presents homosexuality and bisexuality along with heterosexuality as equally valid sexual options and lifestyles.

The training has evolved over the five years and has changed to fit the needs of the callers. The training reflects the proportion and the kind of calls the switchboard receives. The topics include:

The history of sex research
The sexual response cycle
Fantasy
Masturbation
Heterosexuality, homosexuality, bisexuality
Venereal disease
Child and adolescent sexuality
Sex and aging
Lifestyles, including group sex, open relationships, celibacy
Sadism and masochism
Oral sex
Anal sex
Birth control and abortion

Sex therapy
Communication and enrichment

Volunteers have ranged in age from 18 to 62. Many women trained with SFSI for "professional reasons." Among the professionals have been nurses, psychologists, social workers, librarians, teachers, physicians, and many students in the helping professions. They found that their professional training had omitted sex information and that their work required some knowledge of the field of human sexuality.

Some women have seen working with SFSI as both a public service and a contribution to their own personal growth. The personal value gained from SFSI has included comfort with their own sexuality, facility in communication with partners and friends about sexuality, an appreciation of self-sexuality, and an appreciation of and respect for the sexual choices of others.

One third of all callers are under 18 years of age, with equal numbers of men and women. One-third of the callers are women. Eighty-five percent of the callers are heterosexual, perhaps because other switchboards and resources exist for Lesbians and gay men. Approximately 80% of the callers are in a relationship. More callers are in their 20s and 30s than in any other age category. The majority of callers identify themselves as Caucasian. The callers have learned about SFSI from friends, agencies, private practitioners, radio spots and programs, and newspaper articles. Some callers call to talk after their partners have called.

The greatest number of calls from women deal with never having an orgasm or having difficulty having an orgasm. Many callers, both male and female, want information concerning contraception. They want to know the types available; the effectiveness, advantages, and disadvantages of each; the cost; where to get them; and how each method affects sexuality. Communication with partners is a common concern. The callers may have trouble asking for what they want during a sexual experience. Other callers may want to say "no" or "yes" more often and want to know how.

Because each call is unique, the responses and information that a volunteer offers will vary. In general, the response may include:

1. Validation of women's sexuality.
2. Support for her determining her own sexuality.
3. Permission to explore options, make choices, and communicate her needs and desires to her partner(s).
4. Information concerning human sexuality and anatomy and available resources.
5. Structured techniques for changing a specific situation.

Women callers request information concerning Planned Parenthood, VD clinics, public health clinics, private physicians, nurse practitioners, marriage counselors, centers for sexual trauma, couples' groups, and women's groups for consciousness raising, coming out, orgasmic issues, and sexual enrichment.

Women need permission to expand their fantasy life without feeling guilty. They need to know that masturbation is an important sexual option. Women need encouragement to ask questions of the medical profession, since women have a hesitancy about their right to know the workings of their own bodies. In addition, since women have been traditionally taught that "It's not nice to talk about sex," many are reluctant to ask their physicians questions concerning their genitals, their reproductive organs, and their sexuality. Many physicians, perhaps because of their own discomfort with the area of sexuality, make it difficult even for the most confident of patients to ask questions. Finally, doctors frequently do not have the answers.

Women also need to know that any way they have an orgasm is fine. Many women are unaware that the clitoris is their primary sexual organ. They think that their vagina should be as sensitive as or more sensitive than their clitoris. The current statistic is that approximately 30% of women have orgasm through penile thrusting alone and that most women need additional stimulation to have an orgasm. Women have been faking orgasms for so long that they find it difficult to change the pattern.

Volunteers use the word *woman*, even if the caller refers to herself as "girl," to encourage a sense of self-esteem and worth. They encourage independence by giving information, support, and, if needed, a referral, so that the caller can better handle her specific situation.

Chapter 15

Self-Help for Sex

Carol Downer

What would happen if groups of laypeople examined each other's bodies and talked about their health-related experiences? What if they were all women and the part of the body they were examining was their genitals? Shocking? Dangerous? Frivolous? Or a totally new approach to the understanding of female sexuality and reproduction?

In 1971 in Los Angeles, several women, in turn, removed their pants, lay down and inserted a plastic vaginal speculum, looked at themselves with a mirror, and then allowed others in the group to look at their vaginal walls and uterine cervices using a flashlight. Throughout the evening, they freely shared experiences with one another. This type of session, which we named the *self-help clinic*, has been repeated by many groups of women throughout the United States and abroad. Meetings like this continued and, in the next few years, became the basis for the Federation of Feminist Women's Health Centers, which includes centers in Los Angeles, Orange County, San Diego, and Chico, California, and in Atlanta, Georgia, and Tallahassee, Florida.

By breaking the societal taboo of letting our genitals be viewed outside a medical or sexual setting, we have been able to let the feelings of shame (Greek for the genital area is *pudendum*, meaning "shame") fall away and to learn directly about our own bodies.

Since 1971, through participating in self-help clinics, writing and distributing health pamphlets and books, and establishing feminist women's health centers and women's clinics, self-helpers have amassed a new body of knowledge about the healthy functioning of a woman's body, including improved fertility-detection methods, new and safer birth-control methods, natural home remedies for common

CAROL DOWNER • Director, Feminist Women's Health Center, Los Angeles, California.
© Federation of Feminist Women's Health Centers 1979.

problems of well women, and healthy alternatives to estrogen-replacement therapy in menopause.

The women's health movement, for which the self-help clinic is the training ground, has exposed many medical myths perpetrated by male physicians whose only knowledge of women's bodies is derived from medical textbooks, their clinical practices, or personal sexual contact. But of all aspects of women's health, certainly women's sexuality has been the most neglected and misunderstood by the male-dominated medical profession and the related fields of psychotherapy and psychology. Despite some substantial contributions made by William Masters and Virginia Johnson and by Mary Jane Sherfey, whose book, *The Nature and Evolution of Female Sexuality* (1972), is based largely upon Masters and Johnson's work, the first reliable glimpse of women's sexuality in today's society has come from Shere Hite. In the *Hite Report* (1976), which consists of over 1000 responses to a lengthy questionnaire, Hite argued persuasively that women are "sexual slaves," habitually satisfying men's needs during sex and ignoring their own:

> The fact is that the role of women in sex, as in every aspect of life, has been to serve the needs of others—men and children. And just as women did not recognize their oppression in a general sense until recently, just so sexual slavery has been an almost unconscious way of life for most women—based on what was said to be an eternally unchanging biological impulse. . . . Women are sexual slaves insofar as they are (justifiably) afraid to "come out" with their own sexuality, and forced to satisfy others' needs and ignore their own. . . . The truth is that almost everything in our society pushes women toward defining their sexuality only as intercourse with men, and toward not defining themselves as full persons in sex with men. Lack of sexual satisfaction is another sign of oppression of women.

At first, self-help clinics concentrated on the urgent topics of birth control, breast surgery, and alternatives to steroid hormones. But in 1976, in conjunction with writing a book on women's health care, a group of six women in Los Angeles were selected by the Federation of Feminist Women's Health Centers to spend several months studying the female sexual response and the structure and function of the sexual organ. Suzann Gage, an anatomical illustrator and member of the health center staff, brought in thick anatomy books in various languages for the group to consult. We sat on the floor and, using mirrors and flashlights, each carefully examined our genitals and compared them to the illustrations. First we found that although all of us had most of the structures pictured, the variation in size, proportion, coloration, texture, and shape of each component part gave each woman's genitals a markedly different appearance—different from one another, but especially different from the standard drawing. Among other differences, the drawings always show the opening that leads to the vagina as a gaping hole rather than the neatly closed opening that may or may not be visible, depending on the shape (or existence!) of the fourchette, a membranous fold of skin that stretches across the lower part of the opening. (See Figures 1, 2, and 3.)

As part of the study, some of the women masturbated to orgasm while being photographed so that the changes in the sexual organs during the sexual response cycle could be observed. These changes, while not as obvious as those that occur in the penis, are nevertheless pronounced and quite identifiable. Women at the Orange County FWHC also made motion pictures of sexual response. In some instances, the speculum was inserted and kept open throughout so that the changes in the vaginal walls and in the cervix could be seen during the phases of excitement, plateau, orgasm, and resolution.

Careful comparison of living genitals to drawings largely based on dissections of dead tissues, combined with our observations of the sexual response cycle, enabled us to piece together a full description of

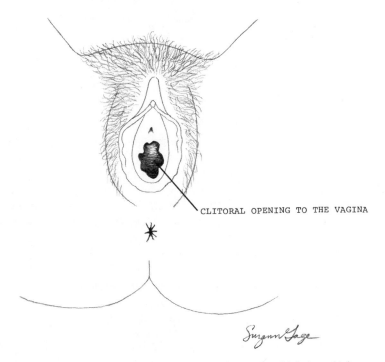

CLITORAL OPENING TO THE VAGINA

Figure 1. Drawn from standard medical text: vagina gaping open; pubic hair on thighs, common to many women, not included.

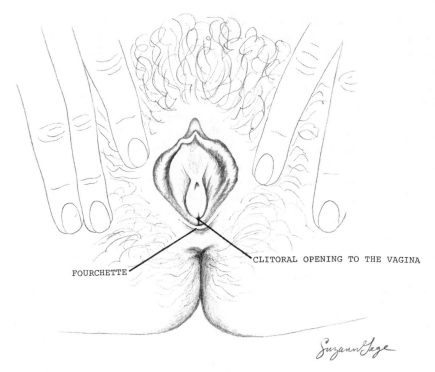

Figure 2. Clitoral opening as it is. To see the entire clitoris, you must separate the lips with your fingers.

the clitoris, the female organ. We learned that the clitoris is an intricate organ located in the crotch below the ischium bones (the bones we sit on), which flare out, forming a triangular space. It consists not only of the hooded glans, the shaft, and the crura, as generally believed, but also of the ligament that suspends these structures from the symphysis (or midline) of the pubic bone; the muscles that bound the triangle; the networks of nerves and blood vessels that branch into the clitoral structures; the spongy erectile bodies, such as the urethral sponge, the clitoral bulbs, and the perineal sponge; and the inner lips, which extend from the hood until they again join and form the fourchette just above the perineum between the clitoral opening to the vagina and the anus. (See Figures 4, 5, and 6.)

In self-examination, the clitoris can be distinguished from the surrounding vulva (the pubic mound and the outer lips) by the fact that it has no hair. The inner part of the clitoris extends to the depth of the hymen, which separates it from the vagina, except along the roof, where a pad of spongy erectile tissue, the urethral sponge, extends back into the vagina. By inserting the index finger and pressing against the ischium bones, the crura (or legs) and the clitoral muscles that extend from the shaft and the pubic bone can be felt as thick rubber bands. By inserting the finger a little deeper and pressing sideways, the soft clitoral bulbs can be felt.

During sexual excitement, the suspensory ligament shortens, pulling the glans and the shaft up under the hood and into the groove of the symphysis. The erectile tissue of the shaft and the crura (corpus cavernosum) fills with blood and becomes bone-hard. As stimulation continues, the muscles begin to tighten, and the soft erectile tissues (corpus spongiosum) of the urethral sponge, the perineal sponge, and the clitoral bulbs swell with blood, causing the vaginal opening to become smaller and to "sweat" and become very moist. (See Figure 7.)

During the plateau phase, erection and muscular tension increase and the inner lips often become bright red or wine-colored from vasocongestion. (See Figure 8.) At orgasm, the muscles (ischiocaver-

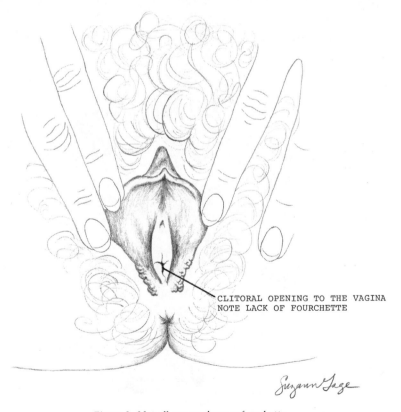

CLITORAL OPENING TO THE VAGINA
NOTE LACK OF FOURCHETTE

Figure 3. Not all women have a fourchette.

nosus, bulbocavernosus, and transverse perineal) contract rhythmically four to eight times at four-fifths of a second. The whole clitoria pulsates as it muscles force the blood from its engorged tissues back into the body. (See Figure 9.) During resolution, the ligament stretches, the shaft returns to its usual position, and muscle tension gradually subsides. This sequence of events closely parallels those that occur in the penis, with its comparable but somewhat differently arranged structures.

In our study, we observed that Masters and Johnson's extremely

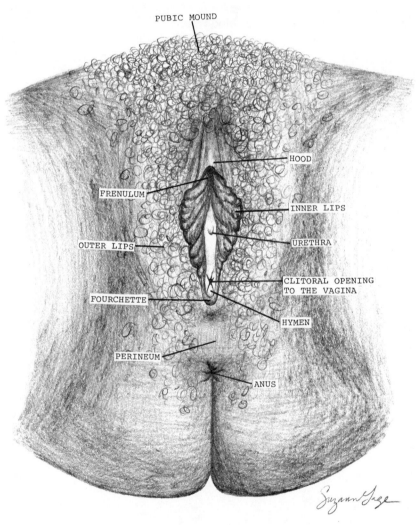

Figure 4. Structure of the clitoris.

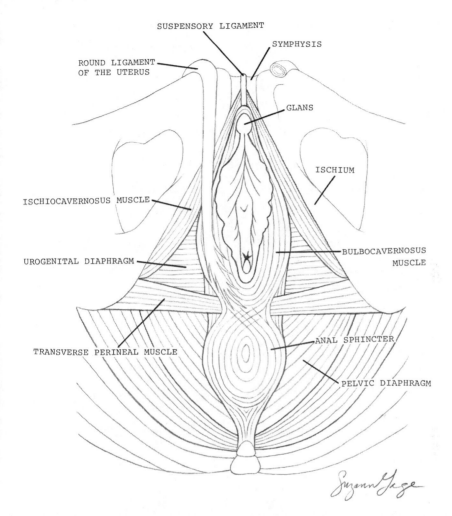

Figure 5. Muscle structure of the clitoris (without overlying layer of skin and fat); one of the round ligaments has been cut away to expose the bulbocavernosus muscle.

important discovery, that the male and the female sexual responses are similar instead of complementary, applies to the structure and the function of the sex organs as well as to the generalized body responses of systemic changes, such as increasing heart rate, rise in blood pressure and respiration, nervous excitation, vasocongestion, and muscle tension.[1]

[1] The vagina, uterus, uterine ligaments, egg tubes, and ovaries—as well as the breasts, indeed, the whole body—are involved in female sexual response. We are merely focusing on the clitoris. For a detailed description of the clitoris, compatible with the observations in our study, see Masters and Johnson (1966, pp. 56, 60–61).

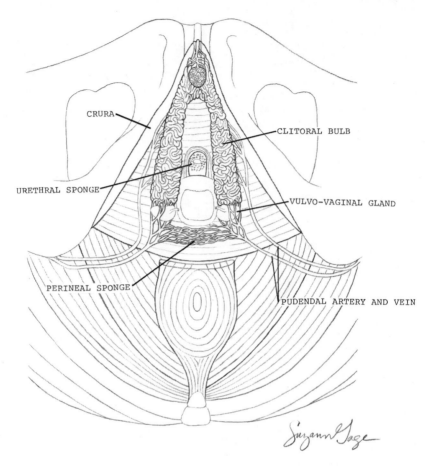

Figure 6. Clitoral muscles not shown so that the clitoral erectile tissue can be seen.

Since the women participating in this project had no access to dis-
section rooms, they were forced to rely on Masters and Johnson, Sherfey, anatomy texts, the drawings of Robert Latou Dickinson (an artist–
physician who interviewed and sketched thousands of his patients in
the 1920s and 1930s), and the observation of their own bodies. Some
people may quibble with the claim that the women discovered "something new" in this study, since all of the structures they identified as
being part of the clitoris can be found described in one anatomy book
or another, especially if one searches back over the last 75 years. In
defense of Masters and Johnson, who failed to describe the clitoris
fully and who instead designated most clitoral structures as being
somehow an extension of the vagina called the "orgasmic platform"

and located in the "outer third of the vagina," the functional unity of the clitoris is totally obscured by the literally fragmented approach that anatomists use. (Feminists will be forever grateful, however, to Masters and Johnson's recognition of the vital role that the glans and the shaft play in orgasm.)

Anatomical artists, first of all, cut out and study sections of tissue and, unless they conceptualize structures as belonging to a unit, do not see them as a unit. Second, for purposes of illustrating certain parts, the artist omits others; therefore, anatomical drawings of cross

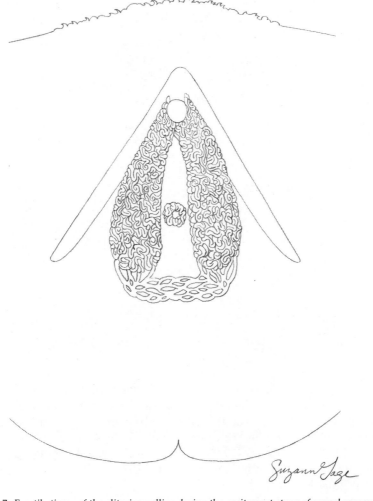

Figure 7. Erectile tissue of the clitoris swelling during the excitement stage of sexual response.

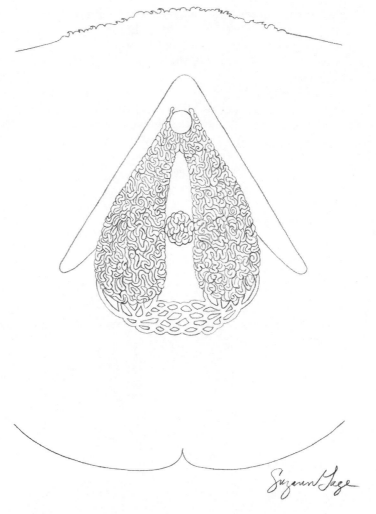

Figure 8. Erectile tissue of the clitoris, more swollen, during the plateau stage of sexual response.

sections of the body seldom show all of the structures. Certainly, no one illustration or set of illustrations we found included all of the clitoral structures. For example, the urethral sponge was missing from all illustrations and descriptions except in three texts: Testut (1931), Toldt (1928), and Netter (1970). The perineal sponge is never pictured; it is merely alluded to in Kinsey's *Sexual Behavior in the Human Female* (1965). (See Figure 10.)

In any inquiry, the best test of theory is how well it fits the facts. As we described our understanding of how the sex organs work in

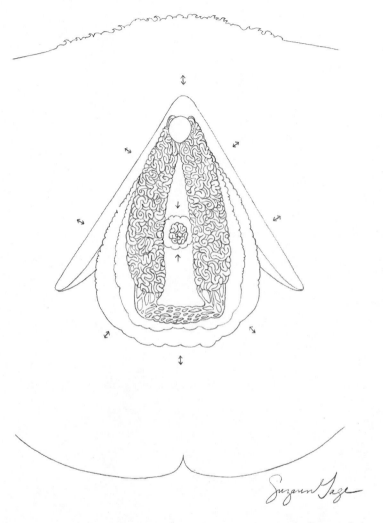

Figure 9. Erectile tissue of the clitoris during orgasm, contracting back to usual size.

self-help clinics, woman after woman has commented matter-of-factly, "Yes, that's how it is with me," not realizing how ignorant the medical profession has been of this simple truth: that the clitoris is an organ as complex and active as the penis. Also, another test is usefulness. After demonstrating self-examination and showing the parts of the clitoris and how it functions, discussions of our sexual experiences become much more concrete and specific. We now have a vocabulary and a conceptual framework to communicate with.

One of the major accomplishments of this group self-study project

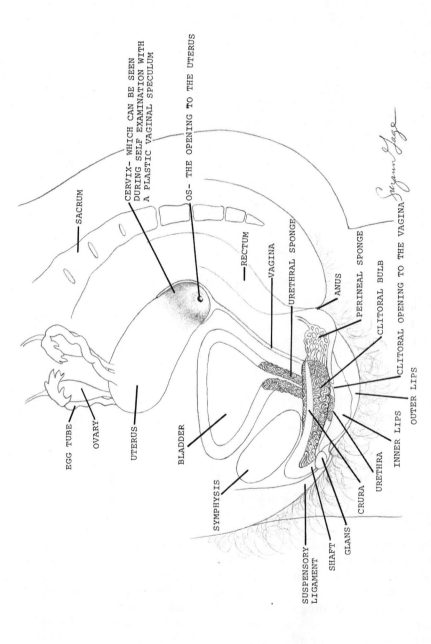

SACRUM

CERVIX— WHICH CAN BE SEEN
DURING SELF EXAMINATION WITH
A PLASTIC VAGINAL SPECULUM

OS— THE OPENING TO THE UTERUS

RECTUM

VAGINA

URETHRAL SPONGE

ANUS

PERINEAL SPONGE

CLITORAL BULB

CLITORAL OPENING TO THE VAGINA

INNER LIPS

OUTER LIPS

URETHRA

CRURA

GLANS

SHAFT

SUSPENSORY
LIGAMENT

SYMPHYSIS

BLADDER

UTERUS

OVARY

EGG TUBE

Figure 10. The urethral sponge, a part of the clitoris, is adjacent to but not a part of the vagina. The figure is schematic: the intestines, among other structures, are missing.

is to put to rest forever the controversy over clitoral or vaginal orgasms. Now that it is understood that the clitoral structures surround and extend into the vagina, the fact that women report pleasurable feelings deep in the vagina in no way contradicts Masters and Johnson's correct if inadequately pursued finding that all orgasms are of clitoral origin. The vagina is involved passively in the orgasm, and the pleasure that women receive from the thrusting of the penis comes from the sensations of the penis rubbing against the erect clitoris.

As part of our research, we gathered accounts of individual experiences. We were more interested in the actual sexual experiences than in feelings about sexuality. We found that some women experience the entire sexual response cycle from the time that they are toddlers. On the other hand, it became clear that many women do not experience orgasm until they are in their 20s or 30s or even later, or never. We found few women who experience orgasm regularly and dependably during coitus. Women agreed with the subjects of the Masters and Johnson study who reported that orgasm from masturbation is frequently stronger than from coitus. Of course, as feminists, we were not very concerned with whether or not the orgasm was obtained during coitus, or by manual or oral stimulation, or with a vibrator. Our aim was not to train ourselves to have orgasms in dull sexual sessions where the *only* clitoral stimulation is from the penis. We found that women usually strive to achieve orgasm during coitus to reassure the partner. In self-help clinics, one of my favorite questions to ask is "Would everyone here who has never faked an orgasm, please raise your hand?" I have yet to see one hand raised.

Other feminists, many of whom participate in self-help, conduct therapy groups for women called *preorgasmic groups*. Rather than viewing women's sexuality solely in the context of heterosexual intercourse, they help women to learn to achieve orgasm through masturbation. These groups use a variety of approaches, but all include group discussion, instruction on the basic facts of the sexual response cycle, and practical tips on how to masturbate to orgasm. Women who participate in these groups have excellent results.

Women in self-help groups not only reexamined the emphasis on a woman's having an orgasm during coitus but reexamined the advice given to couples to aid the woman in achieving orgasm at that time in light of our improved understanding of the structure and function of the clitoris. A typical piece of therapists' advice is to have the woman sit astride the male, in order to bring her glans and shaft into closer proximity to his penis and public bone. While this advice *is* successful in many cases, especially if a couple work together conscientiously with the one goal being the woman's orgasm, it seems probable to us that the success comes more often from the woman's ability to maneuver freely and to control the amount of stimulation she receives and the man's sincere interest in helping her to achieve orgasm, rather than from direct stimulation of the glans and the shaft.

Of course, we talked to women who wanted—indeed, needed—very strong direct stimulation of the glans and shaft, but most seemed to prefer stimulation of the other parts of the clitoris instead. The penis is in good contact with the clitoris at all times in all positions. For example, when the male inserts the penis from behind, the penis is thrusting toward the urethral sponge, which is along the roof of the vagina. Also, many women have said that direct stimulation of the floor of the clitoris, the perineal sponge, gives maximum pleasure.

Misunderstanding the clitoris as merely the glans and the shaft, along with the patriarchal insistence that women rely only on penile stimulation for "normal" orgasms, has led to shocking consequences. Some therapists refer women for female circumcision (clitoridotomy) to have their clitoral hoods removed so that they can be more sensitive to the thrusts of the penis. One gynecologist, James Burt of Dayton, Ohio, has even developed a two-hour operation for surgically redesigning the vagina, referred to as the "reborn Burt vagina." In addition to moving the glans and the shaft closer to the clitoral opening, he narrows and tightens the vagina, cuts the pubococcygeal muscle (which forms the floor of the pelvis and through which the vagina runs), and removes the hood. Some of the women who have this surgery are very satisfied, but others have had problems, such as vaginismus, afterward.

These operations are reminiscent of surgeries and mutilations performed on women's clitorises in the 19th century—and even today in a few countries. As far as we could determine, most of these surgeries were limited to excising the glans and some or all of the shaft (although an operation called *infibulation* can include the inner lips also). Surely these mutilations had a devastating impact on women's ability to have sexual pleasure and to achieve orgasm, but, physiologically, it would seem that since most of the clitoris was left intact, including extensive networks of nerves, blood vessels, erectile bodies, and muscles, orgasm would still have been possible. Masters and Johnson even cite a case where a woman had orgasm despite amputation of the shaft. As for men, those who have had the outer shaft amputated are still capable of having orgasm.

As part of our sex research, we reviewed current sex therapy practices and discussed them in self-help groups. One criticism women have consistently made of therapeutic measures is that often the assumption is made that it is possible for a woman to have a carefree, uninhibited sex life despite the difficulties she faces in a sexist society:

"Oh, sure, just casually lie down in the field of wildflowers and have sex! What about birth control? Or is everybody supposed to use the Pill or IUD?" Or, "Well, I'm forty, and frankly, most men my age or even older just want casual sex with me and they seek out younger women to have even semipermanent relationships with." We came up with a list of institutions, laws, and practices that reinforce women's oppression or sexual repression; our evaluation of this list amounted to a broad-scale condemnation of patriarchal society. Any therapist who tells a woman that "it is up to her" and implies that she is responsible for her "hang-ups" is merely rubbing salt in the wounds inflicted by her church, which preaches the evil of sexuality, especially women's; by schools, which withhold sex education from her, except for perhaps a lecture on menstruation in junior high and another lecture on birth control in high school; and the ubiquitous pornography that degrades her.

Current sex therapy that relies primarily on sex histories and teaching techniques to overcome problems such as vaginismus, inability to achieve orgasm, or inability to maintain an erection seems to be of most help to men and women. Although Masters and Johnson pioneered this type of therapy, their excellent work is tainted with sexism in their use of prostitutes for research and the use of women as surrogate partners.

Like the use of surrogate partners, other tools of the sex therapist are less acceptable to feminists—tools like permission giving, advising, role playing, or setting examples by role modeling and desensitization. Permission giving is the reverse side of the authoritarian coin that has denied people the right to decide their own sexuality. Advising is only as good as the adviser, and our experience is that therapists are as much a part of our culture as anyone else and pass on their own biases and hang-ups; the same criticisms applies to role playing and role modeling. Desensitization involves bombarding the clients with films or tapes of explicit scenes or shocking words to numb them to any feelings of shock or embarrassment. Feminists see a problem with these methods if a woman, in the process of losing her upsetness, also loses her very necessary armor against hurtful influences. Sexist jokes and pornography are more than distasteful; they shame and humiliate women and support sexist practices that cause harm to women.

If sex therapists, male or female, are sincere in wanting to help their female clients, they would be wise to consult feminists, especially those in the women's health movement, to reduce to the minimum their inevitable sexism. Unless sex researchers, counselors, and therapists raise their consciousness about women's oppression, they will perpetuate the models of heterosexuality that suppress women's sexuality. For example, Multi Media Resource Center puts out a series of films showing people having sex. One film starts out with a couple riding their motorcycle on a country road (of course, the man is in the lead, but perhaps that is nit-picking). As they turn down the lane toward their house, they dismount and lie down together among the leaves. The man, Rich, playfully pulls at Judy's clothes. She resists, he persists, and he finally succeeds in disrobing her. Then, in a scene on the sundeck next to their pool, he first applies suntan lotion to her and incorporates it as foreplay, but then he starts teasing her, then chases her and wrestles her down to the mat. He mounts her and embarks on a vigorous (actually borderline violent) coital session. Then, after *his* orgasm, he picks her up and throws her into the pool! When I asked a representative of the organization who made the film, he sidestepped any responsibility for the mock rape format by saying that this was the way this couple had sex and that their aim was not to judge but to record.

As part of their well-woman health-care program, the Women's Choice Clinic of the Feminist Women's Health Center in Los Angeles has initiated a special self-help program where women can learn in groups about the female organs and sexual response. During the group session, which lasts two to three hours, women do self-examination and identify the parts of the vulva, clitoris, vagina, uterus, egg tubes, and ovaries. The phases of the sexual response cycle are presented. Each woman prepares an extensive sexual "herstory" as the group share their experiences and problems. Specific techniques for enhancing sexual enjoyment are demonstrated. The difference between these groups offered at the clinic and at the self-help clinics is that although all self-help clinics talk about sexuality to a greater or lesser extent, and some self-help clinics have chosen to concentrate on sexuality, the clinic sessions offer women the opportunity to come together for the express purpose of learning more about sex.

So a century after Freud asked plaintively, "What do women really want?", women are coming together and overcoming patriarchally instilled and socially enforced taboos to find out what type of sexuality they really want, and of course, from there, it is a short step to demanding that institutions change so that both men and women will be free to express their sexuality to other human beings constructively, joyously, and for mutual satisfaction.

REFERENCES

Hite, *The Hite report.* New York: Dell Publishing, 1976, pp. 419–420.
Kinsey, A. C., Pomeroy, W. B., Martin, C. E., and Gebhard, P. H. *Sexual behavior in the human female.* New York: Pocket Books, 1965, p. 577.

Masters, W., and Johnson, V. *Human sexual response.* Boston: Little, Brown, 1966, pp. 56, 60–61.

Murry, L. Building a better vagina. *Playgirl,* 1977, 5, 40+.

Netter, F. H. *The CIBA collection of medical illustrations,* Vol 2. Summit, N.J.: CIBA Pharmaceutical Company, 1970.

Sherfey, M. J. *The nature and evolution of female sexuality.* New York: Random House, 1972.

Testut, J. L. *Traite d'anatomie humaine* (ed. 8, revised and enlarged by A. Latarjet), Vol. 5: *Appareil urogenital peritoine.* Paris: Doin, 1931.

Toldt, C. *Anatomisher Atlas.* Berlin and Wien: Urban and Schwarzenberg, 1928.

Self-Help in Gynecological Practice

Allen Lawrence and Laura Edwards

When I, as a gynecologist, think of self-help, I think of an individual woman or man helping herself or himself to become a fully functioning "well" person. Not only is self-help valuable in sickness, but it implies feeling healthy and learning what one needs to create that feeling, including where to get information, how to put good health into practice, and finally, how to monitor and face clearly the consequences of decisions affecting health.

My clinical experience has made clear to me that the body and the mind are not separate. They affect each other. The body and the mind are more accurately thought of as a body–mind. As people learn more about their physiology, their understanding of themselves as a whole increases.

Minor problems in women are often relieved, simply, by anatomical instruction or by reliable information about orgasm, birth control, or abortion. On the other hand, a woman with a major or recurrent problem (VD, unplanned pregnancies, recurrent vaginal infection, anorgasmia, etc.) needs guidance to find the root of her problem: Has she "mismotivated" herself"? Has she lost her "healthy image" of herself?

Enlightened physicians such as Dr. Irving Olye (1976) and Dr. Kenneth Pelletier (1976) have pointed out that a mental image of oneself as "sick" can be a fundamental factor in illness. Cancer patients have found that exercises using a visualization of a positive self-image facilitate their recovery. A negative self-image can impede recovery.

Allen Lawrence, M.D. • Director, Caring Parenthood Center and Center for Caring Medicine, Los Angeles, California; and Private Practice, Obstetrics/Gynecology, West Los Angeles, California. Laura Edwards, B.A. • Editorial Assistant to Dr. Allen Lawrence.

Illness can be an unconscious way of solving problems that one may be unable or unwilling to solve consciously.

A woman with a recurrent sexual problem may have a negative self-image that prevents her from enjoying her feelings or seeing herself sexually in a positive way.

I have devised a systematic and objective approach to self-help sexual analysis. I instruct my patient to encounter what I call her "primeval forest." The primeval forest is all of the information that she has collected about sexuality during her growth.

Fear of sex and sexual dysfunctions evolve in part from a multitude of myths and fantasies about men and their sexuality. In our society, women are told to shield their sexuality, for example, "Keep your legs crossed," "Not wearing underpants is a sin," "Men are only after you for your body," "All men are really interested in doing is putting their penises into your vagina," "You'll get pregnant," "You'll get venereal disease," etc.

This primeval forest is a combination of positive and negative experiences and feelings. Recognizing these fears can often help change how a woman thinks and acts. Not all women are able to discover or overcome their particular personal fears by looking at them or discussing them with their gynecologist. These women who are unable to respond to self-help techniques are usually referred for psychiatric therapy. Good therapy can guide them to trust themselves and to recognize and make use of their real feelings.

In self-help sexual analysis, the individual studies her own sexual assumptions, and does some "spring cleaning."

A woman should notice if her partner leaves her confused, disoriented, and feeling dirty or used or whether she is embraced, supported, and feels loved. Then, looking at her choice of partners is the next issue. We examine what I call the "mating dance."

The mating dance is the period between "connecting" and beginning a dating relationship. We speak casually of the unconscious factors in choosing a partner, having good vibes or bad vibes. Some scientific studies (Joy, 1979) suggest that people actually do radiate certain patterns of energy and respond to the "vibes" of others as compatible or not. We may not be able to put our feelings into words, but nonetheless, we *know* the difference.

In the mating dance, my patient and I analyze how she had perceived partners and what kind of positive or negative feelings she picks up about them. Some people are attracted to partners who will treat them badly, will reject them, will not fulfill their needs, and will not support their basic goals in life, while others find themselves attracted to partners with whom they are truly compatible. Much of the choosing occurs on an unconscious level in response to "good chemistry," and if not aware, many women continue to pick nonsupporting partners over and over again.

I try to help my patients think about how they communicate with their partners by a process I call the "soda shop." We look specifically at verbal communication, the sharing of information about each other. (The nonverbal I think of as part of the mating dance.) If two people are unable to communicate effectively, the relationship is definitely in trouble.

Emotional problems may manifest themselves within relationships as sexual conflict and disharmony. To further uncover what is destroying the relationship and why, I look for problems in what I call the "playing field." The sexual part of the relationship may be thought of as a game. It has a beginning, an end, rules, and goals.

Sex has two functions: procreation and recreation. Recreational sex, which means that the motive is not to have babies but to have pleasure, is a kind of game that people play to increase intimate communication. There may be definite rules and regulations agreed upon by the partners. It is a way of expressing feelings and love for another with or without the use of words. I find that the biggest problem arises when two people are sexually involved but have different rules and goals. They are literally playing different games and at the same time wondering why they feel as if they are losing and as if neither the sex nor the relationship is working.

I find that the cause of this major problem in sexual relationships is that the groundwork of the mating dance and soda shop is incomplete. Partners enter the playing field with different sets of rules and different goals. Too often, in the mystical romanticism of courtship, one partner assumes that the other is really different than he or she appears to be or that he or she will change to meet the partner's standards. I hear a woman say, "I don't know what gets into him," or a man say, "I don't know where she is at"—indications that the two are not really listening to each other and that they may be operating according to different rules or goals.

There is a common inhibition from talking about what is sexually exciting or fulfilling. Talking about it might spoil the spontaneity, people think, but it is unrealistic to expect one's lover to read one's mind.

On the other hand, it is impossible to tell a partner what turns one on if one doesn't yet know. I suggest that the couple explore their bodies and communicate to each other what feels good. They should also communicate what they do not like. Exploration should continue to some extent throughout a sexual relationship to keep the relationship fresh and honest. I find that the degree to which couples keep exploring determines the growth and the continuing depth of the relationship.

It is crucial that the couple share the same goals and rules if they are to be happy with one another. Very often, the conflict becomes manifest as a loss of sexual interest. Many people believe that if sex works, it is love and that if sex doesn't work, the relationship is a disaster. If a relationship fails, instead of blaming each other, partners must accept that the relationship no longer fulfils their needs and goals. Each partner should look at the benefits from the relationship. The type of person that was chosen, the quality of communication (spoken and unspoken), and the goals and rules should all be looked at, so that both will know better what to look for in the next relationship. We should continually build on both positive and negative experiences in life. Accusing ourselves or our partners of wrong does not allow us to grow and learn from what didn't work. Leaving a partnership, whether amicably or not, can be a positive learning experience.

Basic Tips for Gynecological Self-Help

1. *The Kegal.* The Kegal exercises were described by Dr. Arnold Kegal many years ago as a self-help technique for women. The Kegal exercises help develop and maintain the anogenital musculature. These muscles serve an important function in intercourse, and they must be exercised to work efficiently. The Kegal essentially consists of tensing and relaxing the anogenital muscles. For the woman who has a fear of sex, learning to control and relax these muscles is the beginning of self-healing. A woman whose pelvic muscles are lax can, by learning to tighten and relax them, have a more satisfying sensation during intercourse.

The Kegal also has great value in reestablishing the strength of the bladder floor, which may preclude the need for surgical repair when stress incontinence is developing.

Practicing the Kegal at any age is a healthy, helpful exercise.

2. *Self-examination of the breast.* One hand holds the breast as the three fingers of the other hand press circularly to feel for lumps or other abnormal growths. Cancer, like any other disease, is more easily cured when discovered early. While some women think of the breast only as a sexual organ, other women find it difficult to think of their breasts as sexual. They complain that they lack sensation in their breasts. If there has been no nerve damage, previous surgery, or physical damage, then a psychological barrier may exist to the enjoyment of breast sensation.

I have seen women in my office with extremely large breasts who have been ridiculed, criticized, attacked, and groped by both males and other females. They react by shutting off their awareness of the feelings in their breasts. I have seen women with breasts so small that they feel self-conscious and do not want the partner to touch or kiss their breasts for fear of ridicule or rejection. I have seen women fearful of their breasts because they get turned on when touched and they feel this response to be dirty or wrong. I have had other patients tell me that they have orgasms when their breasts are touched or sucked.

In this context, self-help examination of the breast allows a woman to discover what kind of stimulation or sensation gives her pleasure or causes discomfort, as well as to look for disease.

3. *Exploration of the male partner.* As well as enlarging her knowledge of her own physiology, it may be helpful for a woman to study the male. Knowing more about the penis and the surrounding musculature and the sensations that he feels may help a woman to please her partner more.

4. *Keeping a menstrual-discharge log.* Some women come to my office with no understanding of how their bodies work, not just in the sexual realm but in all realms. Some come with almost no understanding of the menstrual cycle. Some have no idea where menstrual blood comes from, why menstruation occurs, or what its relationship is to fertility.

Many women complain of swelling; of changes in weight during the month; of changes in their personalities, their emotional needs, and their sexual desires, as well as of spotting and discharge. When I ask such a woman when the change occurs in relation to her cycle, I frequently get a blank stare. Women's physiology is cyclic. Moods, tenderness of the breasts and genitals, crying spells, irritability, hunger, complexion changes, water retention, the inability to focus on work, vaginal discharge, and sexual appetite are all possible symptoms of the variations in hormonal levels during the monthly cycle. Often, all of these troubles as well as menstrual pains may be simply regulated by improving nutrition along with vitamin supplements and a modest exercise plan.

I encourage women to keep a log or a diary of their emotional and physical feelings. Often, such a diary solves many mysteries that have confounded, confused, and worried a woman for years. For example, a mucous discharge occurs about the 14th day of every cycle. The sex drive may be high at this time. Temperature also increases, indicating ovulation, which makes this the most likely time for impregnation.

Thus, if a woman keeps track of her vaginal discharge, takes her temperature every morning before getting out of bed (basal body temperature), and keeps a chart or a log consistently, she will begin to un-

derstand her body's timing; she will become more the master of her
own body.

5. *Self-diagnosis of vaginal infections.* The vagina is equipped with
a reliable self-cleaning system. If something is out of balance in the
body, an infection is liable to develop in the vagina. Emotional problems also increase the susceptibility of the vagina to infection.

By keeping track of her vaginal discharge and learning the various
odors, color, texture, and timing, a woman can learn to spot the three
most common infections: trichomoniasis, yeast, and nonspecific
vaginitis. If she is also aware of VD and its symptoms, she can differentiate simple vaginal infection from VD and initiate methods of
self-treatment for non-VD infections. Suspected VD should always be
checked by a physician. Methods such as douching can easily treat
early vaginal infection. (The best solution for douching is one part
vinegar to two parts water—not only the best douche money can buy
but the cheapest.)

In summation, the woman who uses self-help techniques develops her knowledge of herself. She learns her basic anatomy and
physiology, what turns her on, what turns her off, what turns her
partner on, what turns him off, how to select a partner. She learns
from past experiences when a relationship didn't match her expectations, and she learns something about abnormal conditions of her
body.

As you might see I personally am a proponent of self-help techniques. If women put time and energy into learning about their anatomy and physiology, about the basic fundamentals of medical problems that may especially affect them, and about the proper times to
use and not to use self-help techniques, they help themselves and
their physicians. If the treatment works, they save themselves costly
medical visits. If it does not, the patient is able to give her physician a
responsible and orderly account of her symptoms and to ask intelligent questions about what she is experiencing. In turn, the doctor
is able to make a speedy diagnosis and an appropriate treatment plan.

For me the greatest pleasure as a physician is to have a thoughtful woman come into my office and tell me succinctly and clearly the
problems and symptoms she is experiencing in a language that both of
us understand. Such an account helps me to take a good history, and
to do a more adequate examination. It helps me to give her instructions in such a way that both of us feel confident when she leaves that
she understands the disease process, the treatment plan, and the indications that the plan is working.

"Self"-help is a reality. What is not clear is who is to be responsible for self-help. The physician, the patient, the health educator, the
paraprofessional, the RN—who? Who is qualified to teach it, develop

techniques, and monitor the results, and who is to be responsible for its efficacy? What place have the women's groups that are opposed to the medical profession and its male domination? What help is provided by medial societies that are against any care provided by anyone but licensed physicians or their delegated representatives?

There are as yet no rules or guidelines. In fact, the entire field is up for grabs. Who can and who should provide this care? I see a need for the medical profession to join with the consumers. The movement is toward increasing women's knowledge of themselves and developing their judgment about which professionals are reputable and competent. I would like to see the medical profession and the women's movement sit down together and decide who can provide what. Women, with their newly emerging self-confidence, will decide for themselves where they can best get what they want. Physicians are not trained as educators, and unless medical schools give courses in how to administer self-help, paraprofessionals and radical, liberal, and conservative nonmedical people will find a new career opportunity and fill the void created by the medical profession.

References

Oyle, I. *Time, space and the mind.* Millbrae, Calif.: Celestial Arts, 1976.
Pelletier, K. *Mind as healer, mind as slayer.* New York: Delta, 1976.
Joy, B. *Joy's way.* New York: Tarcher/St. Martin, 1979.

Chapter 16

Young Women and the
Sexual Revolution

Elizabeth K. Canfield

Among the questions most frequently posed at meetings, conferences, and workshops on human sexuality are those dealing with attitudinal and behavioral changes between generations. Are today's young people really different from yesterday's? Will society be able to cope with the new freedoms? Does all the openness about sexuality signal the downfall of civilization? And in the past decade we've constantly been hearing the query, Is there a sexual revolution?

While the scope of this chapter does not permit a thorough investigation of these topics, and definite answers cannot be forthcoming, the intent is to give a personal impression, based on many years' work with college women, of what has been happening to them and with them in the past two decades. The hope is that these briefly discussed observations might facilitate comparisons and offer opportunities for artfully asking further.

In my experience of working with young women, I have found that they welcome questions and are accepting of questioners. They seek accurate, factual information as well as perspective and guidance. They do, however, display quite a bit of uneasiness around those who give facile responses to complex ethical questions. Perhaps the most significant development in our time in history is that we are asking and being asked about matters formerly taken for granted.

It is my personal contention that if indeed there is a sexual revolution, its most important characteristic is choice. The contraceptive age affords an array of options never before available to young women.

ELIZABETH K. CANFIELD • Health and Family Planning Counselor, University of Southern California, Los Angeles, California.

Conversely, it burdens them with the obligation to make choices in areas not previously considered open to decision-making. During my college days, it didn't occur to me that I wouldn't be a wife and mother some day. The bull sessions I participated in reflected the inevitability of these destinies. We would talk endlessly about our plans to finish college, to work as teachers, nurses, social workers, and executive secretaries and maybe, if we had the courage, as journalists, artists, or musicians, until the right man came along; at that time, we would enter a sexually exclusive marriage as virgins, regard our careers as secondary in importance to those of our mates, become economically dependent, and generally "settle down." In the meantime, of course, we would be attractive and popular, lead an active dating life and remain pure. Schoolmates who veered from these norms were regarded as peculiar: those whose virginity was no longer intact; loners who didn't care about going out with young men; those who questioned the validity of the institution of marriage; and women obviously attracted to and more than routinely involved with other women.

Our men, on the other hand, would also finish college, become well established in their chosen careers before considering marriage and all its financial obligations, lead busy dating lives, and become sexually active in order to get their animal urges out of the way and someday bestow upon us the benefits of their sexual experience. To this day, I have been unable to figure out the logistics of this widely accepted standard. If men are to be experienced and women are not, with whom are the men supposed to practice?

Women are asking a related question: Now that greater freedom is possible because both contraception and legal abortion are available, and considering the emphasis on sexual fulfillment for women as well as men, does it not stand to reason that experience would be helpful? Experience is required, they say, in order to obtain the most menial employment; why would the same not be true before entering into a long-term commitment such as marriage?

Not that sexual suitability is the only important component of a workable partnership; but finding out whether one can communicate physically, not to speak of tolerating each other at all over a period of time and beyond dating situations, makes a great deal of sense to the thinking student.

In view of current trends, one is easily trapped into making light of the good old days. But they weren't so "good" (i.e., abstinent) and they aren't so old, as pointed out by Cutright (1970):

> A second possible cause of resistance to the provision of birth control service to young men and women involves the myth of an abstinent past and a promiscuous present. Aside from substantial increases in premarital sex

among young whites with their future husbands, we find no evidence that a change in nonmarital sex of "revolutionary" proportions has occurred since 1940 among either white or nonwhite teenagers.

As is the case with such other social problems as hunger, poverty and racial discrimination recently "discovered" by politicians and social scientists, the problems generated by teenage sexuality have been with us for many years, but we cannot any longer as a society afford to ignore their existence. Hopefully, now that we have acknowledged that teenagers are having sex relations, recognizing that it is no new thing, we may act sensibly and realistically to solve the problems consequent upon it, rather than cling stubbornly to the myth of an age d'or of sexual abstinence or cheer on a largely non-existent "sexual revolution" to topple the establishment.

One popular author referred to sexual decision-making among today's students as a dilemma of not inconsiderable proportion (Hettlinger, 1966). When I first began working in this field some 20 years ago, I recall speaking with a young woman who had waited five months to get into a maternity home. Hers was not an isolated case; somebody was obviously engaging, even then, in activities requiring the services that such an institution offers to unmarried, pregnant young women.

On the other hand, Lorna and Philip Sarrel (1971), well-known sex educators and counselors working as a team at Yale University, reported that only 25% of the students seen in their service had been nonvirgins upon arrival on campus as freshmen in 1971. And under the heading "For Virgins: Male and Female," a guide for students at the University of Pennsylvania contains the following apologia:

> Do not apologize to yourself or anyone. You may even be a part of an apologetic silent majority (that large, discreet group that doesn't talk about the extent or level of their sexual activities)—at least for a while. Premarital sexual activity has almost as many reasons for existing as there are individuals involved, and they are not all negative reasons. (Pierson, 1970)

The same publication contains the reprint of an article by Sidney Callahan entitled: "For Parents: When Chastity Doesn't Make It." These various examples point out the complexity of the way we regard yesterday in relation to sexual values.

It would appear that even in this so-called new age, some people adhere to old ideals and expectations. Virgins constitute an underprivileged group at best; they are supported by unpopular elements such as parents, church leaders, and political conservatives, and they are pressured by peers to discard their prudery and "get with it." Health professionals are frequently called on to reassure these young women that their choice is also healthy and normal.

The young woman's dilemma vis-à-vis virginity is in part responsible for creating a major public health problem: unintentional, often premature pregnancy. One in ten women aged 15–19 (including many first-year college students) becomes pregnant in the United States each

year. Adolescents account for one-third of all legal abortions performed. Three in ten women aged 20 in 1975 had given birth to at least
one child (Zero Population Growth, 1977).

The many hundreds of unintentionally pregnant women I have
seen in my various activities over these past 20 years have confirmed
the theory that in our society sex is not OK, and it follows, therefore,
that planning ahead for sexual activity is also not OK. Even though a
change has occurred in that most young people no longer learn at
home that sex is dirty, they do receive plenty of sex-negative messages, especially in a humorous vein. More often than not, the subject
is entirely omitted in any serious context, beyond the strong message:
Don't! And when it is brought up, it is accorded its most narrow interpretation, one that limits sexuality to the sex act and the inherent
fearful consequences of pregnancy and disease. It is simply not possible to be entirely responsible toward something in which we are not
supposed to be engaged or interested in the first place. Unless major
insights are gained and attitudes change drastically, risk-taking and
gambling must and will prevail, and thousands of young women will
become pregnant inadvertently.

Every student I have ever seen on a college campus has known
something about birth control methods. Every single one had the opportunity of obtaining more information and/or service on campus or
at a nearby family-planning or youth clinic. There is ample proof that
information is not enough; that the nonuse of contraceptives is often a
social and psychological rather than a technological problem (Sarrel
and Sarrel, 1977; Luker, 1975). And it is a problem whether pregnancy
occurs or not.

The guilt felt by young people easily translates into the need for
spontaneity, for considering premeditated sexual activity unromantic
and undesirable, for counting on luck. How often we hear, "I just
didn't think it would happen." This is not to say that if young women
or their partners used birth control methods all the time, all would be
well. Interestingly enough, the so-called sexual revolution has not
been blessed with handy tools for revolutionaries to employ, at least
not in this context. Universally acceptable, safe contraception is far
from a reality, and every day new horror stories appear about the
methods that are available. Many young women as well as their
partners have expressed outrage and desperation about their misfor-
tunes, or those of their friends, with current techniques. Many have
tried to be responsible and have subsequently reverted to chance taking, often as a result of sheer discouragement, sometimes of outright
fear.

Even though much has been said publicly about the new openness, a large number of college women seen in our offices and clinics still obtain their sexual health-care information in a climate of guilt, secrecy, and insecurity. The first questions they bring up often relate to the confidentiality of medical records. Will my parents find out I was here? Who has access to my chart? Also of great concern to them is the reassurance that they are normal—that their peers have similar needs and interests. They fear that they might be different, unique, alone in their struggles with sexual issues or even in their search for accurate information; they seek comfort in the knowledge that this is not the case.

Besides decisions about genital involvement and contraception, the following are other questions most frequently raised by young women seeking health care services.

How does sexual expression fit into my relationship? What does it mean? Formerly, it was clearly understood that women flirted around, fell in love, married, and had babies—in that order, it was hoped. Today's young women may become sexually involved with yesterday's "just friends" or with more casual acquaintances or even anonymous ones, at parties and under the influence of alcohol or drugs. They might also share beds with members of the other sex without erotic or romantic involvement at all—unheard of in the 1940s. There are so many possible categories, combinations, and interpretations that confusion can be considerable as to the definitions of relationships. In a recent Feiffer cartoon, a young man poses the question: "What do you call someone who prefers the same person as a lover and best friend?"

Not long ago, a young couple who had just had a baby completely unexpectedly, since the young woman had taken oral contraceptives the entire time and had been totally unaware of her pregnancy, described their relationship in these words: "We're not in love. We've just been best friends for a long time, but it's not a romantic thing and we have no plans for the future." Whatever the label, they gave the impression of caring a great deal about one another and of being intimate, aware of each other's feelings, self-disclosing, in tune. They evoked the temptation in this counselor to blurt out: "How wonderful to be sexually involved with one's best friend—what a way to celebrate friendship!"

We hear the phrase "just friends" a great deal. Life on the college campus raises many questions about such designations. Counselors, parents, and students ponder the limitations imposed by the language we use. One of the important contributions parents and professionals can make is to encourage careful scrutiny of the expressions we use casually every day—in a spirit of creating awareness, not of criticism. A current book on sex education for parents and children contains a chapter on the most misunderstood and undefinable words and concepts (Canfield, 1975).

The word that arouses the greatest curiosity is love; endless hours are spent in pursuit of definition and understanding. In his guide for young adults, Kelly (1976) aptly described the problem with this troubled, troubling word:

> It seems that the word "love" has become a catchall term in our language. I understand that the Eskimos have fifteen different words to describe different types of the substance we call simply snow. Surely we could use that many different words to do justice to the many aspects of love which we experience.

Closely following concerns about love are those about marriage. Since divorce statistics are widely known and many young women have high school friends whose marriages have ended after a few short years and sometimes several children, they wonder what marriage means and whether they need to chance it. Does it mean permanence? Sexual exclusivity? Serial monogamy? Restrictions of personal freedom? Parenthood? Sameness and boredom?

Possibly the clearest manifestation of the changes brought about by the current evolution of sexual values is the interest in purposeful, carefully considered parenthood as well as nonparenthood and child-free living on a permanent basis. Whereas junior high and high school pregnancies have reached epidemic proportions (Zero Population Growth, 1977), the college woman is more likely to give thought to her readiness for parenthood and is less likely to confuse pregnancy with parenthood. Among the hundreds of pregnant students seen in our clinic over the past years, only a handful continued their pregnancies to term when these had been unintentional; in each instance, moral objection to abortion was the reason. In every case, considerable concern was expressed about adequacy as a mother. Young women all over the country have reacted very positively toward a brochure entitled "Am I Parent Material?" (National Alliance for Optional Parenthood, 1976), a checklist meant to facilitate decision-making about parenthood.

Closely intertwined with these decisions is the entire matter of roles. In regard to parenthood and its many responsibilities, the most frequently asked questions are: Whose career is primary? Who will be the principal caretaker of the child? What is homemaking, and can it be performed by males as well as females? Do homemaking and child-bearing have to be full-time occupations, and must they be deadly?

The shift in parental responsibilities from women to men is reminiscent of the shift in contraceptive responsibility. In times past, male methods prevailed—coitus interruptus and condoms. Gradually, the emphasis turned to women, with the use of diaphragms, intra-uterine devices, and finally oral contraceptives and injectables. Now we may once again observe a trend toward greater male involvement, as male pills and injectables are developed with the aim of reducing sperm production. Thousands of men present themselves, often inap-propriately, considering their ages, for vasectomies. Men are urged to join their female partners in finding birth control information and in pregnancy counseling sessions. Many young women are simply tired of bearing the entire burden of pregnancy prevention, and many men agree and are eager to cooperate.

It goes without saying that the concern with sex roles extends to the realm of sexual communication and negotiation. Increasingly, young women of today feel that they have choices in initiating or declining erotic activities and in expressing preferences (Barbach, 1975). They are demystifying and learning more about their bodies (Boston Women's Health Collective, 1976). Books on masturbation and sexual fantasies are available in college bookstores and are considered helpful aids by counseling professionals, rather than pornographic material to be hidden from public view (Dodson, 1974; Friday, 1974). Not completely obsolete, but fading into the background, is the notion that Mr. Right will come along and unleash the magic of female sexu-ality. Young women are learning to take responsibility for their own sexual response-ability.

Another truly remarkable change to occur in the past decade is the acceptance of variation in sexual expression and lifestyle. This trend may well be the clearest example of the disappearance of automatic as-sumptions and labels. A recently published anthology (Gordon and Libby, 1976) contains no fewer than 14 articles by various authors under the heading: "Variation in Sexual Expression." Here Margaret Mead wrote:

> Today the recognition of bisexuality, in oneself and in others, is part of the whole mid-twentieth-century movement to accord each individual, regard-less of race, class, nationality, age, or sex, the right to be a person who is unique and who has a social identity that is worthy of dignity and respect.

In the same volume, Ira Reiss stated:

> Today young people seem to have more of a "shopper's" attitude toward their sexual lives. They know they will experiment with different kinds of sexual relationships but they also know that they needn't continue any kind of sexuality that they find not to their liking.

Young women are reading these texts and are exploring. "Yes, please" and "No, thank you" are well on the way to becoming equally accept-able, and the options are seemingly limitless. The American Puritan

Ethic (APE) so aptly described by Sherman (1973) may, in fact, be on the way to its eternal rest:

> The American Sex Revolution is over. There are a few isolated pockets of propriety still to be mopped up, but most wholesome, clean-living people have taken to the hills. Tomorrow belongs to us, the Dirty-Minded Americans, and there are more of us than even we dared to dream.
>
> The APE sits shaking his head and licking his wounds, amid the rubble of Morality One. *Deep Throat* is now playing where *The Sound of Music* used to be; movie stars, who once privately chose which parts to be seen in, now choose which of their private parts are to be seen.

In the presence of the current information explosion, the abundance of choices, the awareness that loneliness is often a prime motivator for sexual activity, and the trend toward situation ethics, many of my colleagues and I use a checklist for sexual health care that we offer to young women as a guideline and that has been well received. It consists of five very basic questions:

> Does whatever you do or don't do sexually enhance your self-esteem?
> Is your behavior entirely voluntary?
> Do you derive pleasure and gratification from it?
> Does it start an unplanned pregnancy?
> Does it spread sexually transmitted disease?

Our students have found this checklist helpful and have utilized it as a springboard for further investigation and discussion. We in no way mean to imply that there are not other considerations; we merely suggest that these five major points had best be settled to the best of the person's ability at the time, before she proceeds with the relationship.

These basic questions seem simple enough. A look at them in historical context, however, invites comparison with former times. Self-esteem was neither a term nor a clearly defined concept familiar to the past generation. Personal fulfillment is relatively new as a goal; the notion of pleasure and gratification for women is even newer. These are surely among the major characteristics of the sexual emancipation of young women. As Hunt (1974) stated in the epilogue to his extensive study of sexual behavior:

> The analysis of our questionnaire data shows that profound changes have taken place in the period of roughly a generation since Alfred Kinsey and his associates did their basic fieldwork—changes often loosely referred to as sexual revolution, but which we have preferred to call sexual liberation. We have seen that these changes add up to a major increase in attitudinal and behavioral liberalism, but not a radical break with those cultural values linking sex to love, marriage and family life.

As stated at the outset, these and all other deliberations leave us with more questions than answers. It is amusing and gratifying to contemplate that 20 or 30 years from now, the young women who comprise better than half of the troubling citizenry called "these young people" will look upon their youth as the good old days.

References

Barbach, *For yourself—The fulfillment of female sexuality*. New York: Doubleday, 1975.

Boston Women's Health Collective. *Our bodies, ourselves* (rev. ed.). New York: Simon & Schuster, 1976.

Canfield, E. A skeptic's glossary. In Sol Gordon (Ed.), *Let's make sex a household word*. New York: John Day, 1975.

Cutright, P. The teenage sexual revolution and the myth of an abstinent past. *Family Planning Perspectives*, 1970, *4*, 24–31.

Dodson, B. *Liberating masturbation: A meditation on self and love*. New York: Bodysex Designs, 1974.

Friday, N. *My secret garden: Women's sexual fantasies*. New York: Pocketbooks, 1974.

Gordon, S. *Let's make sex a household word*. New York: John Day, 1975.

Gordon, S., and Libby, R. *Sexuality today and tomorrow*. North Scituate, Mass.: Duxbury Press, 1976.

Hettlinger, R. *Living with sex—The student's dilemma*. New York: Seabury Press, 1966.

Hunt, M. *Sexual behavior in the 1970's*. New York: Dell, 1974.

Kelly, G. *Learning about sex*. Woodbury, N.Y.: Barron's Educational Series, 1976.

Luker, K. *Taking chances—Abortion and the decision not to contracept*. Berkeley: University of California Press, 1975.

Brochure, *Am I parent material?* National Alliance for Optional Parenthood. N.A.O.P., 2010 Massachusetts Ave., N.W., Washington, D.C. 20036, 1976.

Pierson, E. *Sex is never an emergency*. Philadelphia: J. B. Lippincott, 1970.

Sarrel, P., and Sarrel, L. A sex counseling service for college students. *American Journal of Public Health*, July 1971, *61*, 1341–1347.

Sarrel, P., and Sarrel, L. Course work is not enough. *SIECUS Report*, September 1977, pp. 4–5.

Sherman, A. *The rape of the A*P*E**. Chicago: Playboy Press, 1973.

Zero Population Growth. Fact sheet, Teenage pregnancy: A major problem for minors. Z.P.G., 1346 Connecticut Avenue N.W., Washington, D.C. 20036, 1977.

Index